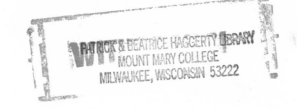

Senior Living Communities

Senior Living Communities

Operations Management and Marketing for Assisted Living, Congregate, and Continuing Care Retirement Communities

Benjamin W. Pearce

The Johns Hopkins University Press
Baltimore and London

© 1998 The Johns Hopkins University Press
All rights reserved. Published 1998
Printed in the United States of America on acid-free paper

9 8 7 6 5 4 3 2

The Johns Hopkins University Press
2715 North Charles Street
Baltimore, Maryland 21218-4363
www.press.jhu.edu

Library of Congress Cataloging-in-Publication Data will be
found at the end of this book.
A catalog record for this book is available from the British Library.

ISBN 0-8018-5961-1 (pbk.)

This book is dedicated to my parents, Robert and Dixie Pearce,
who taught me to respect the elderly, and to my grandmother,
Ellen Pearce, with whom I spent summers during wheat harvest
in my youth, who taught me how to love them.

Contents

The senior living industry has emerged over the past fifteen years as a surprisingly affordable and very attractive living option for many. The senior living product and service concept—properly executed—extends independence, offers lifestyle choices, and provides security and peace of mind.

The industry has evolved in distinct phases. The 1980s constituted the "learning curve" phase. Many mistakes were made as a number of for-profit organizations entered the arena and quickly realized that their products and strategies must be market driven, not situation driven. The late 1980s and early 1990s saw a period of adjustment to true marketplace desires. In the mid-1990s, the industry experienced orderly growth, development, and stabilization. The late 1990s have been a period of transition and industry consolidation characterized by market segmentation, accelerated growth fueled by abundant capital, and the identification of the core market: typically older, more frail seniors. Assisted living/personal care has emerged as a major market niche, in some cases almost a separate industry. Wall Street and the equity markets have recognized senior living as a viable investment option.

It is now time for the industry to achieve increased sophistication by developing and executing proven strategies. This book provides a timely resource and offers a unique and much-needed treatment dealing with the practical application of benchmarking and best practices in the senior living industry. Author Benjamin Pearce provides solid insights into every relevant detail of the successful operations, marketing, and management of both existing and future senior living communities.

Pearce first lays a solid foundation for the senior living business, discussing market positioning and how to set strategic objectives, develop practical management philosophies, and implement leading-edge tactics and best practices in a cost-effective manner. He takes us on a tour of day-to-day, hour-by-hour operations and management, showing how senior living communities should be operated and managed. He sets new standards of "sophisticated simplicity" for how senior living communities can and must perform. Pearce strikes a delicate balance in describing the delivery of quality, value, and high levels of resident satisfaction in a service-enriched environment while also providing useful insights into hard-nosed business strategies that can lead to significant financial success for sponsors and owner-operators of senior living communities.

The timing of this comprehensive treatment of survival, success, and profitability in the senior living industry could not be more appropriate. The industry is entering a period that poses substantial threats and challenges while it also provides opportunities for progressive developers and operators who are willing to focus on details. This book provides those essential details, from cost-effective staffing patterns to the optimal water temperature for the commercial kitchen dishwasher. The book provides a road map for direction and a punch list for executing operational success strategies.

In 1996 and 1997, more than sixteen senior living companies went public, raising hundreds of millions of equity dollars. Most of these companies projected significant levels of market and financial performance to be realized in 1998 and 1999. It is now obvious that some of these companies may not meet their lofty objectives, despite significant capital infusion and aggressive growth initiatives. Other sources of risk capital have also been readily available for growth and development in the senior living industry, including commercial lenders, institutions, pension funds, and real estate investment trusts.

As this book goes to press, there are clear indications of saturation in selected markets; the industry may well be in the early stages of a significant market correction. These evolving trends should be carefully evaluated with a mild sense of urgency. To survive and succeed, operators and sponsors must be on target, doing the right things in the right way at the right time. This book provides comprehensive guidance on the broadest array of relevant issues.

The senior living business involves the challenge of high fixed costs, but also the opportunity for achieving excellent financial results. In Chapter 2, Pearce addresses pertinent accounting fundamentals, important income statement dynamics, and budgeting strategies. He also provides valuable insight into the critical distinction between the accrual basis of accounting and critical elements of cash flow, with direct applications to the senior living business. He integrates the important financial characteristics of the senior consumer, showing the reader precisely how the financial results of a community are actually realized.

Labor is the largest component of fixed cost in a senior living community; the industry is also very management intensive. Chapter 3 covers the total human resource discipline, from developing job expectations and hiring qualified personnel to managing and motivating the workforce. Pearce also provides an excellent analysis of the true cost of fringe benefits, a frequently overlooked or underestimated element of cost.

Annual resident turnover at senior living communities typically varies from 20 percent for independent living to more than 40 percent for assisted living. Hence sales and marketing are critical and continuous processes. In Chapters 13–16, Pearce takes the reader through the complete sales and marketing planning process, from initial planning and feasibility analysis to budgeting, sales training, lead tracking, and successfully closing the sale.

In Chapters 17 and 18, Pearce describes the quantitative and qualitative details of the aging process, leading to a pragmatic assessment of the need for assistance with the activities of daily living. He describes both clinical and human aspects of personal care, again striking a delicate balance between resident dignity and quality of life and the business imperative of developing cost-effective strategies for delivering care.

This book should be required reading from cover to cover for professionals at all levels of the senior living industry. However, the structure of the book allows the reader to consult selected chapters to address specific issues of concern on any given day. For example, one can quickly sharpen one's focus on housekeeping strategies by referring directly to Chapter 10.

Ben Pearce demonstrates that he is not only a talented and seasoned industry professional but also a gifted author. His clear, concise, no-nonsense presentation of complex issues demonstrates the depth of his front-line experience and his access to strong, relevant empirical evidence. He provides readers with tactics and strategies that have been proven effective—there are no unsupported ivory tower theories here.

Jim Moore
President, Moore Diversified Services, Inc.
Fort Worth, Texas

Acknowledgments

I have drawn on many sources for the information covered in this book, ranging from technical books, operations manuals, and my own experience "in the trenches" to discussions and private communications with colleagues. For those who wish to learn more about a specific subject, several important reference works are listed under Further Reading at the end of this book—although I was surprised to discover how very little has been written about operations management in retirement communities.

I thank the many colleagues whose comments on various drafts of the sections of this book have helped to improve its accuracy and have added significantly to its innovation. Although I have endeavored to make this book as complete and as pragmatic as possible, even after working in this business all my adult life I am continually learning new ways to serve the needs of the elderly in better and more efficient ways. I encourage readers who discover errors of omission or who may have a better idea to bring them to my attention so that corrections and inclusions may be made in future editions.

I am indebted to the following colleagues, whose advice, input, and criticisms of various parts of this book have added to its practicality, balance, and fairness: Ralph Bellande; Megan Buffington; Bridget Gibbons; Raymond Goodman for his contribution to Chapter 9; Kittye S. Harman, R.E.H.; Darla Lambertson, R.N.; Cheryl Lucas, C.D.M.; Lisa Carda Pearce, C.T.R.S., for her contribution to Chapter 7; and Vera Taylor for her contribution to Chapter 14. I am especially indebted to Farron Bernhardt and Jim Moore, who reviewed the entire manuscript.

I also wish to recognize the talented executive directors and administrators whom I have been so fortunate to lead. They have provided me success, encouragement, and friendship. Together we have learned the contents of this book, and I offer them my respect, my admiration, and my gratitude: they have brought a sparkle to the eyes of many elderly people.

Finally I thank my wife Lisa and my children Benjamin, Rachel, and Micaela for their patience and support, without which I could not have completed this book.

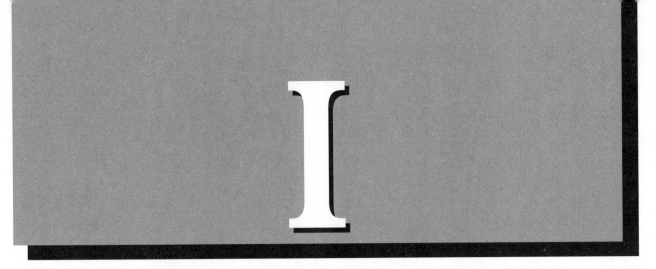

Administration

Introduction

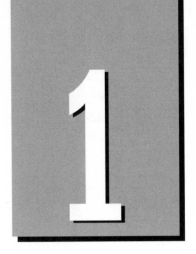

The eighth edition of the *Directory of Retirement Facilities* (1997), published by the HCIA, lists more than 23,000 residential alternatives for the growing senior population, from supervised board-and-care settings to totally independent living communities. The American Association of Retired Persons estimates that the number of senior living communities has doubled in the past ten years and will more than double from present levels before the turn of the century.

The dramatic growth and development of the senior housing business have introduced a number of participants who have learned the complicated task of delivering consistent, high-quality services to elderly persons primarily by trial and error. Many operators have successfully survived the learning curve. For others it has proven to be an expensive and frequently disastrous attempt to capitalize on the growing demand for senior housing—not withstanding the toll on those seniors who bought into the dream and were later entangled in a developer's nightmare of financial difficulties.

INDUSTRY OUTLOOK

Now more than ever before, businesses are seeking new and more efficient ways to operate. The senior living industry has undergone significant change over the last few years that has forced marginal operators out and resulted in the recapitalization of millions of dollars in real estate. The dramatic growth of the industry during the late 1970s was spurred in part by multifamily developers who were unable to thrive when faced with interest rates of 20 percent plus prime and needed the addition of services to make their projects "pencil out." Multifamily developments were made more attractive during this period through the introduction of services that allowed a marginal improvement in the average net income per unit (capitalizing on an economy of scale in overhead) to meet the cash flow requirements of lenders.

Original development assumptions about the size of the market and fill-up rate were grossly overstated, and this has been a significant factor in the cautious attitude of lending institutions. After so many projects had failed, many institutions became reluctant to underwrite new projects until their portfolios of existing projects met certain performance thresholds. Some even opted out of the business entirely. There is still some uncertainty about whether to underwrite the industry as real estate or as a business. It seems that new development is viewed more as real estate, whereas acquisitions are valued on the basis of operating cash flow and revenue multipliers. Even now, as providers are demonstrating a more positive track record, lenders are being very choosy about which type of project to underwrite. They are more attracted to projects that are designed to provide a full continuum of care rather than simply rentals. Members of the senior market are themselves becoming more informed about available options in the industry and are finding more attractive those projects that allow them the greatest flexibility and choice throughout their lives.

Even though the congregate projects of the 1980s are substantially full, there has been a resurgence of interest rate fears, complicated by the recent tendencies of the Federal Reserve to control inflation in the expanding economy. Current operators of congregate communities will attempt to offset the effects of increasing interest rates during the next upward cycle by adding yet another level of services to their communities. This time it will probably take the form of home health care or another form of support services for their residents, designed to increase the average net revenue per unit. This will be a very popular option among the tenants, who will view these services as a cost-effective alternative to nursing home placement that allows them to avoid moving. In addition, many of the residents may qualify for intermittent home health care benefits through Parts A and B Medicare (see Chapter 18 for more details).

The industry has undergone retrenchment, but this has meant less competition and fewer marginal participants. The product concepts, service capabilities, delivery packages, and market planning and sales abilities of the surviving participant have been tested and refined. Prospects for solid growth in the senior housing industry remain very bright, especially in assisted living. The rest of this chapter offers an analysis of growth in demographics within the industry, regulatory issues, the economic concerns of the seniors that the industry serves, the impacts of national health care reform, available financial resources, capital availability and underwriting, lender and investor concerns, and future risks and opportunities for operators and developers.

Basic operations management of senior living communities differs little from one type of senior living community to the next. Other than the provision of various levels of health care, the operational management requirements for running the day-to-day operations have only subtle differences. Where they are material, they are so noted. The intent of this book is to describe operational and marketing strategies widely practiced by the most successful operators in this country today. Operational standards of excellence are detailed in Appendix B. Although the majority of retirement communities provide some form of health care to their residents, regulations governing the provision of care have been well established by the various regulatory bodies and will not be covered herein. I will focus on identi-

fying the best practices employed to operate and market efficiently four types of facilities: independent living facilities, assisted living facilities, congregate seniors housing facilities, and continuing care retirement communities. A preopening critical path for operations from start-up can be found in Appendix D.

Independent Living Facility (ILF)

An independent living facility is a multifamily complex catering to senior citizens. It generally consists of homes, condominiums, apartments, or mobile or motor homes in which residents maintain an independent lifestyle. It offers minimal or no services beyond building and grounds maintenance. Some independent living communities also include subsidized housing that offers rental assistance from the federal government.

Assisted Living Facility (ALF)

An assisted living facility is a type of living arrangement that combines shelter with various personal support services, such as meals, housekeeping, laundry, and maintenance. Assisted living is designed for seniors who need regular help with activities of daily living (ADLs) but do not need nursing home care. ADLs include such common everyday activities as ambulation, bathing, dressing, grooming, self-feeding, and toileting. Units may or may not have full kitchens, although most provide at least a kitchenette. Assisted living facilities may include those termed board-and-care homes, personal care homes, and supervised care facilities. Normally service is provided on a month-to-month basis or through home health agency billings and Medicare.

Congregate Seniors Housing (CSH)

Concregate seniors housing is a multifamily complex catering to senior citizens, with centralized dining services, shared living spaces, and access to social and recreational activities. Many congregate care facilities offer transportation services, personal care services, rehabilitative services, spiritual programs, housekeeping, and other support services. Apartments may rent on a monthly or annual basis, or may have a condominium or fee simple structure.

Continuing Care Retirement Communities (CCRC)

Continuing care communities, also referred to as life care communities, provide a continuum of care, including housing, health care, and various support services.

These communities provide services specified by contract, usually for the balance of the resident's life. The types of services provided range from those in support of independent living to skilled nursing care. Health care services may be provided directly or through access to affiliated health care facilities. Most communities offer a wide variety of contract options. Fees are structured either as a refundable entry fee plus a monthly service fee, as a condominium, as a rental, or as an endowment, and insurance may be mandatory. Residency agreements normally are offered in three versions: extensive, modified, or fee-for-service.

EXTENSIVE AGREEMENT (TYPE A): This contract includes an unlimited amount of long-term care. Residents pay the same rate for care while occupying a nursing unit in the health care center as they would in a residential unit.

MODIFIED AGREEMENT (TYPE B): This contract includes housing, residential services, and amenities. It also covers a specified amount of long-term nursing care per year, normally 30 days. Nursing home fees equal the monthly fee paid in the residential unit during this covered period. After the covered period, residents normally pay the market rate for additional nursing days.

FEE-FOR-SERVICE (TYPE C): This contract includes housing, residential services, and amenities. Residents have guaranteed access to the health care center but pay market rates. Essentially, residents pay only for services used.

▮▮▮ DEMOGRAPHICS THAT WILL DICTATE CHANGE

During the next 30 to 40 years, as many as 55 to 60 million seniors will be making consumer choices tailored to meet their individual needs. By the year 2000, it is estimated that 20 percent of the population of the United States will be over the age of 65.

The statistical picture of America (Figure 1.1) is a vivid portrait of an aging population. In the past twenty years, according to U.S. Bureau of the Census figures, the segment of the population aged 65 and over grew twice as fast as the population as a whole. By 1990, the ratio of elderly persons to those under 65 was one to five. By the year 2010, one-quarter of the U.S. population will be at least 55, as the baby boomers reach for retirement. By 2050, the 55+ cohort, 104.3 million strong, will account for nearly one-third of the U.S. population. In fact, the total U.S. population is expected to increase by one-third between 1982 and 2050, but the over-55 age group will more than double, increasing by 113 percent. Since 1900, the percentage of Americans 65 years and older has tripled (4.1% in 1900 to 12.4% in 1988). Every day 5,000 Americans celebrate their sixty-fifth birthday.[1]

Today people are living longer than ever before. The fastest-growing age group is made up of people 85 and older. In 1940, 365,000 Americans, or 0.3 percent of the population, were age 85 or older. By 1982, the over-85 cohort had increased to 2.5 million, representing 1.1 percent of the total population. This

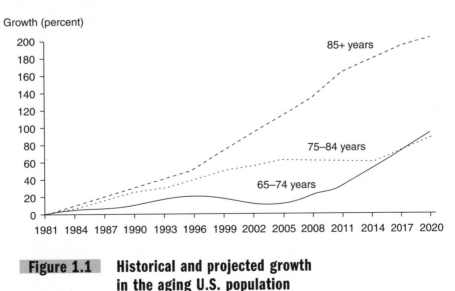

Figure 1.1 Historical and projected growth in the aging U.S. population

Source: Data from U.S. Bureau of the Census

group is expected to reach 5.1 million people (2.5% of the population) by the year 2000 and climb to a staggering 16 million, or 5.2 percent of the population, by 2050.

Statistically, the over-55 age bracket constitutes approximately 50 million people, and the over-65 cohort constitutes approximately 28 million people. It is estimated that this group has a total annual income in excess of $450 billion, almost twice the discretionary buying power of the entire population segment below age 35.

In addition, it is important to understand how seniors spend their income on health care and health care–related services. Statistics compiled by the U.S. Department of Health and Human Services reveal that the elderly are hospitalized twice as often as people under 65, stay twice as long once they are admitted, and use twice as many prescription drugs. Moreover, nursing home use by the elderly has almost doubled since 1966, when Medicare and Medicaid programs were enacted.

As the elderly live longer, their consumption of health care services and products will be weighted more toward increased utilization by the very old. Per capita hospital service spending by the 65-and-over age group is 250 percent higher than spending by those under 65, and spending by the over-85 age group is 327 percent higher than spending by those under 65.

Experts feel that health deteriorates significantly with aging, with the very old becoming increasingly vulnerable to a barrage of chronic, debilitating conditions and diseases. Although only 7.2 percent of those aged 75–84 years are in nursing homes, this statistic almost triples to 20.3 percent after age 85, evidence of the increasing needs of the aged.

The need for personal care assistance for those elderly requiring home management also increases with age. Those seniors surveyed between the ages of 65 and 74 revealed that only 6.7 percent required assistance; however, between the ages of 75 to 84 the percentage increased to 15.7 percent, and for those over 85 it was nearly 40 percent.

The growing number of elderly persons who will require supportive care within the senior living industry will take legislators across the country by storm. The Special Committee on Aging of the U.S. Senate estimates that the number of older persons needing some long-term care services, which was 7 mil-

lion in 1990, will increase to 12 million by the year 2020. The costs associated with providing nursing care for older persons are expected to increase from $37.6 billion in 1990 to $112 billion by the year 2020. Medicaid, which provides 90 percent of public funding for long-term care services has grown in excess of 20 percent per year for the last three years. It is the fastest-growing component of state budgets, and projections indicate that it will soon account for up to 25 percent of state budgets. The Congressional Budget Office reports that by the year 2004 Medicare and Medicaid expenses will lead to a doubling of the national debt. Spending on these programs, if left unchecked, will increase from 16.5 percent of the federal budget in 1994 to 26.4 percent by the year 2003. Figure 1.2 summarizes Part A Medicare payments between 1980 and 1994. Medicare will grow from $158 billion in 1994 to $434 billion, and Medicaid will increase from $84 billion to $250 billion.

▰▰ RECENT TRENDS

It is only a matter of time before legislators will seek to use the largest and most readily available private resource in the country—the approximately $700 billion in home equity owned by Americans over the age of 65—to finance health care costs. The American Seniors Housing Association(ASHA), in its 1994 address to the U.S. House of Representatives Ways and Means Subcommittee on Health, suggested that several tax policies be amended to include incentives for the use of home equity to finance our giant health care conundrum. Among the alternatives are the following:

1. Revise Section 1034 of the Internal Revenue Code to defer the recognition of income from the prior sale of a principal residence to the extent such proceeds are used as an entrance fee for or to gain admission to a "qualified retirement community." Currently one's principal residence, regardless of value, is an asset exempt from Medicaid calculations.

2. Internal Revenue Code Section 121 was recently amended to provide an increase in the exclusion of gain from the sale of a principal residence from $125,000 to $250,000 ($500,000 for a couple). Additional exclusions in the future may be (a) placed in trust for the sole purpose of providing long-term care; or (b) used to gain entrance to an

Dollars (billions)

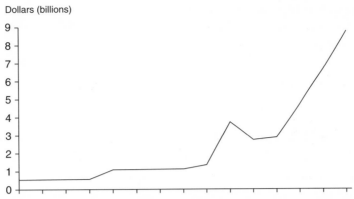

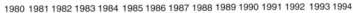

Figure 1.2   Estimated Medicare Part A SNF payments, 1980–1994

Source: Data from Congressional Budget Office

ongoing residence in a qualified CCRC, assisted living facility, or licensed congregate community; or (c) used to purchase long-term care insurance.

3. Provide for tax-free withdrawals from IRAs, 401(k) savings plans, and other qualified pension plans; accelerated death benefits to be paid from life insurance policies on people who are terminally ill or permanently confined to a nursing home; and deductions for long-term care premiums: the higher the age, the greater the deduction. "Rollover privileges should be extended to those who reinvest in regulated IRA type funds, the proceeds of which are used to fund congregate or assisted living residences structured with rental rather than entry fee or endowment programs."[2]

4. Enact into law elder care provisions that would provide tax credits for expenses incurred in providing custodial care for a parent or grandparent in the taxpayer's home. This provision of the Family Reinforcement Act would require a physician to certify that the care receiver cannot perform at least two ADLs without substantial assistance, or exhibits a similar level of disability as a result of a cognitive impairment.

5. Waive the 7.5 percent adjusted gross income threshold for amounts paid for long-term care services, including amounts paid for long-term care insurance premiums for medical care for the taxpayer, his or her spouse, or a dependent. Also clarify that the costs of assisted living services are included in the definition of medical expenses that are presently available for a tax deduction under the Internal Revenue Code.[3] The recently enacted Health Insurance Portability and Accountability Act, effective for the tax year beginning January 1998, provides that the cost of maintenance or personal care services that are required by an individual who is unable to perform at least two ADLs or who suffers from severe cognitive impairment, and who requires supervision to protect him- or herself and others from threats to health and safety, may be tax deductible if such services are provided pursuant to a plan of care prescribed be a licensed health care practitioner. A simple letter from the resident's physician should suffice to prescribe such a plan of care. Meals are subject to only a 50 percent deduction. In the event that an individual does not meet the requirements of the new law, only that portion of the monthly expense that is attributable to medical care may be tax deductible. These costs generally include extended care costs and medications.

Amendments and legislation such as these may ultimately be inevitable if the government is to meet the growing health care needs of America's elderly. Such amendments would have a significant impact on the delivery of senior housing in the coming decade and could potentially offset the incentive for residents to stay in their homes supported by home health care, and encourage them to move into continuing care communities with their life savings and home equity intact. Although the obvious tax advantages of this legislation could have a significant negative effect on rental communities, there will always be people who prefer the flexibility and freedoms afforded by the rental concept.

■■■■■ IMPACTS OF NATIONAL HEALTH CARE

Since Medicare introduced the diagnostic related groups level of care evaluation process, nursing homes have evolved to become subacute and special care providers. When the Omnibus Budget Reconciliation Act of 1987 introduced guidelines to redefine long-term care standards, intermediate care ostensibly became assisted living as we know it today. Federal and state governments have by now so heavily regulated the long-term care industry that the costs of compliance with their own regulations have become prohibitive, as they drown in their own demographics.

As state budgets are stretched to the breaking point by growth in Medicaid spending, states will tighten their control on the certificate of need approval process to limit their liability. The supply of new beds is growing annually at a modest 2 percent (15% annual growth for assisted living). This trend will enable existing nursing home providers to increase their margins slowly in response to the decreasing supply. In addition, nursing home operators today are moving in the direction of specialized care, subacute care, and managed care in order to improve their financial performance.

Washington lawmakers are calling for enhanced matching rates for home- and community-based services and propose to raise the current matching rate by 30 percent. State and federal policy makers have estimated that 20–25 percent of nursing home residents who need assistance with ADLs do not require round-the-clock nursing care. Only those who require acute and chronic care will need to be displaced to skilled nursing environments. Nursing homes will therefore be forced to deal with patients requiring higher levels of care within the same or even lower reimbursement structures (rates are calculated based on prior years' operations) and to compete for staff with flexible government-funded home health care agencies and assisted living communities. The private-pay market, typically consisting of residents requiring lower levels of care (83% of nursing home patients deplete their assets within one year), will ultimately recognize

the inherent benefits, freedom, and economy of less-institutional settings within which they can receive virtually the same care.

The state of Florida is implementing a new law that provides for "extended congregate care" and will enable frail residents to "age in place." Florida lawmakers estimate that extended congregate care will cost half as much as nursing care per resident per month and allow the frail elderly to remain in more desirable residential settings.

Oregon has developed Medicaid waivers to cover assisted living facilities as a way to curb long-term care costs. The cost of the program has averaged about 62.4 percent of the nursing home costs for private-pay patients and 64 percent of the cost for those receiving Medicaid.

The Health Security Act of 1993 would provide assessment and care to those requiring help with three or more ADLs or suffering from severe cognitive impairments. The proposal specifies that the funds must be used in home- or community-based settings such as retirement and assisted living projects. Clearly, the assisted living and home health care business will prosper at the expense of the long-term care industry. We are already seeing dramatic growth in these two related industries proportional to that triggered by the move to congregate housing fueled by rising interest rates in the late 1970s. This growth opportunity may again have the effect of introducing many new players into the industry, who may lack the marketing or operational experience necessary to be successful. The inevitable failures in this growing health care segment will lead to increased regulation and the associated higher costs of compliance. Assisted living appears now to be serving the intermediate care market and even competing for the private nursing home market through innovative, lightly regulated nursing care arrangements (Figure 1.3). In fact, skilled nursing visits are now being provided to the assisted living resident through home health agencies.

Moderate-income residents who do not qualify for Medicaid but cannot afford to pay privately will have access to personal care assistance. This is interpreted to include the assistance that is provided in assisted living in a senior nursing facility setting. However, this approach may prove to be a double-edged sword. If residents could have access to supportive services and home health care in independent living apartments,

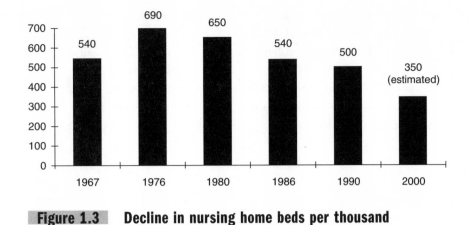

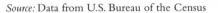

Figure 1.3   Decline in nursing home beds per thousand

Source: Data from U.S. Bureau of the Census

perhaps federal assistance would enable operators to increase the average revenue per unit and residents' financial resources would last longer. On the other hand, the average acuity level in these communities would increase, the average length of stay would decrease, and the units turned over would need to be marketed to a less-active clientele. This could be a very dangerous strategy in the long run. As buildings age, a new developer may come to town with an attractive project, with which existing operators will not be able to compete for independent, active, and affluent prospects. Many retirement communities have been run into the ground by marketing defensively to manage their turnover rather than offensively to build a waiting list as a means of managing their revenue and level of care. (See Chapter 16 for more information on managing stabilized communities.)

STRATEGIC PARTNERSHIPS

Strategic partnerships with hospital systems will play a critical role in fueling the continued expansion of assisted living facilities. The number of Medicare beneficiaries enrolled in managed care plans continues to grow at a rate of over 30 percent per year. Medicare payments currently represent 40 percent or more of a typical hospital system's revenue base, and with this increasing penetration of Medicare risk plans hospitals will increasingly serve as managing agents for low-cost health care offered across a continuum of services.

Assisted living provides services in the middle of the continuum, between home care and acute care settings; it can provide a cost-effective solution to reimbursement and utilization pressures within the managed care continuum controlled by the hospital. As managed

care providers seek high-quality, lower-cost alternatives to home care and nursing home care, the inclusion of assisted living within a hospital system's continuum will clearly enhance the system's attractiveness to managed care payors. In addition, as assisted living residents age in place, they require an increasing amount of ancillary services—such as therapies, pharmacy services, and home care—provision of which will enable the hospital system to utilize its affiliates more fully and extend its services outside the acute care setting. In this way, the system can maximize its revenue potential by controlling market share across the continuum and retain its customer base as their needs change over time.

Joint ventures or other strategic alliances with existing private and public assisted living providers can provide management services while generating significant ancillary referrals to the hospital system. For the assisted living provider, an affiliation with a local hospital system can significantly increase market acceptance within the community, while at the same time allowing access to attractive financing options available to the hospital. For the hospital system, such a partnership can be a very effective use of its excess capital and property, completing the "missing link" in its continuum of health care offerings.

FINANCIAL RESOURCES

A recent survey of 118 lenders and investors sponsored by the National Investment Conference for the senior living and long-term care industries found that commercial banks (39%), mortgage bankers (18.6%), and insurance companies (12.7%) were the most active seniors housing and long-term care lenders in 1994. In 1994, approximately 60 percent of the respondents reported having made loans for seniors housing or long-term care properties, with a median loan amount of $12 million. Lenders reported that their most frequent lending activities for the senior living industry consisted of providing permanent debt for the acquisition of an existing stabilized project (77%), refinancing an existing permanent debt (73.7%), and providing permanent financing on a new project that has already achieved stabilized occupancy (72.9%). Fewer than half reported providing construction and mini-permanent financing for start-up communities.[4]

The availability of financing has traditionally been the primary determinant of the growth rate and direction of senior housing projects. Developers are now becoming much more creative, as some of the nation's largest pension funds have been attracted to the demographically driven senior living industry. Although traditional financing resources remain basically intact, a growing number of new financing vehicles have surfaced now that the majority of the product constructed in the early to mid 1980s has been absorbed. This new availability may spur another growth phase for the industry as established operators can show a positive track record with their existing projects. The following financial resources are among the most popular:

1. **Tax-exempt bonds for 501(c)(3) organizations.** Debt that is normally issued through a government conduit is usually tax exempt. Typical final maturity 30 years, with a level, self-amortizing debt service schedule. There evidently is some flexibility for the issuance of these bonds to for-profit providers.
2. **Individual state financing initiatives.** These are especially common in connection with high-priority senior service delivery systems like assisted living. Industrial revenue bonds (IRBs) have also been available at the local level. These instruments can either be written in the form of level, self-amortizing bonds, or have requirements for balloon principal reductions at regular intervals. Some IRB issues may have minimum low-income requirements and rent caps.
3. **Investment pools such as real estate investment trusts (REITs) and pension funds.** These take an equity position through which they own the real estate and lease it back to an operating company, either in the form of a sale-leaseback arrangement with some rent escalation tied to an increase in revenue or through participating mortgages. REITs are a more expensive vehicle, but they are able to accept higher risks, and as a result returns can be higher. A bank may finance a project at 250 basis points over the yield curve, whereas a REIT will do so at 500 basis points over the curve.
4. **Tax-exempt and taxable bonds.** The Tax Reform Act of 1986 prohibits for-profit developers from financing new congregate projects using industrial revenue bonds. The law does permit the issuance of residential rental project bonds to for-profit owners. Rates are slightly higher than those for 501(c)(3) bonds, and they are subject to the alternative minimum tax; there are limits on volume, and one must obtain an allocation from the home state. There is very strong market demand for unrated tax-exempt bonds that are issued on behalf of nonprofit institutions such as the Massachusetts Industrial Finance Agency (MIFA) or other state finance agencies. To access this financing market, project operators may wish to consider affiliating with health care and religious institutions that can serve as owners, with operators providing management and development services on a fee basis. Tax-exempt mutual funds are currently very aggressive in providing project financing for as much as 85–90 percent of total project costs, with limited guarantee requirements. Interest rates for unrated tax-exempt bonds are currently in the 8.0–8.5 percent range, depending on the credit resources and sponsorship of the project.
5. **Conventional loans by commercial banks and insurance companies.** Commercial banks are slowly returning to the market to finance real estate and health care projects. Commercial lenders are credit oriented and will focus on the capital resources, quality, and experience of the project team. Typical projects will require 20–25 percent in equity and additional creditworthy recourse and lease-up guarantees. Significant advantages of working with a commercial bank are the reduced loan processing time (typically 4–6 months) and freedom from imposed regulatory or construction cost (i.e., prevailing-wage) requirements. Features of their current commercial focus are as follows:
   a. They usually focus on service regionally.
   b. They generally allocate less than 5 percent of their total loan portfolio to health care properties that are currently dominated by SNF loans.

c. As recent industry growth trends favor a more vertically integrated approach, providing an on-site continuum of care, conventional lenders are becoming more reluctant to finance rental communities.

6. **Participating mortgages.** These are loans that share in cash flow or appreciation.

7. **Debt securitization financing for single borrowers with multiple assets that can be cross-collateralized.** Securitization refers to the process by which mortgage loans are combined into pools of $100 million or more to produce rated securities for sale to institutional investors. Ratings range from AAA for the most creditworthy to B for deeply subordinated classes. As the most important underwriting criterion that is scrutinized by the rating agencies is cash flow, Wall Street finances only operating communities and does not provide construction financing. There are joint ventures between commercial banks and other lenders, such as commercial banks and investment banking firms, in which one party will supply the construction financing and the other will provide the take-out financing or securitization. Many lenders are interested in bundling some critical mass of loans, either to diversify their in-house portfolio or to pool the loans for the ultimate sale of interests in the pool to institutional investors. Loan to value ratios of 65–70 percent and debt service coverage ratios of 1.25–1.45 are typical. Loan coupons are set based on a spread over U.S. Treasury securities (typically in the 3.0–3.85% spread range) with a maturity comparable to the term of the mortgage loan.[5]

8. **The Department of Housing and Urban Development (HUD) 232 mortgage insurance program.** This program was created by the National Housing Act in 1959 and was originally designed for nursing homes and intermediate care facilities. However, in 1985 HUD 232 was expanded to include board-and-care homes that HUD defines as "residential facilities that provide room, board, and continuous protective oversight for individuals who cannot live independently, but who do not require the more extensive care offered by intermediate care facilities or nursing homes."

To be eligible for this insurance, facilities may not provide direct medical care. Nearly all assisted living facilities fall under this definition and are, therefore, eligible for HUD 232 mortgage insurance.

The HUD 232 program provides mortgage insurance to help sponsors finance their projects more easily and at a lower cost by providing credit enhancement. Credit is enhanced by the HUD insurance because the insurance guarantees that the federal government will repay the loans if the borrower fails to meet the mortgage payments. The insurance is available for mortgages for new construction, purchase of facilities, rehabilitation of existing structures, or mortgage refinancing.

The major drawbacks of the HUD program are the uncertainty regarding application processing time (currently estimated at 12 months) and the ability to secure project approvals in a timely manner. Most regional offices of HUD are significantly understaffed and cautious about underwriting assisted living projects. In addition, construction contracts must be written at prevailing wages rather than as less costly open-bid jobs.

Despite its drawbacks, the benefits of the HUD 232 financing program are significant. It can be particularly useful to providers of assisted living because there are no low-income criteria; the program can be used by facilities that plan to charge market rents.

Financing under HUD 232 is nonrecourse. Funds must be borrowed for a 30- to 40-year period at fixed interest rates. Regulation of operations is minimal. Equity requirements are 10 percent for new construction plus additional support for working capital and start-up. HUD will recognize the appraised value of the land owned by the sponsor as counting toward the 10 percent equity contribution.

9. **Private funding sources.** Wall Street has discovered the assisted living industry. With estimated annual revenues of $14 billion, the industry is expected to grow dramatically to $30 billion by the year 2000. Two years ago there was only one publicly traded assisted living company; today there are sixteen. In 1996, assisted living companies raised 19 percent of the total amount of capital obtained in the entire health care industry, compared to 6.9 percent in 1995 and less than 1 percent in 1994. The industry showed phenomenal growth during the past year, with many top operators more than doubling their bed capacity. Companies that went public in 1996 generally used 1998 as their benchmark year for performance. During that year, as actual results fell behind

projections, the industry experienced considerable consolidation. (See Appendix C for a complete list of financing alternatives.)

LENDER AND INVESTOR CONCERNS

As they analyze prospective investments, lenders and investors are primarily concerned with the management of risk. Because of the preponderance of failed projects in the 1980s, lenders grew very wary of the industry, requiring high equity contributions, while buyers began to demand high internal rates of return to support expected market yields. The market had run the course from aggressive and speculative to conservative and risk averse.[6] Operators who have established a reputation for consistently meeting investment expectations and absorption projections in the past will have a better chance of securing acceptable rates and loan ratios from lenders. The following twelve points outline the most significant concerns of lenders and investors:

1. Developer or sponsor experience and track record, and management depth.
2. Project concept viability and long-run exit strategy.
3. Aggressive market area definition and assumptions.
4. Implied market penetration rates.
5. Aggressive/optimistic fill-up and absorption forecasts, with appropriate financial reserves (typically, capital and operational reserves of 30–35%).
6. Competitiveness of project based on existing and future competition.
7. Cost containment or value engineering, minimizing operating expenses and maximizing returns on capital expenditures.
8. Project affordability and perceived value in the eyes of the senior consumer.
9. Long-run actuarial integrity.
10. Level and validity of presales.
11. Capitalization rates. These have gone up because of the perception of increased risks associated with financing seniors housing. Generally, as the health care component of the project increases, so does the capitalization rate (Table 1.1) because of the higher management intensity as well as the increased costs and risks associated with consistent compliance with government regulations. (See Chapter 2 for a detailed discussion of capitalization rates.)

Table 1.1 Capitalization Rates by Level of Care

Level of care	Capitalization rate (percent)
Congregate seniors housing	10.5–11
Assisted living facility	11–12
Continuing care retirement community	11–14
Senior nursing facility	13–16

12. Debt service coverage ratios (DSCRs). These have increased for seniors housing from 1.2 to 1.3 and even 1.35. (The DSCR is calculated by dividing the net project cash flow by the debt service. A DSCR of 1.25 means that for every $1.00 in debt service, the project produces $1.25 in cash flow.)

CAPITAL AVAILABILITY AND UNDERWRITING

Many projects that were developed in the 1980s have now changed ownership or management. Many of the industry's troubled facilities (owned and managed by inexperienced or undercapitalized firms) are being transferred to industry professionals and firms that have developed expertise in all phases of determining market and financial feasibility, planning and design, marketing and sales, and management operations. Investors' aversion to seniors housing has been justified, and lenders will remain cautious until the failure rate of their underwriting falls more closely into line with the risk assumed. The following underwriting issues are still faced by developers after 15 to 20 years of successful operation in this industry:[7]

1. **Absence of an industry track record.** Many defaults in the 1980s were due to erroneous marketing assumptions. Developers aggressively predicted that seniors 65 years of age and older would move to communities from as far away as 15 miles. However, operators found their communities actually being filled by seniors 80 years of age and older who, for the most part, moved from only 5–7 miles away. Underfunding of marketing and operating deficit reserves was based on unrealistic fill-up expectations. Further consolidation favoring successful operators with well-performing portfolios will serve to establish more refined underwriting evaluation criteria.

2. **Is it real estate or is it a business?** Investors are more comfortable with office, retail, industrial, and apartment investments. The degree of management intensity has often been an excuse not to invest. Investors have come to realize that the greatest opportunity for profit in seniors housing acquisitions will be produced by adding services and improving operational and marketing efficiencies.

3. **Lack of expertise in seniors housing.** Investors' in-house investment personnel or advisers and consultants have not been knowledgeable enough to analyze developers' projections properly. In the past, experience has been gained through reactive evaluation of failing or nonperforming projects. Recent trends indicate that lenders are turning to competent industry consultants, in addition to their own staffs, to perform due diligence analysis prior to making loan commitments. The industry is relatively new, and traditional multifamily investments have been more predictable and better understood. Lending opportunities will continue to improve as lenders develop more sophisticated underwriting and creditworthiness.

4. **Disappointing historical results of seniors housing investments.** Poor past performance—attributable to flawed market assumptions, underfunding of marketing, poor sales ability, unrealistic lease-up projections, and inadequate operating reserves—has resulted in unsatisfactory cash yields and writedowns in investment value. Successful projects are motivated by market forces, rather than by site availability.

5. **Success of alternative asset classes.** Poor real estate portfolio performance has deflected real estate capital to better-performing asset classes, including stocks, fixed-income instruments, venture capital, and private placements. Wall Street has embraced assisted living. Some companies are trading for twenty times earnings.

██████ LEGAL AND LEGISLATIVE REGULATORY ISSUES

Legislators, state agencies, and particularly those charged with safeguarding consumer rights have noticed the growth of the elderly housing industry. A number of states have enacted, or are in the process of enacting, legislation designed to regulate senior housing developments and subsequent operations. Typically, life care or continuing care retirement communities face the greatest exposure to regulations; however, many states are taking steps to introduce and adopt regulations for assisted living communities.

Many state regulatory agencies have imposed definitions of what constitutes assisted living or continuing care retirement communities and have implemented rules for such living arrangements. Great diversity exists, and states are primarily concerned with ensuring that prospective residents have adequate, accurate information with which to make decisions about joining and remaining in a community. Some states have established precise regulations governing the development and operation of such communities. Still others have imposed legislation, failure to comply with which can subject owners and management to civil or criminal penalties. Scenarios for state regulations governing senior housing development can be summarized as falling within four major categories:

1. **Preopening request.** The community may be requested to have state certification and to disclose certain financial information to the prospective residents. Some states also impose a minimum presale occupancy requirement before granting a permit to begin construction.

2. **Contracts between the residents and the community.** Regulations may address the form and content of the resident contract, promotional materials, resident rights, resident councils, liens, and terms of withdrawal from the community.

3. **Health care request.** The community may be required to obtain a certificate of need (CON). This involves an extensive and expensive approval process wherein the developer is required to demonstrate that a market need actually exists for the project within the chosen geographical market location. Many states have enacted CON legislation to control the supply of nursing home beds so that excessive supply will not result in competitive practices that could potentially compromise quality of care. Because Medicaid is the single fastest growing component of many state budgets, the CON process has also been used by legislators to limit states' potential liability.

4. **Financial requirements.** Regulations may call for escrow deposits before and after occupancy, reserve requirements, performance bonding, annual audits, and restrictions on fee adjustments and refunds.

The retirement community must also comply with regulations not specific to the industry, such as zoning and building codes. Depending on its source of permanent financing, the community may be subject to further requirements, such as minimum low-income qualification for a percentage of its tenants (as required under many industrial revenue bond financing rules).

FOUR MAJOR CONCERNS FOR SENIORS

Understanding the characteristics and concerns of the market it serves is critical to the success of any business. Not only does this understanding optimally position the provider to market to and serve its existing clientele, but it also provides the insight needed for future planning. Major concerns for seniors facing the decision to move to a retirement community are as follows:

1. **Future inflation.** Seniors typically underestimate their current cost of living by $400–$500 per month. They may forget about real estate taxes and other costs that are not paid on a monthly basis. When exposed to retirement community pricing, they are subject to sticker shock, for their biggest fear is to outlive their savings.

2. **Realization of the declining value of their existing homes and transferring assets.** Seniors have always thought their homes were worth more than prevailing market conditions would suggest, and they therefore conclude that now is not the time to sell. This is especially true if a senior is subconsciously looking for ways to delay the difficult decision to move to a retirement community. In addition, Americans have traditionally used real estate as a vehicle to transfer inheritance to their children and thus protect their largest asset from taxation upon their death. Their children inherit the "stepped-up" basis or fair market value of the home and therefore avoid the capital gains tax on the original purchase price of the home.

3. **Future health care costs.** Seniors worry about health care and related costs, but they may rationalize that somehow they are likely to be covered by Medicare or their complex supplemental insurance policies. Many of their children also share this belief. Nationally, Medicare covers only about 3 percent of nursing home costs.

4. **Living with dramatically lower interest yields in their conservative savings portfolios.** In the early 1990s, inter-est earned on seniors' cash or cash equivalents plummeted by 50 percent or more compared to returns in the mid- to late 1980s. Returns dropped from 8 percent in 1991 to 4 percent in 1992 to 2½ or 3 percent in 1993. After accounting for Social Security payments and other noncash investments, seniors in the $30,000 annual income category derive up to 50 percent of their income from cash or near-cash investments. Many seniors have watched in horror as their monthly disposable income has declined in the face of ever-increasing health care costs, even as their health declines with age.

FUTURE RISKS

Responding to and addressing the concerns of investors and lenders will require that most developers and subsequent operators incorporate pro forma safeguards and contingencies into their projections to get them approved. These margins of safety may ultimately bridge the gap between the success or failure of a single project or an entire company:[8]

1. A well-conceived community should not rely on more than 4–5 percent of the age- and income-qualified prospects as a penetration rate to reach stabilized occupancy. The higher the penetration, the longer the expected fill to stabilization. Communities with 10 percent or higher penetration may take more than 24 months to reach this threshold.

2. Bottom fishing for troubled projects may not always be a success strategy. Deep-discount or "fire sale" communities will not automatically transform themselves into future success stories. Many troubled communities may have been overvalued and undercapitalized, based on unrealistic fill-up projections. These same communities may have been developed by inexperienced operators who may have incorporated other fatal flaws, involving design, location, and product or service mix, into their projects. Experienced operators may or may not be able to overcome these obstacles and attain success. Many acquisitions are currently being purchased for replacement value.

3. Developers must build first-class projects that are appropriate for the geographic location and that are value engineered. They must strike a balance between not spending capital dollars unnecessarily and prudently investing where the returns are the

greatest. All development must be built around what the primary market prospects can afford. The economics of community enhancements must also be closely scrutinized. For example, for every $10,000 *per unit* of capital savings (or expenditure), the impact on the resident monthly service fee is approximately $95 (assuming a 9% cost of capital, a 1.2 DSCR, and achieving 95% stabilized occupancy). Operators must focus pragmatically on where to save capital and where to invest prudently to provide the best value for the residents. Is the financial decision prudent considering the $95 per month impact it will have on the residents?

■ FUTURE OPPORTUNITIES FOR DEVELOPMENT IN THE INDUSTRY

Even during this period of rapid expansion in the industry, there are still opportunities for developers with insight into their local marketplaces to grow and compete effectively. The following strategies are being employed by successful operators to strengthen their market position:

1. Adding assisted living to complete the continuum of living arrangements for an existing community, as well as developing a freestanding assisted living community, perhaps with a home health care provider.
2. Bringing state-of-the-art independent living with a continuum of care to areas that have gradually evolved to require need-driven catered living owing to the aging in place of residents.
3. Developing new start-up projects in underserved markets offering a full continuum of care (CCRCs).
4. Taking advantage of evolving private-public partnerships and affinity groups, especially with respect to managed care.
5. Purchasing existing full or nearly full rental communities from banks or other institutions willing to write down or recapitalize the asset to meet one's investment criteria.
6. Developing a relationship with an existing provider who has a favorable track record of successful development and who could capitalize on the company's reputation and management.
7. Converting existing functionally obsolete properties in strong market areas to full-service retirement centers offering a continuum of care.

■ Development Opportunities for Assisted Living

ADVANTAGES

1. Market penetration rates required from age- and income-qualified seniors for a typical project range from 1 to 4 percent. (Demographic data should be adjusted to include only single-occupant households and exclude populations already institutionalized.)
2. Market awareness of the concept has increased. Assisted living has been embraced by senior consumers and their families, as well as professional referral sources and legislators, as a cost-effective alternative for the 15–20 percent of nursing home residents who are primarily private-pay patients. In 1995 it was estimated that 5.4 million people would need assisted living. This number is expected to increase by 30 percent to 7 million people by the year 2005.
3. Assisted living is a welcomed resource for adult children (ages 45–60) who are trying to deal with the needs of aging parents. These people are decision influencers and prefer the residential alternative of assisted living to skilled nursing settings.
4. Assisted living has a synergistic fit with existing independent communities. When added to an existing campus, the concept draws upon many resources already in place and further amortizes existing fixed overhead. This high-impact revenue enhancer can add positive annual cash flow after debt service of $4,000–$7,000 per unit. It is also an effective response to aging in place because it maintains the integrity of the independent segment of the senior population.
5. Assisted living can successfully compete for traditional private-pay nursing home patients. The market is rapidly expanding as skilled nursing facilities move toward subacute care and specialized care. The light-care private-pay segment will expand in the future, and well-positioned freestanding operators will take advantage of this. As a rule, the cost of providing assisted living care services to light-care patients is only about two-thirds the cost of providing similar services in a skilled nursing facility. In reality, assisted living providers are delivering a need-driven product that can be adapted to the market. Nursing home operators are confined by government mandates that are based on a medical model, and by the delivery and compliance costs associated

with it. Table 1.2 compares the cost of assisted living with that of skilled nursing in three states.

6. The care of residents with dementia is growing, and some providers may direct all of their resources to providing this type of care in a more cost-efficient setting, such as assisted living.

7. Current Medicaid funding is allocated 57 percent from the federal government and 43 percent from the states. This relationship could change, forcing the states to enact legislation designed to expand the delivery of services to lower levels of care. Several states have already established moratoriums on the CON process to halt the construction of additional skilled nursing beds.

8. As managed care becomes more widespread, physician groups will increasingly control health care dollars. Medicare risk programs will encourage physicians to look to assisted living communities with respite or transitional care units, rather than the traditional acute care or skilled nursing environments, for the rehabilitation of certain classes of patients, such as those who have undergone knee or hip replacements or are in need of stabilization.

9. Some community hospitals are paid a daily rate when a health maintenance organization (HMO) controls the length of a patient's stay. After surgery, the HMO encourages the physician to discharge the patient to a lower-acuity setting for recovery and rehabilitation. Although there are significant variations in the spectrum of care provided in lower-acuity settings, the common challenges of managing this care highlight the need for a seamless delivery system.

CHALLENGES AND RISKS

1. In most states, varying levels of assistance in daily living can currently be offered with limited levels of regulation. As this market cools as a result of increased supply (on which there are currently no CON restrictions), market saturation and increased regulation are inevitable. Projects that are likely to withstand the test of time are those that (a) are well conceived and backed by experienced, "brand name" operators, (b) are tightly integrated into continuum-of-care companies, and (c) have a realistic exit strategy. Regulators do understand that the business is designed to promote cost containment, and states are moving toward spending Medicaid dollars for the delivery of these services in the assisted living arena. They therefore have a strong incentive not to overburden the industry with onerous regulations.

2. Projects should be conceived and operated today in a manner that regulators might enforce in the future.

3. It will be risky to draw comparisons between the current demand for nursing home beds and projected alternative demand for assisted living. This comparison will be misleading because as much as 50–70 percent of nursing care may involve Medicaid reimbursement, whereas assisted living is a private-pay market. Many seniors in the service area may not be able to pay privately for assisted living.

4. New facilities always draw the most attention, even from residents of other nursing homes and retirement communities. Reverse effects can also transpire with older developments. Turnover rates can be as high as 50 percent annually; marketing plans must be geared with this in mind. For a 90-unit project, this translates to 45 units per year.

5. The average pricing of assisted living is usually about 66–75 percent of prevailing nursing rates in the area. The maximum level of consumer affordability for privately paid assisted living is typically 80–85 percent of cash flow disposable income applied to the monthly fee.

Table 1.2 Assisted Living: Low-Cost Providers in Three States

	Michigan	Pennsylvania	New York
Assisted living	$1,909	$2,340	$2,390
Home health	$5,323	$3,600	$2,760
Nursing home	$3,534	$4,125	$5,170
Cost of assisted living versus skilled nursing	−46%	−43%	−54%

Source: Assisted Living Today (Summer 1995): 13.

Financial Qualifications—Private Pay

Independent (@ 75%)	$2,200 × 12 = $26,400 $26,400 ÷ .75 = $35,200 per year or $2,933 per month
Assisted living (@ 85%)	$2,800 × 12 = $33,600 $33,600 ÷ .85 = $39,529 per year or $3,294 per month

An independent resident leasing a unit for $2,200 per month would need to have an annual income of $35,000 to qualify. An assisted living resident would need approximately $39,500 in annual income to qualify.

The long-term strategy must be to keep development costs and overhead to a minimum and strike a balance between spending capital dollars and building value as it is perceived by the residents.

6. Concerns about the availability of funding for home care may ultimately act as a deterrent for people to leave their homes and move into a group residential setting, where costs can be more easily controlled by economies of scale.

7. As competition increases in this rapidly growing environment (Figure 1.4), projects will find it difficult to maintain full occupancy. Profit margins that today average around 40 percent will be harder to achieve, and they will parallel the downward trends already experienced by congregate operators. Steep price competition, the development of more affordable models, and the need to add more intensive services to meet residents' expectations will drive down operating margins across the country. A report entitled *Selected Seniors Housing Transactions,*

recently published by the American Seniors Housing Association, states that average operating profit margins have generally decreased from a high of 55 percent in 1985 to 30 percent in 1993, with an overall average of 37 percent.[9]

8. Nursing homes may bifurcate licenses to include assisted living units within their skilled nursing facilities, or convert partial or entire wings from skilled care to custodial care and assisted living.

Development Opportunities for Continuing Care Retirement Communities

ADVANTAGES

1. CCRCs represent a major industry growth area that is compatible with and likely to benefit from health care reform.

2. They address the continuum-of-care needs and sensitivities of today's informed senior market. They are also well suited to the more affluent and sophisticated clientele that can afford them.

3. CCRCs may provide opportunity for significant tax advantages if Internal Revenue Code Section 1034 (rollover) and Section 121 (exclusion of gain) are amended to include these types of properties. An

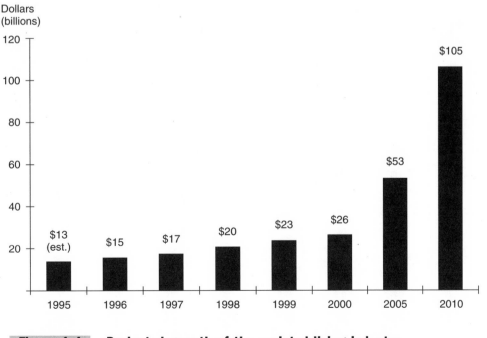

Dollars (billions)

Year	Dollars (billions)
1995	$13 (est.)
1996	$15
1997	$17
1998	$20
1999	$23
2000	$26
2005	$53
2010	$105

Figure 1.4 **Projected growth of the assisted living industry**

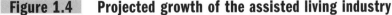

Source: Data from Dean Witter

additional segment of the homebound elderly market will then have a financial incentive to move out of their homes. Currently 94 percent of America's elderly have their health care needs provided for at home.

4. Lenders and investors recognize the inherent value of CCRCs as a business investment rather than as real estate.

5. State governments are looking for ways to defray their expanding health care budgets and may facilitate development and financing of new construction.

6. CCRCs structured with a nonprofit operating entity will benefit from the aging in place of their residents and unit turnover. Resident responsibility for operating expenses will minimize disruption and costs.

7. There are few current regulations limiting expansion in these market segments. CONs will be awarded more freely for the development of CCRCs than for freestanding nursing homes.

CHALLENGES AND RISKS

1. The lengthy development process—up to three years—is complicated by the involvement of multiple regulatory agencies.

2. Appropriate sites with sufficient acreage and optimal location will be increasingly difficult to find and expensive to buy.

3. Performance and value are more closely associated with the accuracy of actuarial predictions than with traditional operational skill and efficiency.

Legislators, investors, and lenders nationwide are headed in the most prudent and politically popular direction for elderly health care. We will see a dramatic growth in the development of CCRCs, freestanding assisted living facilities, and home health care over the next ten years. As inexperienced or undercapitalized operators enter these developing arenas, future consolidation of this new wave of development can be predicted. Although well-established, competent operators will surely benefit from this trend, lending institutions and investors have become more sophisticated in their underwriting criteria, having already felt the sting of the consolidation in congregate developments during the 1980s.

NOTES

1. Based on data from the U.S. Bureau of the Census, 1990.

2. *Seniors Housing: The Market-Driven Solution to Long-Term Care* (Washington, D.C.: American Seniors Housing Association [ASHA], 1994), 12.

3. *Seniors Housing Update* (Washington, D.C.: ASHA, 1994), 2.

4. "Incentives for Long-Term Care Insurance: Elder Tax Credit," *Selling to Seniors* 95-1 (Jan. 1995): 7.

5. R. Anthony, "Capital Markets Financing for the Small Borrower," *Spectrum* 8(5) (Sept. 1994): 29–32.

6. *Selected Seniors Housing Transactions* (Washington, D.C.: ASHA, 1994), 5.

7. W. H. Elliot, J. L. Beck, and D. S. Schless, *Seniors Housing Finance: Trends and Prospects* (Washington, D.C.: ASHA, 1992), 21.

8. J. Moore, "Strategic Industry Focus Needed," *Contemporary Long-Term Care* 16 (March 1993): 24, 94.

9. *Selected Seniors Housing Transactions*, 5.

Financial Principles

2

The successful operation of a retirement community largely depends on the executive director's ability to balance the financial objectives of ownership with the interests of residents and the employees who serve them. These are often conflicting interests, and achieving resident satisfaction while maximizing return on investment and adding value to the project are the trademarks of a seasoned executive director. In this chapter I attempt to familiarize management with how various ownership structures might evaluate the performance of a retirement community and offer some general guidelines. I do not discuss the many complex financing vehicles or partnership organizations.

It is important for senior management personnel at the community level to be comfortable with their respective budgets and to have a basic understanding of the financial principles affecting community operations. The average executive director and middle management supervisors, with little or no training in accounting, usually find it difficult to make sense of company financial statements. However, if one studies their form and function and learns the meaning of a few accounting terms, these statements are not hard to understand and reveal a great deal about the community's financial health and how individual departmental performance affects the big picture. The first step in learning about the financial principles of the seniors housing industry begins with an understanding of the various types of ownership.

TYPES OF OWNERSHIP

There are three basic types of ownership common to the senior living business: proprietary (with and without entry fees), nonprofit–tax exempt, and nonprofit–taxable. A brief review of the advantages, disadvantages, and general financial considerations of each follows.

Proprietary

Projects with proprietary ownership are commonly referred to as for-profit communities. Generally they are sponsored by a privately owned corporation or a publicly traded entity. In publicly owned companies, equity is normally divided into common or preferred stock, held as retained earnings, or distributed to stockholders' equity accounts. Profits may be distributed as dividends. Private companies are generally capitalized by a group of investors or through private funds and are under no obligation to publicize financial results other than to their investors. The owner or each partner will have an equity account to which profits are distributed for withdrawal. In both cases, investors will expect a return on their invested dollars much the same as one would expect interest on money in the bank, the fundamental difference being the amount of return and the corresponding risk on the investment. The primary operational advantage of proprietary ownership is in the degree of control of the real estate and the ongoing operations.

Proprietary developers have historically concentrated on the construction and operation of congregate and assisted living projects, leaving the continuing care communities (CCRCs) in the domain of nonprofit sponsors. In recent years, however, the proprietary interests have entered the CCRC arena in larger numbers, mainly because of the evolution of the market. Seniors have become more educated about their living choices and have communicated loud and clear to developers that they are primarily interested in options. The communities that provide the most choices and lifestyle alternatives are becoming increasingly attractive. There will always be a market for congregate projects, however, for those seniors who prefer the flexibility offered by the rental arrangement. They see congregate living as an acceptable and cost-effective alternative to nursing home placement and, most important, may not feel comfortable about investing any of their hard-earned capital in a project just to move in.

As the newly developed community fills, it will first reach a break-even point for operations. This is the point at which revenues collected from residents equal the cost of operating the community. The next break-even threshold will be reached when revenues increase to the point where they equal the cost of operations plus debt service. After this point is reached, any surplus cash flow will first be earmarked for capital improvements and then used to refinance construction or pay down working capital loans. Construction and working capital loans normally bear a higher interest rate than the permanent loan that will replace them because of the inherent risk factors. The longer they remain outstanding, the greater the interest expense born by the project. Permanent mortgage financing will normally replace construction financing after the operating net income of the project is sufficient to cover the debt service of the permanent loan by about 10–20 percent. Therefore, for each month that occupancy fails to reach this threshold and the construction loan remains in place, the project incurs a higher interest expense than was projected in the financial pro forma, and in essence experiences a construction cost overrun.[1] At this point in the project the investor still has generally not seen any return on investment. The investment flow is used to pay down short-term working capital, and it could easily be two years before the project produces any real return. This is known as the *discounted payback period*

(DPP) and is the time required to recover the original investment plus working capital contributions from the present value of the project's future cash flows. The cumulative shortfall balance is a year-end or month-end balance of the negative cash flow. Over time, as the community fills, this balance should equal zero. At the point at which operations cover debt service and capital improvements, the investment flow will begin to show signs of reversal and offset the cumulative shortfall balance.

All future investment flows must be converted to their present value to provide a basis for comparison with other alternate opportunities for investment. Return on investment for the project will be spread over the number of years that the investor maintains ownership. In order to determine the value of these future returns today, we must consider the time value of money. This process assumes that $1 today is worth more than $1 in the future because interest can be earned by investing today's dollar. The determination proceeds by calculating the present value of the projected future cash flows of the project. The *present value* (PV) converts future cash in and outflows to their present value using the project's cost of capital as the discount rate. The *net present value* (NPV) is the cost of the investment subtracted from the present value of the future cash flows. The NPV represents the dollar amount that the project will return after factoring in the cost of capital. Simply put, the DPP is the number of years it takes for the cumulative present value of the investment to equal zero.

The investor's *return on equity* (ROE) is calculated by dividing the community's cash flow by the investor's equity contribution. Generally the investor will compare this return (including the time value of money during the fill-up stage), upon stabilization of the community's occupancy, to the opportunity cost or return in an alternate investment. Return on equity will generally increase with the occupancy of the community, as the fixed costs of the operation will be absorbed by the initial tenants and the variable costs of additional tenants once the property has exceeded 90 percent occupancy are marginal. As cash flow is calculated after debt service, any increase in the interest rate of adjustable rate financing will have an inverse effect on the investor's return. This can be particularly devastating if management is unable to pass the increased costs on to the residents, who are generally on fixed incomes. *Return on assets* (ROA) is calculated by dividing the project's cash flow by the total asset value (total project costs, including land, buildings, and furniture, fixtures, and equipment) less accumulated depreciation. ROA will always be less than ROE unless the project is not leveraged.

Another measure of financial return is *internal rate of return* (IRR). This measure is widely used by investors to evaluate the net return. The IRR is calculated by a process of iteration to find the discount rate that equates the present value of future cash flows (normally 5- or 10-year periods) with the cost of the investment. The IRR must be greater than the cost of capital (greater than the interest rate on the borrowed funds) for the project to add value to the company. Most investors will calculate their pretax IRRs on a leveraged and an unleveraged basis, that is, before and after debt service. The leveraged IRR will of course always be greater.

If the flow of cash is negative or does not cover all current obligations, the owner may need to convert some other assets to cash, secure short-term or long-term financing, or bring in additional investment partners. The owner in a private company will increase her investment, but a public company may sell a new issue of stock. Most primary lenders consider this working capital as the owner's "risk money" and will expect her to raise it rather than ask the lending institution to supply it.

Nonprofit—Tax Exempt

The nonprofit organization exists by a charter issued by the secretary of state of the incorporating state and must function within the definition of the charter. The preponderance of nonprofit retirement communities have been designed after the model of a continuing care retirement community. The typical nonprofit CCRC is not owned by stockholders or a private corporation but rather by its members. Normally the organization is sponsored by a nonprofit affinity group such as a religious order and governed by a board of trustees. In most cases, one or more of the resident members of the community sit on the board as either voting or nonvoting participants. The board is normally responsible for setting overall policy and delegates the day-to-day operations to management. The system works best when the board provides management with the flexibility to run the property,

and management in turn demonstrates a willingness to tap into the expertise and business acumen of the various board members. The CCRC industry by definition operates in the face of considerable external competitive and regulatory pressures as well as internal organizational issues.

Newly developed communities are generally required by state regulations to meet presale thresholds prior to receiving construction approval. The proportion of the advance fees collected that can be used to fund construction of the community will vary by state. Most states will require the escrowing of resident advance fees during the development period and occasionally even after start-up. Generally presale levels in excess of 75 percent indicate a reasonably rapid absorption of the community upon opening. Presale levels less than 50 percent suggest a weak market and are cause for serious concern. Entry fees are normally shielded from the Internal Revenue Service, and some states allow ad valorem tax exemption as well as favorable sales tax and payroll tax treatments. These projects also may have access to favorable borrowing sources, such as tax-exempt bonds, which can carry very attractive rates.

The disadvantages of the nonprofit community is that control is vested in a board of directors who are typically well intentioned but without financial resources, industry-specific operational experience, or personal investment. Currently the residents are unable to pass through any rollover of capital gains and are not able to recognize the benefits of any real estate–related deductions. In addition, as the cost of the operations is directly borne by the residents, any increases in debt service are passed directly through. On the other hand, there is significant peer pressure to minimize the expansion of services and resulting expenses, and this can have a moderating effect on resident demands.

Some life-care communities have come under criticism where fee calculations have not been based on sound actuarial data. Communities that have structured operations in such a manner as to rely on the advance payment of entrance fees to partially offset operational losses have, on reaching stabilized occupancy, found themselves without adequate turnover to cover the operational shortfalls. This is especially true in communities that have introduced home health care to residents in their apartments in an effort to minimize obligations to provide care in the more expensive skilled nursing component.

Surplus cash from operations is normally used to fund capital improvements or resident reserve funds, or it is invested. The accumulation of significant amounts in the reserve can jeopardize the community's 501(c)(3) nonprofit status and subject the organization to taxes. Therefore, management must carefully balance the operation to maintain its nonprofit status while still planning for the future cash requirements of debt service, capital improvements, and growth in operating expenses. The latter is especially important for newer communities with a substantial nursing home component that when fully occupied will add significant operational expense to the community.

Nonprofit—Taxable

Nonprofit taxable operations typically are designed in the form of cooperatives or condominiums. These operations will provide certain real estate advantages to their members such as rollover of capital gains and pass-through of real estate taxes and interest. In addition, real estate taxes and surcharges are reduced owing to investment in the membership fee that is not producing income. In addition, residents can participate in the appreciation of their units and retain control of their assets. To many seniors who are used to a lifetime of home ownership, these structures have very attractive advantages.

The disadvantages include the requirement of typically higher financial thresholds to qualify and involvement in substantially more complex residency agreements. In addition, condominiums and cooperatives normally fall under the auspices of the state real estate commission and exist at the complicated interface among tax laws, real estate laws, and CCRC regulations (where they exist), some of which may be in conflict.

The operation is generally governed by a board of directors composed of members, the developer, and outside local interests. The board normally hires a management company to oversee operations. Normally the developer will structure the program such that its own management company is awarded the management contract; however, most states will limit the term of these contracts to a maximum of three years. Surplus cash flow is either used to fund capital improvements or invested.

OPERATIONAL BUDGETING

The annual budget process is one of the exercises most universally dreaded by middle management, and it is generally thought to be overwhelming. It does, however, provide management the opportunity to evaluate individual operations annually for efficiency, form, and function. Putting into place a system of financial planning not only makes it more likely that financial targets will be reached but also facilitates more accurate cash flow planning and forecasts. Accurate financial forecasts enable owners to make informed decisions that could result in acquiring financing at lower rates or distributing greater returns to investors. Essentially the goal of the budget process is to forecast whether or not the expenses of running the business (cash outflows) will exceed revenues collected from the residents and what is to be done to cover the projected deficit or, conversely, how the surplus will be distributed. The budgeting process itself can be helpful by revealing areas in the operation where the setting of measurable goals would be especially beneficial to all participants.

Budgeting Revenue

Budgeting revenue is normally done using projected monthly average revenue per unit. In this way census projections for the year can be multiplied by the average revenue per unit to obtain the total expected unit revenue for each month of the budget period. Average revenue per unit should be calculated from existing tenants based on prior period actual results and then adjusted for expected rent or monthly service fee increases. It is important to calculate these figures for each different unit type. This can be done by isolating the revenue for each unit type and simply dividing by the total number of units that were occupied for the previous full month. It is important to recognize that the resulting figure, when used for budgeting purposes, implies that the number of units budgeted at the average revenue per unit assumes that those units are to be occupied and producing revenue for each and every day of the month. In other words, the budget will not account for prorations on the units that may be occupied for a partial month in cases in which the tenant did not start paying rent on the first day of the month for move-ins, or end payments on the last day of the month if he moved out before this date. Some operators simply do not allow prorations for move-ins or move-outs and require prepayments on move-ins and notice periods for move-outs. This is the best arrangement to minimize lost revenue days, but it may not always be enforceable.

Projections for rent or monthly service fee increases should be made for the month in which they are expected to occur. Remember to account for legal notice requirements to the residents as may be applicable or required under local landlord-tenant legislation. Some operators raise fees for all residents once per year at the same time, rather than at the anniversary date of the residency agreement. This can be accomplished only if the fee increases are universally applied. Under this scenario management always runs the risk of an organized protest among the residents, especially in for-profit operations. If management has not done an adequate job of laying the groundwork for managing residents' expectations about their pending fee increases, it may find itself on the defensive if residents do not feel the fee increase is justified. Conversely, if management elects to increase fees on the anniversary date of the residency agreement, the opportunity to apply different increases to similar apartments without the risk of any collective action is greatly reduced. In addition, when only a few of the residents' renewals become due each month, the task of dealing with individual concerns privately is more easily managed.

Interest rate factors will play an important role in determining the relative cash effects on the residents' investment returns and the project's debt service. For example, for a resident to qualify financially to live in a congregate community, most operators require that the monthly service fee be no more than 70 percent (85% for assisted living) of the resident's monthly cash flow disposable income. Therefore, for a resident to afford a monthly service fee of $2,100 per month, or $25,200 per year, he will require $36,000 ($25,200 ÷ 0.70 = $36,000) in annual income from investments and social security. Assuming a 7 percent annual return on his investments, the resident will require approximately $514,285 ($36,000 ÷ 0.07 = $514,285) in assets to produce this income (not including Social Security payments). Every 1 percent increase in interest rates will have a $5,143 annual positive effect on the income produced from the assets, or $428 per month (not including compounding). For a 250-unit community valued at $20 million with a 75 percent loan to value and financed with $15 million on a floating rate note, the same 1 percent increase in interest rates will cost the owner $150,000 more in interest expense per year. Divide this among 250 residents and the $50 per month fee increase required just to cover the increase in interest expense will amount to 2.4 percent, not including normal increases in operating expenses. Clearly, in this example the resident's ability to absorb the community's increase in debt service and operational expenses in an expanding economy will be adequate. As interest rates decrease, however, residents' earnings can fall dramatically, and the community may need to consider refinancing as a vehicle for underwriting the ever increasing cost of operations, as the residents' ability to absorb these increases will be significantly limited.

Budgeting Expenses

The development of an annual budget is generally a process of evaluation of each expense account of the general ledger against community historical results, industry standards, and assumptions as outlined in the original financial projections or pro forma. For new communities, the first budget is generally built from these projections in combination with industry standards in the absence of historical data. Each year thereafter as the community matures, actual operating results help to refine the budget's accuracy.

For mature projects, historical data are generally collected and then annualized and compared to financial projections and ownership objectives. During the fill-up stage of the project, however, the budgeting process is referred to as "zero based," that is, built without the use of historical data or from scratch. Some companies build their budgets every year using the zero base method, arguing that calculating the cost of delivering services based on prior-period results compounds any existing intrinsic inefficiencies of the system. Reviewing each department budget line item from scratch each year can be a more involved process, yet it may uncover areas that can be trimmed. After all, the costs of operating the community are ultimately borne by the residents, some of whom may not be well equipped to manage continuous annual increases.

When constructing budgets, it is important to separate those expenses that are not dependent on changes in community occupancy (fixed) from those that will vary according to occupancy (variable). There will be fixed and variable expenses in each department. For example, food and beverage fixed expenses would include the chef's salary, cooking utensils, kitchen equipment and operations, and utilities. Variable expenses that will generally increase proportionally with occupancy include those for food, cook staffing, and supplies.

Department heads who track their monthly expenditures with a declining-balance ledger can simplify budgetary compliance. This is simply a ledger sheet or spreadsheet listing at the top each expense category along with its corresponding monthly budgeted amount. As materials or supplies are received, the department head codes each invoice or packing slip item to the appropriate account and enters it into her ledger. The expense is subtracted from the monthly total budget to determine the remaining amount of budgeted dollars in each category. As the month progresses, the department manager will have an accurate picture of the amount of money remaining. As the budgeted amount in each category becomes exhausted, additional orders can be placed for receipt in the following month. In this way, the department head does not have to wait until the financial statement comes out to determine if her department expenses are over or under budget. The declining-balance ledger is an excellent planning tool, and its use should be standard procedure for all department heads, especially new hires.

Nonprofit communities will by definition have the objective of balancing expenses with revenues, plus perhaps a small surplus to cover a reserve fund and any unexpected contingencies. They are generally able to provide a greater level of service to their residents for the same or lower monthly fee structure than their for-profit counterparts. This is partly because profit considerations are not taken into account during their budgeting process, but their tax-exempt status will also shelter them from real estate and sales taxes, and most communities are self-managed by a board of directors or sponsorship. Consider a large 350-unit CCRC with an annual budget of $9.4 million in total operating expenses. Costs for taxes and management could easily total $1.3 million annually. The difference, then, between a for-profit and a nonprofit operation represents a 14 percent savings to the residents of the nonprofit community for an equivalent service package, not including the premium for profit and risk.

Many owners are now including clauses in their management agreements to specify performance thresholds based on the community's EBITDAR, defined as net income excluding interest expense (net of interest income), taxes (federal, state, local, and property), depreciation, amortization, and lease expense (property and capital leases). This approach segregates noncontrollable expenses from operations and allows targeting as a percentage of revenue or minimum dollar amount to cover debt. The EBITDAR calculation reflects the true operational expenses and is not subject to fluctuations in interest expense (especially for variable-rate financing). Using EBITDAR net income, owners can establish a predebt value for the revenue stream created by the property using capitalization rates. See the section on "Capitalization Rates" for a detailed discussion on project valuation.

Industry standards for budgeting expenses are detailed in each respective departmental chapter in this book. The relationships are presented as ratios for variable expenses and itemized for fixed expenses, where appropriate, for a typical 200-unit congregate community. These figures can be adjusted upward or downward according to community size and occupancy. Clearly, the development of a community budget and allocation of financial resources will vary greatly according to state regulations, labor markets, community size, competition, service package, and, most important, owner philosophy. Alternatives for various levels of service and quality are offered for management consideration throughout the text.

■ FIXED ASSET CAPITALIZATION

Fixed asset capitalization, also known as capital improvement, is a process of addressing the current and projected physical needs of a property, establishing the costs of maintaining or modernizing it, and creating a strategic plan for addressing the needs within financial constraints.

Some financing vehicles require the maintenance of minimum replacement reserves. The adequacy of these funding levels should be reevaluated over time to identify the optimal reserve through an interactive process. These normally involve rather substantial amounts of capital that may not otherwise be required after the identification of need through the capital planning process.

Clearly understanding current physical needs and anticipating longer-term requirements can help managers control their cash planning, making the most of advantageous credit opportunities and avoiding unnecessary refinancing in unfavorable markets. In other words, asset managers who employ a comprehensive capital planning process can be well served by addressing capital concerns with property resources while the opportunity exists. Owners, managers, and maintenance staff who engage in this planning process together can integrate their objectives into a workable program. Capital planning is a valuable diagnostic tool to prioritize often limited resources in managing the community's current and long-term physical, financial, and human requirements. See Chapter 12 for a complete description of how to develop a comprehensive capital replacement plan.

ACCOUNTING OVERVIEW

The following brief accounting overview is designed to familiarize management with some basic accounting principles and how they apply to operations management in retirement communities. Whether the community objective is to achieve a profit from the operations or merely balance revenues with expenses, it is important to understand the accounting of the community's finances.

Several governing bodies in the accounting profession are dedicated to defining generally accepted accounting principles (GAAP) by setting up accounting standards and rules.[2] These groups publish formal statements and pronouncements on how to handle all kinds of accounting issues, and their publications serve as the authoritative sources on GAAP-basis accounting. The guidelines followed here are generally the most current information provided by the following texts: (1) The Financial Accounting Standards Board (FASB) Statements of Financial Accounting Standards; (2) FASB Interpretations; (3) The American Institute of Certified Public Accountants (AICPA) Accounting Research Bulletins; and (4) The Opinions of the Accounting Principles Board (APB).

Accounting Methods

There are two primary methods of recognizing revenues and expenses: the *cash* basis and the *accrual* basis. It is important to understand what the accrual basis of accounting is, as well as the difference between these two methods of accounting.

The *accrual basis (or method) of accounting* recognizes revenues in the period they are *earned,* that is, when a

good has been sold or a service rendered, and recognizes expenses in the period they are *incurred,* that is, when a legal liability exists. This means that transactions are recorded as earnings and expenses happen, regardless of whether any cash is involved at the time.

The *cash basis (or method) of accounting,* in contrast, only accounts for cash receipts and cash expenditures, not revenues and expenses. Thus transactions are recorded only when there is a flow of cash into or out of a business. For example, when a guest is served a $12.00 guest meal in the dining room, the business has *earned* the $12.00 for that meal. The resident who hosted the guest will pay for the meal next month. Under the *accrual* method of accounting, the business will record or accrue the meal *this month* as a revenue and a balance due (account receivable) from the resident; in contrast, under the *cash* method of accounting, the business would not get to recognize that the meal was served until *next month* when the resident pays for it.

The retirement housing industry lends itself very well to the accrual basis of accounting, as residents normally are charged and pay for their services on a monthly basis. The expenses of delivering these services are also budgeted monthly and yield a clear picture of the financial balance of the operation.

General Ledger

A *general ledger* is the final accounting record of the financial condition and results of operations of a business. All financial business activity is categorized by account codes and recorded in the general ledger. The general ledger keeps track of all account balances as well as the transactions coded to each account. There are two major types of general ledger accounts: *balance sheet accounts,* which keep track of the company's financial condition in the categories of assets, liabilities, and equity; and *income statement accounts,* which keep track of the company's operating results in the categories of revenues and expenses.

ASSETS. *Assets* are items of value or use that a company owns at a given point in time, which usually help the company produce earnings. Assets also include properties and claims against others that may be directly or indirectly applied to cover liabilities. Each company employee is also an asset. Although an employee is not an asset that is "owned" by the company, he or she does help generate earnings for the business and provides valuable services for the company. Examples of other assets are cash, accounts receivable from residents, the facility building, the facility van, and kitchen equipment.

Depreciation is the allocation of cost over the useful life of an asset to determine the true cost of operation. Depreciation recognizes the deterioration or depletion in value of an asset over a given period of time or over the life of the asset. Some assets may be considered to have some salvage (residual) value at the end of the depreciation period. Depreciation does not mean that an item is worthless once it has been depleted, only that the item's cost has been allocated to its estimated useful life. Accounting for depreciation is normally based on the cost or purchase price of the asset plus installation expenses, if any. Normally retirement community assets are depreciated using the straight-line method. This calculation is based on the cost less the salvage value, divided by the years of useful life.

Under the tax-based accounting method, the property is depreciated over 25.5 years, an approach that will render a higher calculated depreciation amount and in turn reduce the tax liability. The tax-based method recognizes income as it is received, or what is known as "constructive receipt." Conversely, under GAAP, income is recognized for income tax purposes as it is earned. The depreciation period is 40 years, which results in a smaller depreciation amount and a higher taxable income.

LIABILITIES. *Liabilities* are legal obligations a company has to others at a given point in time. The point in time usually used to measure these balance sheet items is the end of a month. Examples of liabilities are accounts payable to vendors, loans from the bank or another company, payroll payable to employees, and prepaid rent from residents.

EQUITY. *Equity* is the net worth of the company or business. By definition it is the net of assets minus liabilities.

REVENUES. *Revenues* are amounts that have been *earned* during a specified period of time, or that have already been paid or have a legal right to be paid. The term *revenue* is associated with the accrual basis of account-

ing. Do not confuse revenue with a cash receipt. Cash receipts are the physical collections of money from people who have rented apartments or purchased goods or services from the business. The process by which cash is received in the same period that revenue is earned is called a *cash sale*. Cash received before the period when revenue is earned is called a *prepaid item* and is categorized as a liability, because the business still has a legal obligation to provide a product or service to the resident. If cash is received after the period when revenue is earned, the business is said to be collecting on a *balance due* or *accounts receivable* item, which is an asset, because the business has a claim against the resident to pay for the services and has a legal right to collect it.

EXPENSES. *Expenses* are the costs of operating and owning a business during a specified period of time. The term *expense* is associated with the accrual basis of accounting. Do not confuse an expense with a cash payment. Cash payments are the physical payments of money to people who have provided, or will provide, goods or services to the business. The process by which cash is paid in the same period that the expense was incurred is called a *cash purchase*. Cash paid before the period when the expense is incurred is called a *prepaid expense* and is categorized as an asset, because someone else has a legal obligation to provide the business with the goods or services requested. If cash is paid after the period when the expense was incurred, the business is said to be paying an *accounts payable* item, which is a liability, or a legal obligation to pay someone else. By paying, the business settles a claim the other party had against its assets (cash).

Costs of operating a business can either be expensed or capitalized. All expenditures for new assets and permanent improvements can be capitalized if they increase the value of the property *and* clearly have a benefit that extends three or more years *and* generally have a minimum purchase of $200 per invoice with a unit cost of at least $50 *and* do not fall within the classification of repair and maintenance. Expenditures that are capitalized will not be expensed and therefore will not appear on the statement of profit and loss; rather they become a balance sheet asset and are subject to depreciation. Expenditures made for the purpose of keeping the property in ordinary, efficient operating condition, which do not add value or appreciably extend the useful life of the asset, are repair and maintenance expenses. Employees involved in requesting or approving expenditures should understand the characteristics of these expenditures in order to classify them properly as capital or expense. The facts and circumstances surrounding the expenditure often determine whether it is capital in nature or an ordinary expense. Therefore, all requests for purchase should be accompanied by complete descriptions and justification from the department head. In most cases, expenditures that can be capitalized should be. Expenditures such as these are generally not planned for in the operations budget but are dealt with separately in a fixed-asset capitalization budget.

By knowing what information is included in the general ledger, and how to read the general ledger, you can keep track of the progress and status of your business. By reviewing the general ledger every month, you will see the final product of all the individual transactions you record, approve, or handle every month. The general ledger is a comprehensive tool to help you monitor the strengths and weaknesses of your financial decisions and their results.

It is important to review the general ledger because it can help you identify transactions that may have been recorded in error to a wrong account code. These errors, if left uncorrected, would misstate the results of operations at the community and perhaps its financial condition.

In any business accounting function it is critical to set up systems that provide for a *segregation of duties*, that is, for accounting procedures to be carried out by more than one employee. Tasks are split up and assigned to each employee in a way that creates a system of checks and balances for everyone's work. Typically, the tasks can be categorized into three types of functions:

1. **Custody of assets.** This function controls, has physical access to, and is responsible for the maintenance of a given set of company assets, such as cash.
2. **Recording of assets.** This function keeps the records of what assets the company should have on hand at a given time, based on approved paperwork and information from (3) below.
3. **Review and approval of assets.** This function reviews the actual assets on hand with (1), matches the related paperwork to the assets, and approves the paperwork and information for use by (2). It also reviews the

records being kept by (2) and compares them to the actual assets being handled by (1).

If the records and actual assets do not coincide, the employees in each function must check their work, report their findings to each other, and resolve the problem.

Retirement housing facilities can be set up with various organizational structures. For example, some may have an executive director, office manager or bookkeeper, and office staff, whereas others have resident manager couples, who fulfill the roles of director, bookkeeper, marketing director, and so on. Because of the different titles and roles, it is important to identify functional roles for these employees that will provide the necessary segregation. Adequate internal controls must be designed and maintained to help protect company assets from errors and irregularities.

One of the greatest side benefits of dividing tasks in this way is that each employee involved in the cycle must be aware of what the other employees' duties are. Ideally, every employee involved in the cycle becomes cross-trained to carry out someone else's duties in case of illness, vacation, or turnover. Another equally important side benefit is that segregation of duties can promote an atmosphere of teamwork. Each person is motivated to do his best work, knowing that his peers are relying on its accuracy and integrity and are checking one another's work against it.

An *audit* is a formal review and evaluation of a company. There are two types of audits, each with a different focus or purpose. A *financial* audit is performed on a company's financial records for a specified period of time. The purpose of a financial audit is to determine whether a company's financial condition and results of operations are stated fairly in the financial statements in accordance with GAAP. An audit by an independent (external) certified public accounting firm would be considered a financial audit. An *operational* audit is also performed on a company's financial records or on general departmental operations, but the purpose of an operational audit is to determine whether a company has been operating according to its prescribed policies and procedures. An operational audit also evaluates whether those policies and procedures promote operating standards that are adequate to comply with GAAP. An internal audit would be an example of an operational audit.

■ FINANCIAL ANALYSIS

Financial information to be analyzed varies among companies; however, return on investment and value are two key indicators of performance. In for-profit operations, these indicators are both intrinsically linked to cash flow. *Cash flow* is simply the actual inflow and outflow of cash. It is the heartbeat of any business. It is determined by first subtracting operating expenses from gross revenues to calculate gross operating profit or loss. From gross operating profit are subtracted depreciation, amortization, taxes and insurance, and debt service to calculate net operating income, also referred to as pretax income. Finally, noncash expenses such as depreciation and amortization are added back, and out-of-pocket expenses such as principal reduction (if any) and capital expenditures are subtracted, to yield cash flow. Exhibit 2.1 summarizes the normal calculation of cash flow.

There are essentially two types of cash flow: cash flow from raising and investing capital (also known as non-operating revenue) and cash flow from operations. The two components are combined to produce the cash balance—either positive or negative. As explained earlier, cash received during the year does not necessarily represent the year's total gross revenue, as the funds (while recognized as earned under the accrual-basis accounting method) may not all be recovered from the residents or their estates. Similarly, cash disbursements do not mea-sure total expenses for the year since some products will remain in inventory at year end. In other words, cash inflows and outflows may not necessarily equate to the total respective revenue and expenses for the community. The size of the company's assets (e.g., inventory, accounts receivable) and its liabilities (e.g., loans, bills payable) reveals its financial condition. This information is presented in the *balance sheet*. The balance sheet summarizes the assets and liabilities for one year as recorded on the last day of the income statement period.

Capitalization Rates

The *capitalization rate* is an indicator commonly used to determine asset value based on a single year's cash flow before interest, depreciation, amortization, and taxes, but after a management fee (EBITDAR). Normally the higher the capitalization rate, the greater the investment risk. Buyers who have a declining appetite for risk are requiring higher initial cash-on-cash returns to attract capital because of the limited prospects for future earnings and increased property values. Generally, the higher the level of care, the greater the degree of management intensity and the higher the capitalization rate. Capitalization rates are integrally composed of a number of key factors, such as loan to value ratio, prevailing lending rate, ratio of equity to value, and equity return. Exhibit 2.2 summarizes the calculation of the capitalization rate.

Exhibit 2.1   Income Statement and Cash Flow

	Gross operating revenue
Less	deductions and adjustments (e.g., rental allowance)
Equals	**total income or revenue**
Less	total departmental expenses
Equals	**gross operating profit or loss**
Less	depreciation
Less	amortization
Less	interest expenses
Less	other property expenses (taxes and insurance)
Equals	**net operating income (pretax income)**
Add	depreciation
Add	amortization
Less	capital improvements
Less	principal reduction
Equals	**cash flow**

Exhibit 2.2   **Calculation of Capitalization Rate**

70% Loan to value ratio $\times$ 8.75% lending rate = 6.01%

30% Equity to value $\times$ 20% equity return = 6.00%

Capitalization rate = 12.01%

Assume cash flow before debt service, depreciation, and taxes = $3,800,000

Value of community at 12% capitalization rate = $3,800,000 $\div$ 0.12 = *$31,666,666*

An inverse multiplier of the capitalization rate can reach the same conclusion:
1 $\div$ 0.12 = 8.33 $\times$ $3,800,000 = $31,654,000

Capitalization rates can also be used by management to estimate the effects of revenue and expenses on the value of the community. Even a modest combination of $50 per unit per month in increased revenue or decreased expenses yields $10,000 per month, or $120,000 per year, for a 200-unit project (200 $\times$ $50 $\times$ 12 = $120,000). The enhanced product value is more than $1 million using an 11 percent capitalization rate ($120,000 $\div$ 11% = $1,090,909). As a general rule, every $1 savings in expenses or increase in revenue yields $10 in increased value to the community using a 10 percent capitalization rate ($1 $\div$ 10% = $10). In other words, expense management by department managers has a tenfold effect on enhancing the value of the community to the owner. Conversely, managers who carelessly overspend their budgets will decrease the value of their community for the owner in the same proportion.

A break-even point analysis on operating expenses only and operating expenses plus debt service (principal plus interest), not including depreciation, can be very useful in determining the number of occupied units needed to reach certain investment performance thresholds. It is important to note that the ratios of loan to value affect the break-even point analysis relative to the level of leverage and debt service on the properties. The first break-even point will be reached when revenues cover operating expenses. Industry averages will range from 49 to 67 percent. Property taxes, location, and type of community will also affect this margin. The second and more important break-even point is reached when operating revenues equal operating expenses plus debt service.

This point is generally lower for congregate communities, then increases with the level of care provided. This factor will vary according to the relationship of debt service to the number of units and revenue generated from the unit mix. For a 100-unit assisted living community, this break-even point with debt service should be reached at approximately 80 percent occupancy. Projects with higher break-even points either are operated inefficiently or carry too much debt. Projects that are overburdened with debt may, for example, be highly leveraged or expensively built. As a general rule, it is important that a community operating at stabilized occupancy have a capitalized value equal to or greater than its debt service balance. Projects that fall short of this target are probably not worth their debt service balances and will cost equity to liquidate.

Another method to calculate the value of a community is its *gross revenue multiplier*. This is derived simply by dividing the sale price by the annual gross revenue. This measure will generally fluctuate with the capitalization rate. It is perceived to be more reliable because gross revenues are easier to calculate than net operating income, especially considering the wide variety of operational models employed by different owners and managers in the industry. In the preceding example, if the sale price was $32,000,000 and the gross revenue was $7,800,000, the gross revenue multiplier would be 4.1. The higher the multiplier, generally the more efficient the operation and the higher the revenue trends. Conversely, a low multiplier may be an indication of an inability of residents to absorb increases in operational expenses.

A number of methods and ratios are commonly used to evaluate financial performance and value. The information needed to calculate these ratios is drawn from the major financial statements that the community produces: the balance sheet, revenue and expense statement (profit and loss), and cash flow statement. These financial statements are generally prepared according to the AICPA guidelines and according to GAAP. Normally the ratios are presented as a percentage of 100, and the period analyzed is usually one fiscal year, but it could be as short as one month. In 1990, the AICPA published two reports that standardized the industry's accounting practices regarding the presentation of external financial statements: *Audits of Providers of Health Care Services* and *Statement of Position 90-8.* These were summarized by Fitch Investor Services and are reprinted in Exhibits 2.3–2.6 with their permission.[3]

Debt Service Coverage Ratio

The *debt service coverage ratio* (DSCR) measures the ability to service debt from two sources: DSCR operating and nonoperating income activities, and cash flows from receipt of advance fees and deposits, less any refunds. Income-related numbers derive from the revenue and expense statement, advance fees from the cash flow statement. Thus the ratio combines dollar amounts from audited financial statements that are based on both accrual accounting and cash accounting.

The DSCR is more easily understood when it is dissected. The denominator, maximum annual debt service, is straightforward. However, the numerator is known by several names, including *net available for debt service, net revenues available for debt service,* or simply *net available.*

The calculation of net available adds in actual cash from advance fees (if any), net of refunds, and subtracts noncash revenue associated with the amortization of advance fees. Thus the amortization portion is correctly excluded from net available because it involves no cash flow. By using this method to calculate coverage, the ratio accurately measures the community's ability to service its debt. A DSCR of 1.25 means that for every $1.00 in debt service, the project produces $1.25 in cash flow. Exhibit 2.3 summarizes the calculation of the DSCR.

Exhibit 2.3   Calculation of Debt Service Coverage Ratio

Excess (deficit) of revenue over expenses
Plus interest expense
Plus depreciation expense
Plus amortization expense
Minus amortization of deferred revenue from nonrefundable advance fees (if any)
Plus proceeds from advance fees and deposits (if any)
Minus refunds of advance fees and deposits (if any)

Equals **net available**

DSCR = Net available ÷ maximum annual debt service

REVENUE AND EXPENSE RATIOS

Operating Margin

The operating margin reflects that portion of total revenues retained as operating income, and it relates solely to operations. Because CCRCs have an option in how they present contributions, this ratio can fluctuate. This ratio is also referred to as *operating profit margin.* For example, a 250-unit community fully occupied with $7,800,000 in gross revenue and $4,000,000 in net operating expenses will have a net income from operations of $3,800,000. The operating margin then is the ratio of $3,800,000 to $7,800,000 or 48.7 percent. The operating margin can also be calculated by subtracting the *expense ratio* from 1 (1 − 0.513 = 0.487).

Operating Ratio (Expense Ratio)

By subtracting out noncash items such as amortization of debt issuance expense, the operating ratio determines if ongoing cash revenues sufficiently cover ongoing cash expenses. The ratio also measures the adequacy of periodic service or monthly fees. When it is more than 100 percent, the ratio may indicate a reliance on receiving advance fees to cover operating expenses. *Operating (expense) ratios* are a useful tool to determine overall operational efficiency. They are an expression of the proportion of operating expenses to gross revenue. Operating expenses should include management fees, but should be net of depreciation, real estate taxes, capital improvements, and debt service. For example, a 250-unit community fully occupied with $7,800,000 in gross revenue and $4,000,000 in net operating expenses will have an expense ratio of $4,000,000 ÷ $7,800,000 = 51.3 percent. To approximate net operating income from an expense ratio and gross operating income, take the gross operating income × (1 − expense ratio). In our example, $7,800,000 × (1 − 0.513) = $3,798,600. Expense ratios will vary with the size of the community, underlining the importance of economies of scale. In for-profit communities of under 200 units, an expense ratio of 70 percent may indicate a well-run operation; however, as the number of units increases to 250, an expense ratio of 60 percent may be more in line, and if there are more than 300 units, ratios of 50–55 percent are considered appropriate. Nonprofit communities will have operating ratios close to 100 percent.

Total Excess Margin

The inclusion of nonoperating revenue in the equation provides a total picture of performance.

Exhibit 2.4 summarizes the calculation of revenue and expense ratios.

LIQUIDITY RATIOS

Current Ratio

The *current ratio* is easily calculated by taking the community's total current assets and dividing by its total current liabilities. Most lenders demand at least a 2:1 ratio: for every dollar of debt or liability, there are $2 of cash or assets. Ratios vary from industry to industry, and Dun & Bradstreet publishes the current ratios for a wide range of businesses. The ratios will vary depending on such broad factors as composition of current assets, inventory turnover rate, and credit terms. If a community's current ratio exceeds 5:1 and consistently maintains such a high level, the company would have an unnecessary accumulation of funds that could indicate financial mismanagement. Conversely, a current ratio much below 2:1 in this industry could be cause for serious concern for the operation's liquidity and ability to service short-term obligations. This ratio is not as useful in measuring a CCRC's cash position because its board-designated cash and investments are typically presented as noncurrent assets under the heading "Assets whose use is limited by board for capital/investments."

Other Useful Ratios

The following two calculations, although not true ratios, are defined here because they are used in determining several ratios:

Exhibit 2.4 **Calculation of Revenue and Expense Ratios**

Operating margin

$$\frac{\text{Income (loss) from operations}}{\text{Total revenues}}$$

Operating (expense) ratio

$$\frac{\text{Total operating expenses} \quad \textit{Less} \text{ depreciation expense} \quad \textit{Less} \text{ amortization expense}}{\text{Total Revenues}}$$

Total excess margin

$$\frac{\text{Excess (deficit) of revenues over expenses}}{\text{Total revenues } + \text{ nonoperating revenue}}$$

Daily operating revenues: Total revenues, minus amortization of deferred revenue from nonrefundable advance fees (if any), divided by the number of days in the period, usually 365.

Daily operating expenses: Total operating expenses, minus depreciation expense, amortization expense, divided by the number of days in the period, usually 365.

Net Days in Accounts Receivable

Net days in accounts receivable indicates, in days, the average length of time it takes to collect accounts receivable. Senior living communities normally bill monthly fees in advance. Typically the biggest component of receivables is Medicaid.

Days Cash on Hand

Days cash on hand measures, in days, all cash and investments deemed available to cover daily expenses. The ratio indicates an organization's ability to withstand short-term disruptions in cash receipts. Because the board of trustees or owner commonly imposes this limitation and despite their presentation as limited, these

funds theoretically are available for any use, including payment of debt service if necessary.

Average Days in Current Liabilities

Instead of a "days in accounts payable" ratio, which measures vendor accounts payable, Fitch Investor Services calculates *average days in current liabilites* because this ratio measures the average length of time elapsing before all current liabilities are met. Users should examine the working relationship between net days in accounts receivable and this ratio.

Cushion Ratio

The *cushion ratio* measures cash deemed available in relation to maximum annual debt service. If principal amortization is not structured to produce level debt service, using maximum annual debt service prompts the user to investigate how the balloon payment will be funded.

Exhibit 2.5 summarizes the calculation of liquidity ratios.

Exhibit 2.5   Calculation of Liquidity Ratios

Current ratio

$$\frac{\text{Current assets}}{\text{Current liabilities}}$$

Net days in accounts receivable

$$\frac{\text{Accounts receivable (net)}}{\text{Daily operating revenues}}$$

Days cash on hand

$$\frac{\text{Current assets: cash}}{\textit{Plus} \text{ assets whose use is limited to capital improvements or investments}}{\text{Daily operating expenses}}$$

Average days in current liabilities

$$\frac{\text{Total current liabilities}}{\text{Daily operating expenses}}$$

Cushion ratio

$$\frac{\text{Current assets: cash}}{\textit{Plus} \text{ assets whose use is limited to capital improvements or investments}}{\text{Maximum annual debt service}}$$

CAPITAL STRUCTURE AND CASH FLOW RATIOS

Debt Service Coverage Ratio: Revenues Only

The *debt service coverage ratio for revenues only* is directly related to the DSCR discussed earlier. It reflects the community's ability to service its debt, but only through operating sources. The cash received from net advance fees, a "financing" activity, is intentionally not included in this calculation. When compared to the DSCR, this ratio measures the degree to which the community relies on net advance fees to service its debt. This ratio is expressed as "times covered" or "× ____."

Debt Service as a Percentage of Net Operating and Nonoperating Revenues

Debt service as a percentage of net operating and nonoperating revenues indicates the percentage of all "cash-generating" revenue applied to the maximum annual debt service. It excludes amortization of deferred revenue from nonrefundable advance fees (if any).

Debt Service as a Percentage of Operating Expenses

Debt service as a percentage of operating expenses indicates the percentage of operating expenses applied to the maximum annual debt service burden.

Reserve Ratio

The *reserve ratio* measures the strength of an organization's available cash position relative to its long-term debt.

The next two items, although not capital structure ratios, are included here because they may be leading indicators of future capital needs:

Percentage of plant fully depreciated: Accumulated depreciation, divided by gross total property and equipment.

Average age of plant: Accumulated depreciation, divided by depreciation expense. This result is expressed in years and may indicate the possible need for future capital expenditures.

Long-Term Debt as a Percentage of Total Assets

The *ratio of long-term debt to total assets* reflects indebtedness as it relates to all assets owned. It indicates the relative strength or weakness of a community's capital structure.

Debt-to-Capitalization Ratio

The *debt-to-capitalization ratio* measures leverage and capital structure in relation to net equity or fund balance. It reflects the strength of the equity or net asset base.

Exhibit 2.6 summarizes the calculation of capital structure and cash flow ratios.

INTERPRETING FINANCIAL STATEMENTS

Ratios are helpful but must be used with caution. One ratio alone does not import much information. Ratios are not in and of themselves proofs, but rather clues, providing a basis on which to form a judgment. Suspicion of an unfavorable condition might be aroused by an unsatisfactory ratio. Conversely, the conclusion that a community is financially strong may be confirmed by compiling a series of ratios. It is also important to note that the significance of a ratio may vary among different forms of ownership. In analyzing a for-profit community, for example, particular emphasis is laid on the operating or expense ratio. In a nonprofit community, this ratio is somewhat meaningless.

In their empirical analysis of continuing care retirement communities, Powell and Winklevoss caution that "the drawback of ratio analysis is that even though they may be useful for setting minimum standards, they are heavily dependent on a component that can remain constant over time (debt service), whereas other elements are increasing for inflation. This results in unusually high ratio values in future years. Therefore, taken alone, ratio analysis can present a misleading picture of the community's financial picture."[4]

Ratios calculated from a community's financial statements for only one year have limited value. They become meaningful, however, when compared with other ratios *internally,* that is, with a series of similar ratios for the same community (or company) over a period, or *externally,* that is, with comparable ratios for similar companies or with industry averages. When comparing ratios externally, it is important to ensure not only that the communities are similar, but also that the basis used to calculate each ratio is the same.

A trend is shown by selecting a base date or period, treating the figure or ratio for that period as 100, and then dividing it successively into the comparable ratios for subsequent periods. Analyzing trends in these ratios and in the actual operational revenues and expenses is useful because changes year to year can be easily identified. This approach is also much simpler and lends itself

---

Exhibit 2.6 **Calculation of Capital Structure and Flow Ratios**

Debt service coverage ratio: Revenues only

$$\frac{\text{Excess (deficit) of revenues over expenses}}{\text{Maximum annual debt service}}$$

Excess (deficit) of revenues over expenses
Plus interest expense
Plus depreciation expense
Plus amortization expense
Minus amortization of deferred revenue from nonrefundable advance fees (if any)
———————————————————————————————
Maximum annual debt service

Debt service as a percentage of net operating and nonoperating revenues

Maximum annual debt service
———————————————————————————————
Total revenues
Minus amortization of deferred revenue from nonrefundable advance fees (if any)
Plus nonoperating revenues

Debt service as a percentage of operating expenses

Maximum annual debt service
———————————————————————————————
Total operating expenses

Reserve ratio

Current assets:cash
Plus assets whose use is limited to capital improvements and investments
———————————————————————————————
Long-term debt
Less current maturities

Long-term debt as a percentage of total assets

Long-term debt, *less* current maturities
———————————————————————————————
Total Assets

Debt-to-capitalization ratio

Long-term debt, *less* current maturities
———————————————————————————————
Long-term debt, *less* current maturities + Unrestricted fund balance

---

to clearer interpretation than the alternative two-step method of calculating percentage changes from year to year.

Whether proprietary or nonprofit, each individual owner will have different financial performance expectations. It is most helpful for the executive director and her direct supervisor to understand each other's objectives fully. An operation works best when the needs and interests of the owner are held in balance with the expectations of the residents and employees.

NOTES

1. *Selected Seniors Housing Transactions* (Washington, D. C.: American Seniors Housing Association, 1994), 15–16.
2. P. R. Delaney, B. J. Epstein, J. R. Adler, and M. F. Foran, *GAAP: Interpretation and Application of Generally Accepted Accounting Principles* (New York: John Wiley, 1993).
3. E. C. Merrigan, *Rating Guidelines for Nonprofit Continuing Care Retirement Communities. Fitch Health Care Special Report* (New York: Fitch Investor Services, Inc., 1994).
4. A. V. Powell and H. E. Winklevoss, *Continuing Care Retirement Communities: An Empirical, Financial, and Legal Analysis* (Homewood, Ill.: Pension Research Council, 1984), 176.

Management and Human Resources

3

The secret to stable and consistent operation rests in the hands of the on-site employees and in management's ability to minimize turnover. The retirement housing industry is a "people" business, and those operators who recognize the importance and value of their long-term staff will ultimately be more successful. My roots are in the nursing home business, where there is a hierarchy among the staff that is comparable to that in the military. The acquisitions program at the company for which I worked was aimed at troubled facilities, most of which experienced similar management problems. It usually was not the sponsor's or owner's lack of commitment to good-quality care, but rather the politics of management on site, that led to turnover problems in the ranks, which translated into problems with the consistency of care.

At the very bottom of the totem pole is the certified nursing assistant (CNA). It has always been a mystery to me where that name came from; if anything, the nurses are assisting the CNAs, who really do all the work. Many of them are poorly educated and unskilled, and they have their share of personal problems. The CNA job is without a doubt one of the toughest there is, tantamount to indoor manual labor. It is emotionally and physically draining, and the pay is usually poor. Many people higher up in the ranks look down on the CNA. Those few who escape through education and training to become licensed practical nurses or supervisors rarely look back.

So what keeps CNAs in their jobs? In fact, there is a lot of turnover in these positions, usually more than in any other position on the property. Those who stay either are totally committed to their patients or are locked into their job because of benefits or other reasons. CNAs cannot simply be motivated by the pay they earn. If they are given the right amount of supportive management and recognition, they will stay. Over time a symbiotic relationship will develop between patients and their CNAs. Patients will tell the CNAs how much they appreciate them, comment on their appearance, help them through their personal problems, and even love them. Each becomes a support system for the other, and it is then in the CNAs' best interests to care for their patients. In return, patients will receive the best quality of care that the assistants are capable of giving. It is human nature for people (especially caregivers) to bond with each other; in the right environment, it happens naturally. Managers that recognize the importance of bonding between the caregivers and their patients can create such an environment and enjoy much lower turnover and a higher commitment to the quality of care. It all begins with a resolution to hire the best-quality people in the marketplace.

HIRING PERSONNEL

The single most important decision that we make as managers is the hiring decision. The quality and character of those in whom we place our trust to select and manage our employees will absolutely determine the success of our business. Most managers find the hiring and firing process among the most difficult aspects of their job. What they learn over time is that if they spend more time selecting the right employees for the job, the firing process can be minimized. Inexperienced managers often will hire the first qualified applicant who comes along so as not to prolong the agony of the search and interview process. It is much more difficult and time-consuming to find the right person for the job, but in the long run doing so will make the manager's job easier. It will always take less time to conduct a thorough hiring process than to terminate a bad hire legally.

Employers should seek out applicants who genuinely show an interest in the elderly and like being around older people. Because of the personal nature of this business, it is critical to find caring people who are in part personally motivated by their direct contact with seniors. In this way, close personal relationships can develop and the caregiver can begin to bond with the residents. Residents have a way of overlooking flaws in the operation if they are surrounded by staff members who sincerely care about them. However, residents will be quick to point out each and every shortcoming of the operation to employees who are only working at the community to collect a paycheck and do not make an effort to develop personal relationships with them.

Managers who hire caring employees and create an atmosphere of warmth and kindness will make the delivery of their services much simpler to manage. Managers who recognize the value of bonding between their employees and the residents will see over time a sense of community and family develop within their project. The employees are the support system for the residents, and ultimately the residents reciprocate, through recognition and encouragement, becoming for many employees the only source of support and self-satisfaction they may have in their lives.

Advertising

Help-wanted advertisements should be placed in the local papers, normally by Thursday afternoon to run on the following Saturday and Sunday. If the hiring need is urgent, management might also consider running an ad on Tuesday and Thursday as well. Newspaper classified ad clerks will always try to get an advertiser

to commit to a week-long run and could charge you for one unless you specify specific days. Normally it is a waste of money to run an ad every day, and your ad will quickly become stale.

Ad copy should be imaginative, witty, clear, and concise. Make it appear as though the company is growing and is a fun place to work. Many qualified people who are already employed routinely scan the Sunday classifieds to learn about new companies and growth opportunities and to compare wages. Abbreviate only when necessary, as overuse of this device can make the company appear cheap. Always include a contact name, such as "Ask for Molly," to add a personal touch. Watch the use of phrases. Marilyn Moats Kennedy, in her *Career Strategist* newsletter, explains that some people might read "fast-growing company" to mean "it's a sweatshop." A "lean" organization could be interpreted as one that has "been through budget cuts, a reorganization, downsizing, or all three." And a "prestigious" firm could be one that "hopes you'll accept the afterglow from its reputation in the place of money."[1]

Never use the same ad for two consecutive weeks, unless it is prepared in camera-ready form and includes artwork. This format may even be more economical for a high-profile company with several openings. Always ask the ad clerk for a tear sheet of the ad, the cost, and the number of lines. Keep track of the responses and keep a library of the ads that give the best results and build on them.

An advertising agency can be useful in developing a quality shell ad for placement in the classifieds. The agency will qualify for discounts on their media buys from the newspaper, and a portion of these discounts can be passed on to the community in the form of rebates or services such as writing ad copy, coordinating the layout of inserts, and placement. Display advertisements developed using desktop publishing can significantly improve response rates and are routinely developed at no charge by agencies. Once the relationship has been established, the community need only place a call to the agency with its request, and the agency will incorporate the ad requests directly into a predesigned corporate template and send the camera-ready artwork directly to the newspaper. The newspaper then bills the agency for the media placement, and the agency in turn bills the community at the discounted rate.

The Interview Process

The interviewing process is a challenging one. In a short period of time, you must develop a rapport with a candidate and evaluate whether the individual is capable of performing the essential functions of the job, fitting the profile that management requires and the residents will accept, blending into the current team environment, and delivering the results you are looking for in a professional and caring manner. This process must be accomplished in a way that presents a favorable impression of the community regardless of whether the candidate is excellent or disappointing. Recruitment specialists agree that some of the most successful managers are those who hire and surround themselves with high-quality, self-confident people who will in turn hire the same type of people to work for them. The end result is an organization built on strength and confidence from the bottom up.

Interviewing to fill a management position is an especially difficult task. Most résumés will detail accomplishments and work history but tell you nothing about the person's people skills and management abilities, when in fact the manager is hired to manage. Most people will gravitate toward what they perceive themselves to be best at. Normally this involves the actual mechanics of doing the job. Most candidates can tell you in great detail *how to do the job,* but what they really need to be telling you is *how to get the job done through others.* Inexperienced managers will almost always revert to the mechanical aspects of their jobs when the jobs become difficult, in an effort to conceal their management shortcomings. This normally happens at the most inconvenient of times, underscoring the vital importance of hiring *experienced* managers in the first place. There is no easy way to evaluate a candidate's management skills in a short interview or on paper. Anyone can put on his or her best act for the one or two hours that it takes to interview for a job. In fact many managers are so anxious to get the hiring process over with that they fall victim to the "tell them what they want to hear" routine from job applicants. Managers are well advised to understand that among all the decisions they will make, everything else pales in comparison to the hiring decision. Once made, it is not easily reversed; other employees and the residents whom they will serve are depending on the manager to make the right choice.

PREPARING FOR THE INTERVIEW

The interviewer's ability to take maximum advantage of the limited time available with each candidate depends on her preparedness for the interview process. In addition to receiving specific training in interview skills, the interviewer can prepare for the interview in advance. To begin with, she should establish a clear idea of the selection criteria that will be used to evaluate the candidate. She should also be familiar with the specific requirements of the position for which the candidate is applying.

The key to reviewing a résumé is the ability to recognize what information is there as well as what information is *not.* The interviewer should fix clearly in her mind the candidate's name and background highlights so that the interview questions can be personalized. This personal touch will build rapport as well as allow the interviewer to focus on relevant data.

Omissions or unusual information on the résumé or application are signals that the interviewer may need more evidence before reaching a decision. Important pieces of information to note when reviewing a résumé include the following:

- Appearance of the résumé, correct use of vocabulary and grammar and syntax
- Degree program(s) completed, or relevant course work
- Level of scholastic achievement
- Relevant extracurricular activities versus "filler" intended merely to impress
- Work experience relevant to the senior housing industry
- Time gaps or periods of unemployment or spotty school attendance
- Reasons for leaving jobs
- Job-related health problems
- Language proficiencies
- Availability to start
- Descriptions of former positions as accomplishments rather than duties performed

The next requirement in preparing for an interview is to have a clear idea of the traits and abilities that will be needed for the individual to be successful in the new job. The following traits, skills, and abilities are well matched to the demands of employees working with seniors:

Personal traits: Appearance, initiative, enthusiasm, creativity, maturity, tenacity, common sense, flexibility, and *warmth*.

Abilities and skills: Communication skills, interpersonal skills, organizational skills, work experience, leadership ability, and education.

The following set of working definitions for these traits, abilities, and skills should provide the interviewer a better understanding of what to look for in a candidate:

Appearance: Able to create a positive first impression based on appropriate standards of dress and grooming; displays a self-confident demeanor that is friendly and capable.

Initiative: Actively attempts to influence events to achieve goals; self-starting rather than passively accepting. Generates alternative solutions to problems and initiates action beyond what is necessarily called for.

Enthusiasm: Projects a positive mental attitude and maintains a high level of activity. Displays a cheerful, helpful, service-oriented attitude.

Creativity: Generates or recognizes imaginative, innovative solutions in work-related situations. Demonstrates ability to implement an ordinary idea with extraordinary style and flair.

Maturity: Able to reflect on and learn from experiences. Projects self-confidence based on an accurate self-assessment of strengths and weaknesses. Can exercise patience and self-control in difficult situations. Demonstrates awareness of social, ethical, and legal norms in job-related activities. Able to balance work priorities and personal priorities.

Tenacity: Shows willingness and drive to work through difficulties in order to achieve goals, as well as perseverance in maintaining high standards of excellence.

Common sense: Exercises sound judgment, develops alternative courses of action, and makes decisions that are based on logical assumptions and reflect factual information. Calmly exercises resourcefulness when faced with an unexpected challenge.

Flexibility: Demonstrates ability to adjust readily to new and changing circumstances. Maintains adaptability in varying environments in which tasks, responsibilities, or people are constantly changing. Able to switch to a new or different way of doing something to accomplish a goal.

Warmth: Describes peers and former residents in terms of endearment and compassion. Is motivated by the development of interpersonal relationships and is a good communicator. Seems to be relaxed and friendly, is engaging. (This is the most important characteristic for employees who will be dealing directly with the residents. Residents will immediately spot an employee who is not genuine, and they may at times feel threatened by them. As residents age, they experience a heightened sense of vulnerability, so it is important to surround them with warm and caring employees.)

Communication skills: Expresses ideas clearly and appropriately and demonstrates active listening skills when interacting with others. Is patient when communicating with elderly persons and does not interrupt when someone is talking. Written communications demonstrate appropriate vocabulary and correct grammar and syntax.

Interpersonal skills: Demonstrates ability to meet people easily and build rapport quickly. Shows consideration for the feelings and needs of others. Puts people at ease; smoothly and successfully gets along with a variety of people at all organizational levels.

Organizational skills: Plans a logical course of action or establishes a system for self and others to accomplish goals. Properly allocates time, personnel, and resources to meet production objectives and deadlines.

Work experience: Possesses relevant job experience that demonstrates interest in the senior living industry. Has demonstrated effective work relationships with peers and supervisors. Has the ability to apply and transfer insights from one work environment to another. (A pattern of dissatisfaction with working conditions, superiors, or coworkers may be an indicator of instability in the applicant.)

Leadership ability: Utilizes appropriate interpersonal styles and methods in guiding individuals (subordinates, peers, and superiors) or groups toward task accomplishment without relying on the power of authority or position. Earns the respect of coworkers and subordinates through demonstrated results. Takes an active interest in helping others to achieve their goals. Sets high standards of performance for self and inspires others to achieve.

Education: Has completed relevant course work and achieved an adequate level of scholastic attainment. Has demonstrated similar levels of effort and motivation in achieving school-related goals as well as work-related goals.

CONDUCTING THE INTERVIEW

Interviewing requires a great deal of effort, concentration, and practice. Gathering the same general background data from each candidate and remembering what each candidate said may appear to be an awesome task, yet it becomes much more manageable when a standardized and rehearsed technique is consistently used. The following five-step plan can form the basis for a thorough interview in which the maximum amount of information can be exchanged in the limited time available.

STEP 1: Building Rapport

This step involves creating an environment that puts the candidate at ease and establishes a warm conversational tone from the very beginning of the interview. People will communicate better when they feel relaxed. The interview itself is a stressful event at best, and most people are forced to step outside their own comfort zones when they communicate about themselves and their accomplishments. The interviewer must recognize this and actively strive to set the candidate at ease and begin to build trust. Only candidates who are comfortable with the interviewer will be willing to open up and share positive and negative information about their past experiences.

Greet each candidate with a warm and pleasant smile and a firm handshake; look the candidate in the eye and let her know you are sincerely interested in spending time with her. Once the applicant has been invited to be seated, the interviewer can use additional small talk to start the conversation flowing. The important thing is to get the applicant talking about herself. Most people will open up when the conversation turns to a subject that may be their hobby or involves personal experience, children, or something of which they are particularly proud.

As soon as the candidate is relaxed, the interview can begin. By mentally preparing a transition statement in advance, the interviewer can, after the sense of rapport has been established, move smoothly into the information-gathering stage without appearing abrupt. The transition statement should politely signal to the candidate that the "official" interview is about to begin and let the candidate know what to expect. Experienced interviewers can accomplish this transition without missing a beat.

STEP 2: Gathering Information

Some information about a candidate, such as level of social skills or verbal expression, can be easily observed in the interview. The interview itself is a "behavioral sample" of what can be expected from the candidate, and the interviewer must then dig for the evidence. A good way to inform the candidate that references will be checked is to start the interview by asking him to answer the questions the way he expects his references would answer them. The purpose of the information-gathering phase is to ask questions that

1. Gather behavioral examples of past job and school experiences related to the selection criteria.
2. Keep the candidate talking and maintain rapport.
3. Avoid legally inappropriate areas.

Ask broadly based or open-ended questions to steer the candidate to the information that is needed. For example: "Suppose you begin by telling me about your last position. I would be interested in how you chose the company and what you liked best and least about your former job." (See Chapter 14 for more on gathering information and asking probing questions.) The interviewer should concentrate on the candidate's story, picking up significant clues, analyzing their meaning, and making mental notes of any inconsistencies or voids that should be touched on in follow-up questions.

Follow-up questions directly follow from the information the candidate shared in response to a broadly based question. These more focused questions are designed to gather specific examples of behavior and encourage the candidate to share more details or feelings. For example: "That's interesting—tell me more," or "Why did you make that decision?" or "How did you react when that happened?" Even a silent pause can be used effectively as a follow-up question, provoking the candidate to share more information in an effort to break the silence. If there is obviously more to be said by the applicant on an issue, the interviewer can simply pause, looking at the candidate expectantly for several seconds, until the candidate realizes that she should elaborate. It is important for the interviewer to be a good listener and allow the candidate to do most of the talking. The interviewer should avoid interrupting the candidate or changing the subject abruptly. The interviewer should always be alert to nonverbal communication from the candidate; nonverbal behavior can provide real clues to comfort levels and the legitimacy of information that is being discussed. (See Chapter 14 for tips on improving listening skills.)

The interviewer should give the candidate his undivided attention, maintain constant eye contact, and paraphrase statements made by the applicant if they are unclear. The interviewer should be aware of personal opinions and how they are expressed and gauge them against the philosophy of the organization and compatibility with the team.

Several types of questions should be avoided when interviewing, some because they will not yield useful information and waste valuable time and others because they delve into legally inappropriate areas. Title VII of the Civil Rights Act of 1964 requires that selection criteria for job applicants be "job related." Any questions asked in a selection interview that directly or indirectly uncover information about the following areas are specifically prohibited by law: age, race, national origin, religion, marital status, dependents, child care concerns, housing, health status, type of military discharge, arrest records, sexual preference, willingness to work weekends, and any information from minority or female applicants not routinely requested of white or male applicants. Exhibit 3.1 lists some sample interview questions for candidates applying for management positions.

Exhibit 3.1   Sample Interview Questions for Management Candidates

I. Education

1. How did you become interested in this field?
2. What courses did you particularly enjoy or excel at?
3. What courses were a challenge for you?
4. Did you participate in any clubs or organizations?
5. How did you finance your education?
6. How has your education prepared you for this position?

II. Experience

1. How has your experience prepared you for this position?
2. At this point in your career are you satisfied with what you have accomplished? Have you realized the career goals that you set for yourself?
3. What are your most important career accomplishments?
4. Have you ever been promoted?
5. What features of your previous jobs have you liked?
6. Describe your best boss and your worst.
7. What is the best piece of constructive criticism that you ever received? What did you do with it?

III. Motivation

1. What interests you most about the position we have? The least?
2. What are your short- and long-term planning objectives?
3. Apart from benefits and compensation, what would you look to gain from or develop in this role?
4. How would you describe success?

5. What is the most important decision you have ever made?
6. What is the biggest disappointment you have suffered recently?
7. What do you look for in a position?
8. Why do you want to leave your current position?
9. What kind of references would you receive from your former employees?
10. What would you like to do better?
11. As your new boss, what should I learn from your former boss on how to motivate you?

IV. Personality

1. What is the greatest risk you have ever taken?
2. What do you look for in the people you hire?
3. How would your coworkers describe you? Your subordinates?
4. Describe the professional profile of someone whom you admire. What are some of their professional skills that you would like to incorporate into your own professional style?
5. You have been asked to write a book on managing people and are limited to five chapters. What are they entitled?

V. Compensation and benefits

1. What is your current rate of pay? Are you eligible for bonuses?
2. Are you satisfied with your current compensation?
3. How frequently were increases given?
4. What benefits do you currently receive?
5. Are you satisfied with your benefits?
6. Are you paying any portion of your employee benefits?

STEP 3: Selling Yourself and the Company

Most job interviews should involve a mutual exchange of information. If the job applicant is a high-quality person, she will want to associate with a high-quality operation and supervisor. The shrewd interviewer will recognize that highly qualified people will require a high-quality work environment with a company that recognizes and values the individual contributions of each of its employees and actively seeks opportunities to keep its top performers properly challenged, motivated, and rewarded. Top candidates will be looking for a long-term relationship with an employer and will evaluate the company's standards, especially turnover. Companies that demonstrate a commitment to solving problems rather than "firing them away" will create a culture of trust within their current employee base. Ultimately, the company's reputation (good or bad) will determine the type of employee who will work there. Top people have a tendency to gravitate to organizations that treat their employees as assets and teach their managers to respect and motivate their staffs. Walt Disney World in Orlando, Florida, receives 65,000 unsolicited résumés per year for its 200 annual job openings. Satisfied employees are your best advertisement for new staff.

There are only a limited number of top people in the workplace. These people are normally treated well by their employers and are usually comfortable in their current positions. To attract these people away from competitors, your organization must demonstrate distinct advantages. Wages and salaries play only a small part in attracting people; the real motivators are work environment and growth opportunities.

The interviewer should take time to explain the mission of the company and how the company has grown by building on the strengths of its employees and their commitment to that mission. Examples of employees who have overcome adversity and turned challenge into achievement that ultimately strengthened the company will create a sense of belonging for job applicants. Success stories will build a desire to share in the company's success and motivate top candidates to want to join.

The interviewer should also describe specifically the expectations of the position for which the candidate is applying. The better the understanding of the job requirements, the more likely the candidate will be successful once hired for the job. The new employee should not encounter any surprises once hired. Many applicants will need an explanation of what assisted living or congregate housing is, including a description of services offered and the company's management philosophy. This can help the applicant to understand the job duties and performance expectations.

It is generally better to hire someone who is slightly *underqualified* for a position, and who can then be trained and molded, rather than to hire someone who may be overqualified for the job and who may feel that he is settling for something less than what he wants or feels he deserves. It is much easier to motivate someone who is feeling challenged in the job than someone who may feel bored.

For new communities, benefits should be kept somewhat lean but competitive. Cash flow from the operation will be short until the building fills, so management should at first be conservative with benefits. After the community has been open for a few years, additional benefit layers can be added to promote longevity for employees who may be approaching the maximum wage rate for their positions.

Finally, it is important to stress the considerable rewards afforded to those who serve the elderly. Senior living employees are uniquely empowered to influence their residents dramatically and make a real difference in their lives. As seniors become increasingly challenged by their own aging, their inability to perform formerly routine tasks can become a source of stress. Much of this stress is internalized; this can make them very vulnerable to depression. Ample research has demonstrated the mind's capacity to influence one's health—both positively and negatively. If left unchecked, depression and despair can inhibit recovery from illness and lead to hopelessness and even, ultimately, premature death. A caring staff can help seniors accept their own aging and cope with everyday difficulties. Often close personal relationships can reverse the depression and exert a genuinely recuperative effect. Time and again, employees in senior living communities enjoy the self-satisfaction of giving seniors back their lives. This can be the single most effective motivating factor of all, for self-satisfaction can never be bought with a paycheck.

STEP 4: Closing the Interview

The manner in which the interviewer concludes the interview is very important to the candidate's overall impression of the company. It is important to thank the candidate for the time spent together and be encouraging but noncommittal. Inform the candidate about the next steps, when you expect to reach a decision, who will contact her, and whom to call if she has any further questions. Verify her phone number, and let her know that references will be checked.

Often the true measure of the quality of a company is the caliber and experience of the people who seek employment with it. Few things that a manager can do will better reflect the high quality of the organization than sending a personal note. I always send a personal note to each applicant, thanking them for the interview. The note normally says that their qualifications and background are most impressive, that we are flattered that they have included our company in their employment exploration, and that we look forward to the possibility of working together. Not only can this simple gesture communicate the quality level of the organization, it may also create within the applicant a desire to belong. Impressing an applicant in this way can often strengthen the manager's negotiating position at the time of hiring while setting the stage for a positive first encounter.

If the interviewer does not intend to pursue the matter further, he should let the applicant know why. There are many legitimate reasons for declining applicants, including the following:

1. The applicant is qualified for the position, but other applicants may be better suited to the team.
2. The candidate's abilities to perform the duties of the position properly do not meet the community's skill requirements for the position.
3. The applicant has sensory, mental, or physical handicaps that would interfere with or prevent the applicant from properly performing the functions of the job.
4. The applicant has insufficient education or experience to meet the set requirements of the position.
5. The applicant has provided false information on the application or résumé.

STEP 5: Evaluate the Candidate

At this time, the interviewer will begin to evaluate all of the information collected to determine if the candidate possesses the traits necessary to be successful in the position for which she has applied. The eval-

uation process will draw upon information from the candidate, information collected from the interview, and information about the candidate from former employers and coworkers. The hiring decision is a gamble at best; there are many more marginal applicants looking for jobs than top-quality people, and the odds are against you. The best you can do is make an informed decision, for a decision made in haste can create conflict within an established team and be time-consuming to reverse. In addition, a bad hire can be a poor reflection on the manager and embarrassing to the company.

The best predictor of future job performance is past job behavior, and reference checks are the most reliable way to verify impressions, authenticate the information the candidate has presented, and help predict if the candidate will be successful in the job if hired. References can either confirm the interviewer's instincts that the candidate will meet the demands of the position or uncover information about the person that does not match up with that provided during the interview. The candidate should be asked to provide the name and phone number of at least one subordinate, one peer, and one superior. Often the measure of the quality of an employee is in how that person treats people at all levels in the organization. Managers who treat their subordinates and their supervisors differently may be inconsistent in how they manage the many functions of their jobs. References that are not checked adequately can often put the organization at risk of hiring a problem employee and cause the interviewer to pass up others who may deserve consideration.

Formulate questions in advance of making contact with an applicant's references. Questions asked of a candidate's subordinate should include inquiries about sense of fairness, job knowledge, attitude toward employees and the company's management, supervisory skills, and interest in the growth of employees. Questions for a peer might address teamwork issues, involvement in company politics, demonstration of willingness to share credit for accomplishments, and whether the candidate was successful in the job. The nine tough questions in Exhibit 3.2 are adapted from a book entitled *Robert Half on Hiring,* by Robert Half, founder of one of the country's largest recruiting firms.[2]

Reference checking is a time-consuming and often frustrating process in today's litigious business environ-

| **Exhibit 3.2** | **Nine Tough Questions** |

1. How does he compare to the person who's doing the job now? Or, what characteristics will you look for in his replacement?
2. If she was so good, why didn't you try to rehire her? Or, why didn't you try to induce her to stay?
3. When there was a particularly urgent assignment, what steps did she take to get it done on time?
4. None of us is perfect at everything we do; please describe some of his shortcomings.
5. Have you seen his current résumé? Let me read you the part that describes his job with your organization. (Stop at each significant point and ask the reference for a comment.)
6. Not all employees like all other employees. With what kinds of people did she have difficulty?
7. On average, how many times a month does he take off for personal reasons or sickness? How many times a month did he come in late or leave early?
8. Who referred her to your company? (Could it have been a relative or a customer or client?)
9. When she was hired, were her references checked thoroughly? Who checked these references, and what did her references have to say?

ment, for many employers hesitate to be candid in giving references, fearing lawsuits by an ex-employee.

Hiring former employees or promoting from within the organization is the best and safest method. The individual will already be well known to the organization, and it is good for morale for employees to see top performers singled out for promotion. The practice sends a message throughout the entire organization that there is a future for those who can apply themselves and that everyone has the chance to share in the success of the company. Recommendations from friends and acquaintances can also be a source of qualified candidates, although it is still a good idea to check references regardless of who may have recommended the candidate.

Checking references is not an easy task, especially if the reference is unable to confirm the interviewer's impressions of the candidate from the résumé and interview. Most people have established work patterns during their careers. An employee's long-term behavioral patterns are rarely changeable; do not

assume you can manage an unsatisfactory applicant into a good employee. Most behavioral problems follow people from one job to the next; if they had difficulties with their former employers, they are at risk of having the same difficulties (or worse) with you.

Do not expect anything to fit perfectly. Most people will be very general when offering comments about an employee's past work history; ask references to explain any broad generalizations. When you are hearing only glowing accounts of the employee's past performance, ask the reference to cite specific examples to support those accolades. Do not make up your mind about a candidate *before* the references are properly checked, even if there is pressure to do so.

When hiring employees who will have direct contact with seniors, it is advisable to speak with former residents, the president of the resident council, or another unrelated senior to test perceptions regarding the candidate's attitude and approach toward the elderly. Seniors will generally be the most candid and can provide the customer's perspective—the most important one of all.

The Criminal Offender Record Information System (CORI) includes records and data compiled by a criminal justice agency that relate to the nature or disposition of criminal charges, arrests, pretrial proceedings, other judicial proceedings, sentencing, incarceration, rehabilitation, and release. The Criminal History Systems Board restricts access to this information to those individuals or businesses for which it has been determined that the public interest in disseminating such information clearly outweighs the risk to security and privacy. This information is collected and controlled by each state, although federal databases also exist. Once certified, a management designee can access the system for as little as $10 per employee to screen current and otherwise qualified prospective employees and volunteers who will have the opportunity for unsupervised contact with the elderly and infirm in their homes, a category that technically includes senior living communities. The consistent utilization of the CORI system will help management minimize the risk of criminal activity among employees and is strongly recommended. It is important to notify current employees that all staff members who work with residents in the privacy of their apartments will be subject to a CORI check, and new hires should be notified at the time of the interview.

Finally, do not be afraid to reject your last candidate and start the process all over from the beginning; wait for the *right* candidate—sooner or later she will come around. It is far better to be slightly short-handed or ask other department heads to pitch in than to hire the wrong person for the job. The residents will understand; after all, they are paying for, and expect, the best.

Once a job offer has been accepted, the newly hired candidate should be sent a hiring letter to confirm the terms of employment. The letter should welcome and encourage the new employee, as well as confirm the title, salary, commencement date, and review schedule. It should also state the direct supervisor's name and include a job description that can be signed in duplicate and returned. Finally, the letter should restate the company's objectives. For example: "I am looking forward to this new partnership and to the significant contribution that I know you will make to our overall operations. Let's work together to make [the company] the preferred provider, the choice employer, and the standard by which excellence will be measured in the senior living industry. . . . If you have any questions or need further clarification, please feel free to contact me. Otherwise, please sign and return the second copy of this letter to confirm your acceptance of this offer. Welcome!"

Even the best of research can result in a problem after the employee has been hired. In such a situation you might want to call a few of the same references again: "Remember me? I'm Ben Pearce. I called you about six weeks ago in connection with a reference that you gave regarding Joe Slow, and we hired him." Ask the reference for additional clarification about the employee's problem. When confronted with a specific complaint, the reference is likely to be much more candid and offer some solutions on how to manage the behavioral issue. At the very least, the reference will think twice before offering such an enthusiastic endorsement in the future.

In many areas of the country, the competition for qualified and competent staff takes precedence over competition for resident prospects. It is a good idea to develop a one-page summary fact sheet outlining the employee benefits offered by the company. It is also a very nice touch to develop a "summary of benefits" brochure for your community that attractively presents the benefit plan. This can be accomplished very inex-

pensively with most word processing programs and printed, front and back, on preformatted paper. Colorful two-sided paper specifically formatted for brochure development with word processors can be found in most print shops or through companies such as Paper Direct.[3] The finished brochure can be folded to fit into a no. 10 business envelope.

It is important to manage employee expectations of company-provided benefits. The benefit plan should be perceived as an added value and part of the total compensation package. One good way to accomplish this is to develop a "compensation summary" worksheet for each employee. This worksheet can be developed using any spreadsheet program. It is intended to calculate the dollar value to the employee of each benefit; it can be prorated for part-time employees. In this way, when the hiring letter is sent, it can be accompanied by a worksheet detailing the cash value of the total compensation package. The prospective employee can see that, although the starting wage may be a bit low compared to other employers, the *total value* of the compensation package reflects a much higher dollar figure. These summary sheets should also be prepared annually for all employees at raise time to remind them of the value added in their benefit package or to minimize the negative feelings resulting from changing benefit plans. Exhibit 3.3 shows a representative compensation summary for a full-time employee.

■■■■■ PERFORMANCE EVALUATIONS

The evaluation process is fraught with anticipation and anxiety for everyone involved. Going through this procedure together each year provides managers and employees an opportunity to review and evaluate the process, allowing for a greater understanding of its need and importance. Yet managers often conduct performance evaluations with one goal in mind: how can we get through this without having to tell this employee how we really feel?

The evaluation process provides an opportunity to evaluate an employee's work performance from a manager's point of view and the manager's ability to manage from the employee's point of view. It creates a forum in which managers and staff should discuss opportunities, goals, and expectations; overcome objections; and voice concerns. The end result should be a positive exchange of information leading to a clear-

Exhibit 3.3   **Total Compensation Summary**

Employee: Executive director
SSN#:   000-00-0000

Cash compensation		**Per hour**
Base salary	$55,000.00	$26.44
Bonus	2,500.00	
Total cash	57,500.00	

Benefit value	
Medical	2,400.00
Dental	204.00
Life insurance and accidental death and dismemberment	115.50
Long-term disability	269.50
Sick days	1,692.31
Personal days	423.08
Holidays	2,115.30
Vacation	3,173.08
Bereavement	634.62
Tuition reimbursement	1,000.00
Employee assistance program	30.00
Child care reimbursement	360.00
401(k) retirement plan	1,100.00
	10,797.89

Employer contributions	
FICA—Social Security	4,207.50
Federal unemployment	440.00
State unemployment	1,650.00
Worker's compensation	2,310.00
	8,607.50

Total benefits costs/contributions	22,124.89
Total cash compensation	57,500.00
Total cash plus benefits	**$79,624.89**

Your total benefits package equals an additional   14%   of your annual salary.

Health insurance

Several health insurance plans are available to choose from. For **executive directors,** the first three months of premiums are fully paid by the employer. The employee contribution is dependent on the plan you choose and whether you need individual or family coverage.

Life insurance

In the event of your death, your beneficiary will receive **$55,000.00.** This insurance is provided at no cost to you.

Long-term disability insurance

Long term disability insurance is provided as a source of income protection. This coverage will provide you each month **$2,750.00** (60% of salary) beginning 90 days after the onset of the disability.

Absence benefits

			Vacation			
Holidays	Personal	Sick	1–2 yrs	3–5 yrs	5+ yrs	Bereavement
10 days	2 days	8 days	10 days	15 days	20 days	3 days

The total value of your time-off benefits (holidays, personal days, sick days, and vacation) is **$7,403.85.** This amount is included as part of your regular annual income.

cut set of goals and objectives for continued staff development. As managers, we are empowered to be leaders and teachers, providing specific guidelines and opportunities for growth and personal influence on our growing organizations.

Any meaningful evaluation process must be ongoing. Each employee is entitled to regular and consistent feedback. The process should explore and evaluate certain themes or trends in an individual's performance, highlighting those that are positive, providing an action plan for correcting those that are not, focusing on future growth, and establishing priorities. The annual merit evaluation should be the culmination of this process rather than a discussion of new issues. It is not the time for surprises.

If the employee's performance has been proactively managed throughout the year by providing recognition and support for accomplishments and redirection when needed, the evaluation meeting should be a positive experience for both parties. Even a distinguished performer should receive feedback on areas needing improvement and should be given goals and objectives for continued development.

Performance evaluations are useful not only as an annual evaluation tool but also as a means for managers to clarify expectations. Many times performance issues arise because employees become mired in details and lose sight of their priorities. The performance evaluation process can help manager and employee alike to regain their perspective and redefine the essential priorities of the position. When employee performance problems start to arise, they are often a good indicator of some bigger issue. The performance evaluation is one of the best tools at the manager's disposal to get things back on track.

Performance evaluations that are expected to be negative are normally the result of poor management. An inexperienced manager avoids confronting performance issues, hoping things will improve. Yet procrastination will only lead to a deterioration of the situation and result in hard feelings. Breakdowns in communication between the supervisor and the employee almost always degenerate into conflict, ultimately leading the manager into a hopeless situation that can result in the employee's termination. Managers must not be allowed to "fire their problems away." It is much easier and cheaper in the long run to manage performance than to start from scratch with a new employee. Managers should be taught to look for solutions to problems.

Persons working for more than one supervisor should attend an evaluation session with the supervisor of the department for which they work the greatest percentage of their time. (However, input from the other supervisor(s) should be sought out and utilized during the review process.) All evaluation forms should be reviewed by the department head and the executive director before being discussed with staff members. In this way the executive director can understand the strengths and vulnerabilities of all the employees and use this process as an opportunity to help each supervisor clarify expectations for the staff. The executive director can also take the time to reemphasize the importance of the evaluation process and coach each supervisor on how to achieve the desired results.

Performance Appraisal Guidelines

Giving employees feedback through performance appraisals is fundamental to good management. Like most management skills, constructive evaluation requires a great deal of preparation, concentration, and practice. Summarizing information about an employee's strengths and areas for improvement covering every aspect of the job is for most supervisors an agonizing task. Most of our time is spent handling the day-to-day issues that arise and performing the essential duties of our positions. Rarely do we take the time to relax and communicate with our employees regarding how they actually feel about their jobs: their perceptions about work flow, residents, other employees, and the company. Over time, professional managers learn that the appraisal process can be a welcome respite from the daily grind and one of the most effective uses of their time. Performance appraisals should be well thought out *in advance* and should encompass the following key components: (1) preparation, (2) appraisal discussion, (3) giving feedback, (4) listening, (5) establishing agreement, (6) discussing performance improvement, and (7) closing.

STEP 1: Preparation

Being prepared for the meeting is very important. How you begin sets the tone for the entire session. The appointment should be made well in advance so that the supervisor and employee have ample time to prepare for the discussion. It is a good idea to distribute a "self-appraisal" form that will provide the employee an opportunity to evaluate her own performance as well as begin to set future goals. The completed form should be returned to the supervisor before the meeting.

The meeting should be scheduled in a private place free from interruptions. It is important to schedule enough time for each employee so that neither party feels hurried. Avoid interrupting the appraisal to take care of business. After an appointment has been set it should not be canceled, and the meeting should start on time, thus communicating to the employee the importance that is attached to the process and demonstrating respect.

The employee's personnel file should be reviewed before a written appraisal of job performance can be performed. The supervisor should be familiar with the contents, especially areas for improvement that were previously noted. The supervisor should be prepared to discuss any negative areas and also to review accomplishments. Striking a balance between positive and negative feedback demonstrates fairness by management and the validity of the process.

The supervisor should be able to anticipate and answer several questions from the employee:

- How am I doing?
- Where do I go from here?
- What are my major skills?
- In what areas do I need to improve?
- What do I need to do to improve?

STEP 2: The Appraisal Discussion

It is a good idea to begin the meeting with a discussion of the purpose of the performance appraisal and what the supervisor hopes to accomplish during this meeting. The supervisor should stress that the process is not intended simply to report to the employee on her performance, but to open up lines of communication in both directions. In order to accomplish this, the supervisor will need to take some time to set the employee at ease. Most people find it difficult to talk about performance; the evaluation process is at best a bit intimidating. The supervisor should set the stage early for a relaxed discussion.

Before reviewing the evaluation form itself, the supervisor should initiate an informal discussion about the employee and the job. How does the employee feel about the job, the department, the supervisor, and

coworkers? In this way, the employee can begin to feel comfortable talking about himself. The supervisor can begin discussing the performance of the department in general and discuss areas of potential growth. The supervisor should also explain the evaluation process and what it is intended to accomplish.

The supervisor can start by reviewing each item on a *blank* evaluation form and discussing her views about it. An employee may want to challenge some of the supervisor's negative perceptions on each topic of the evaluation form. This can be done later; first the employee needs to understand all the criteria. The supervisor should then allow the employee to discuss his views, or what each evaluation criterion means to him. Sometimes it is easier to ask the employee for a personal evaluation of how he is doing relative to the criterion. If the employee is led to feel that he is not here to be criticized, he will tend to be more objective and honest with the supervisor—and himself. However, if he thinks he is going to be disciplined as part of the evaluation process, he will become defensive and even argumentative. This is the hard way to evaluate performance. It is much easier to be fair and honest with employees, showing concern and a genuine desire to look for solutions, than to provoke an argument, during which no one listens and nothing is accomplished other than driving employee and supervisor even further apart. If the supervisor has done her job throughout the year by giving continuous feedback (managing the employee), then the evaluation process should be nothing more than a summary of solutions and corrections, along with recognition for positive contributions. The employee should, likewise, feel free to share his views and to help the supervisor understand how to manage the department and its employees more effectively.

STEP 3: Giving Feedback

It is important to be sensitive to *how* to give feedback to an employee; this is just as important as *what* the supervisor tells him. If what is said results in defensiveness, then little will be communicated, and chances are that no behavior change will occur. Employees will often want to "cut to the chase" and determine their final rating. Instead, the supervisor should methodically cover each area, building justification for the outcome. Explain in detail what the expectations of the job are in terms that are as specific as possible. It is up to the supervisor to take the guesswork out of good performance. Most people want to do a good job; they need and deserve to have an explanation of what excellence is.

Supervisors should characterize an employee's work in terms of the performance standards that have been established and *never* evaluate personality. Criticizing someone's personality almost always evokes defensive reactions. Most people cannot change their personality, and an employee will recognize that if this is his shortcoming in the eyes of his supervisor, his long-term prospects with the company are limited. Behavior is manageable; personality is not. The supervisor should also not allow the employee to redirect the focus to community problems that do not affect the employee's personal performance.

Remember: the performance appraisal should present a balanced view of the employee's performance. It is important to give feedback about strengths as well as weaknesses. Never withhold high ratings if they are deserved, for they encourage people to strive even harder and build their self-confidence. Good news inspires employees to do even better, and effective managers will gain employee commitment by helping their employees to feel like winners. Although positive feedback is a strong motivator, the balance of positive to negative statements must reflect the overall performance of the employee. It never helps to gloss over the evaluation process by offering only praise for the employee. Naturally it is easier to give someone good news than bad; we all fall into that trap. Often managers will seek to terminate a problem employee, only to discover outstanding performance evaluations in the employee's personnel file. Supervisors should be honest with themselves and the employees they are evaluating. Most people are aware of their vulnerabilities, and they deserve feedback that will enable them to overcome them and grow as professionals.

STEP 4: Listening

Listening is the key skill in all performance appraisals. The very act of listening communicates to the employee that her opinions are valued and worthy of consideration. A manager who does not seek the opinions of his employees is a fool. After all, they are actually doing the job—who better to advise management on how it might be done better or more efficiently? The most obvious way to get the employee talk-

ing is to begin by asking *what, how, where,* and *why.* For example, "How do you feel about improving ———?" Open-ended questions and follow-up questions will solicit information on attitudes, commitment, and understanding of the job. The supervisor will in turn need to demonstrate some flexibility and sincere interest.

Some tangible evidence of acceptance is always helpful in encouraging the employee to speak out. The evaluator should nod his head, smile encouragingly, and punctuate the employee's statements with "yes," "good idea," "I see." Reassurance is particularly important if the employee is saying something that may be anxiety-producing for him.

Paraphrasing is another useful method of encouraging others to talk and demonstrating that the supervisor is listening. The supervisor can restate in her own words what she thinks the employee is saying. Capture the essence of the thought and repeat it. Normally the person will pick up on the restatement and continue talking, giving more information.

The ideal time to be silent is when you ask a question. The employee knows it is his turn to talk. If the employee delays in responding, then the supervisor knows he is trying to decide what to share. Another time when silence is useful is when the employee finishes a statement. Wait a few seconds before going on; the employee may be hesitant about telling you something else that is important. Be patient and allow the employee to express his thoughts.

STEP 5: Establishing Agreement

Listening without arguing is a major factor in helping people accept feedback. If the supervisor does not agree with the employee on any particular area, she should clarify the areas of disagreement and summarize. If the employee disagrees with the observation, let him voice his feelings. Make every attempt to resolve the conflict by giving specific examples of performance. Look first for small things on which both parties can agree in order to build consensus.

The supervisor should make every attempt to focus on the issues. In the face of criticism, many employees will strike back, attacking a manager's style, personality, likes, and dislikes. The supervisor must be on guard to resist the temptation to become defensive as well.

The supervisor should not allow herself to be backed into a corner by an errant employee. If she is too quick to give in on one point, the employee will pick away at others. However, if the employee raises a valid concern, the supervisor should be prepared to admit the misunderstanding and correct it. Ultimately, the supervisor needs to use her judgment on the various points of discussion and remember that the purpose of the evaluation meeting is to clarify expectations and manage the employee's performance in a fair and consistent manner.

STEP 6: Discussing Performance Improvement

The employee should be involved as much as possible in determining which areas are in need of improvement. The supervisor must be careful not to intimidate the employee by addressing too many areas at once. It is preferable to prioritize and develop action plans for the most important areas. The best way to achieve prioritization is to ask the question, "What is the negative impact on the operation if nothing is done to improve the situation?" The supervisor should pick her battles and focus on major areas of improvement that would be visible to the residents and to other employees or that would affect the quality of the services rendered.

An action plan should focus on specifics, avoid broad generalizations, and stick to the issues. The action plan should attempt to define and clarify the expectations for the job. It should paint a vivid picture of what an employee needs to do to be successful in his job rather than document his failures. The plan should be clear and specific enough to reduce the expectation to a choice: the employee can either choose to follow the plan and be successful in his position, or choose not to follow the plan, a decision that can be used to justify termination. The plan should establish specific goals and target dates for achieving them.

The law protects employees from discrimination and wrongful termination. The federal Equal Employment Opportunity Commission (EEOC) will provide employees with free counseling and arbitration in the event they choose to file complaints. The first thing an EEOC investigator will ask is whether the employee was treated fairly. A record of proactive action plans that confirm management's efforts to influence the employee in a positive manner prior to termination and demonstrate that the employee *chose* not to respond can help avoid a negative EEOC determination or possible legal action. Employers who get into legal trouble

with their employees have normally either done an inadequate job of communicating expectations to them or made a bad hire in the first place. It is simply good business to treat people fairly.

A word of caution: Performance appraisals should never be used to pressure an employee, to find an excuse for discharging someone, or to bully an employee into a behavioral change. To do so will cause employees to fear the process rather than perceive it as a useful management tool. It is up to management to motivate employees to want to deliver good service and equip them to do so, not threaten them if they do not.

STEP 7: Closing

The closing of the performance appraisal meeting is as important as the opening. Conducting it properly will maximize the possibility of obtaining improved performance. The supervisor should do the following:

- Ask the employee to recap his understanding of the major areas discussed in the review and plans for achieving them. This will give the supervisor the opportunity to determine if the employee has understood the points communicated.

- Ask the employee for his overall feelings about the review. If they are negative, encourage him to say more. You do not have to agree—merely granting the employee the right to express negative feelings will be helpful in dissipating them.

- Ask the employee to sign the appraisal form. If the employee refuses to sign, the supervisor should remind him that his signature merely confirms that the appraisal discussion occurred and does not necessarily confirm agreement with the points raised.

- *Do not discuss merit increases during the appraisal.* Although increases are based on performance, all increases should be communicated at a later date on approval from management. Supervisors who promise specific increases or even a range without approval can seriously jeopardize their credibility in the eyes of employees.

- End the review on a positive note. Everyone will benefit from a well-executed performance review: the employee, the supervisor, the residents, the company.

- Most importantly, make a commitment to follow up and actively participate in the employee's success. The extent of management's commitment to making this process a worthwhile, positive, and honest discussion will be measured in the overall success of the company.

Compensation

Before calculating merit increases, management will need to complete a local wage and labor survey. This information will make management knowledgeable about the local labor market and ensure that its rates of pay are competitive. To begin with, the community should attempt to define the meaning of *competitive*. Does it want to pay at the top of the scale, as do start-up operators or troubled facilities, or at the low end of the scale, owing to good reputation, desirable location, or stability? Paying a competitive wage is critical if the community wants to attract and retain employees. If entry rates are standardized, there will be a higher perceived level of fairness in overall wage administration and fewer exceptions. Few things contribute more to a sense of employee dissatisfaction than the perception of favoritism or inequality in compensation rates. Wage standardization also helps avoid legal complications and employee–labor relations issues such as "equal pay for equal work."

The most important source of information is, of course, one's primary competitors. Wage and salary data should be collected on each position in the community, from dishwasher to administrator. The best way to collect this information is for the bookkeeper from your community to place a call to the bookkeeper of each of your competitors. The bookkeeper should fully explain to his competitors that he is conducting a wage and salary survey of communities in the area and offer to share the information with them as well. Normally, a bookkeeper will willingly share the information if the arrangement is to be reciprocal, but if he is hesitant, offer to have the executive director make the call to the competitor's executive director. Information requested should include entry rate per hour, amount of incremental increases at 30 or 90 days, shift differentials, employment inducements, and benefit levels, if possible. The information should be compared to the current rate and actual average rate for each position in your community. Factors influencing the validity of competitors' information—such as union versus nonunion shop and degree of comparability in business and product quality—should also be taken into consideration. Once the new entry rates have been

established, there should be no exceptions. Adjustments for current employees may be appropriate and can be handled through the performance evaluation process so that they can be seen as tied to performance rather than market conditions.

Although it is important to pay competitive wages, work environment and community reputation are key factors considered by potential applicants as well as existing employees. Quality employees will rarely leave to go to a competitor for a few dollars more if they are satisfied in their jobs and believe they are treated fairly and valued by management.

Other sources of compensation information can include the local newspaper classified section, the state department of wage and labor, specialty retirement housing surveys such as those conducted by *Retirement Housing Business Report*,[4] or trade associations such as the National Association for Senior Living Industries (NASLI).[5]

Mature communities that are well managed and consequently enjoy low employee turnover are often faced with the need to establish maximums for hourly positions. It is standard practice in the industry to establish this limit, often referred to as the "red circle," as no more than 25 percent higher than the established minimum. The maximum rate is then increased if the minimum rate is increased to avoid wage compression. When employees do reach maximums, several options may be available to continue to reward them. These can include

- An annual bonus based on performance. This can be equivalent to the budgeted percentage increase for the community but paid in a lump sum while the base rate remains frozen.
- Additional absence benefits, such as vacation or personal days.
- Company-paid health insurance or dental insurance premiums.
- Company contributions to retirement plans.
- Creative scheduling.

Calculating Merit Increases

It is helpful to establish guidelines for outstanding, competent, and acceptable performance categories and use ranges, not a flat percentage, (e.g., 4–6%). The high end of the scale should be chosen in order to place the individual's salary at an appropriate position in her salary range with respect to length of tenure, performance, and the salaries of other employees in the same or similar positions.

Employees should receive a prorated share of their merit increases depending on length of service with the company. For example: employees with 3 months of service will receive 3/12 of a share; employees with 12 or more months of service will receive a full share. This strategy helps to avoid wage compression and promotes fairness. For example:

"Jane Doe" is a concierge. She has been with the company for ten months. Her present salary is $7.00 per hour. She has been rated as a competent employee and will receive a 4 percent increase.

The computation is as follows:

$7.00 per hour × 0.04 (percent of increase) = 0.28

0.28 divided by 12 shares = 0.023

0.023 × 10 shares (based on 10 months of service) = $0.2 per hour increase

A computer spreadsheet can be developed to prorate employee raises automatically based on hire date. The total compensation increases can then be calculated by department or for the entire community for comparison to the budget. Normally flat percentages are used to adjust the total payroll budget of the community for annual merit increases. The prorating method enables the total merit increase dollars available to be allocated so that the community can proportionately reward longevity and performance.

Annual increases at midyear can also be effective in minimizing the cost to the community. Giving employees their 3 percent annual raise in July will only cost the project 1.5 percent for the fiscal year. This impact is further reduced by prorating new hires.

■■■■ EMPLOYEE OPINIONS

Soliciting employee opinions about the operation is an essential element of good management and communication. No one knows better than the employee doing the job how it can be done better, and employees will also have valuable perceptions about management, training, resident satisfaction, benefits and compensation, and the company image. Collecting and analyzing employee opinions can not only help measure employee satisfaction, but also communicate

to middle management the company's expectations on how staff is to be treated and managed. Companies that solicit regular feedback from their employees also tend to find that managers will communicate better with them and treat them with more respect. The very process communicates to staff that management values their opinions and makes them feel as though their opinions are considered when management goals are evaluated. It builds more of a team atmosphere within the operation when employees feel they have some influence in the overall success of the community. Employees who share in the success of an operation have a vested interest in the company and begin to feel they have helped build something rather than just worked their shifts and collected their paychecks. Feelings of accomplishment can never be bought with a paycheck. Employees *at all levels* need to feel a sense of purpose when they come to work.

Surveys should be conducted at least annually (or more frequently if a problem develops), and management should expect 100 percent employee participation. Management should call a general meeting of the employees to go over the survey instrument and explain the importance of total participation. When asked for our evaluation of something, most of us tap into our short-term memory, and the results of a successful employee event or recent wage increase may positively or negatively skew the results. The surveys should be distributed during a neutral time of year. It should be stressed that the survey is intended to summarize the employees' opinions over the last year (or whatever period of time has elapsed since the last survey), and they should be cautioned not to evaluate only their most recent encounter with management. Furthermore, employees should be asked to ensure that their completed surveys objectively represent their *personal opinions* and not what they may have heard from other employees or residents. Surveys can be distributed at an all-employee meeting along with a stamped, addressed envelope. Encourage the employees to fill out the survey at the end of the meeting to discourage collaboration, and serve refreshments. Surveys should be tabulated off site, either at a corporate headquarters or using a consultant, if for no other reason than to guarantee the participants' complete anonymity and confidentiality. If there is a high negative response rate to questions dealing with the degree of openness and trust in management, then this same lack of trust will carry through to the survey responses themselves. On the other hand, if there is a high level of employee confidence in and endorsement of management, the staff will want to tell the world about it.

The survey instrument should be designed with two objectives. First, it should solicit opinions on such matters as job satisfaction, supervision, management, resident satisfaction, compensation and benefits, company image, and overall satisfaction. Second, the survey should be used as a training tool to reinforce the company's expectations of how managers are to supervise and manage their employees. Management has the ability to communicate its overall mission and values to all employees through the types of questions asked, so great care should be exercised to ensure that the survey is asking questions consistent with how the company is managed. The survey should be translated for the benefit of those for whom English is a second language. It sends the wrong message when the employees, whose opinions are supposed to be valued, are forced to struggle to understand the survey.

Employees must be convinced that management will act on the results of the survey; otherwise the process will achieve nothing more than damaging its own credibility in the eyes of employees and even residents. Any combined positive response level less than 80 percent, or any increase in combined unfavorable response level greater than 10 percent, should automatically trigger a plan of correction, which should be formulated by the department head and her direct supervisor within 30 days of the tabulation of the survey. Plans of correction that are SMART—specific, measurable, attainable, responsive, and time measured—will be the most effective. This should not be an exercise that simply identifies existing problems with general recommendations that are "ongoing." Department heads should call all their employees together to brainstorm so that everyone can be part of the solution. Plans of correction should describe the area in need of improvement in specific terms, detail a solution, assign a responsible party, and target a completion date. Some companies are very reluctant to publish the results of their surveys, citing fears that some specific results may add fuel to arguments by special-interest groups and affect employee morale. A survey of any nature will *raise* the expectations of the population served. When employees give their valuable input, it is with the clear expectation that management fully

intends to respond positively, quickly, and thoroughly to the issues and concerns raised. If management is unwilling to commit itself to feeding back survey results to the participants, and to addressing the survey findings as quickly as possible, it is better not to do the survey at all. Conversely, positive results from an employee survey can be a powerful recruitment tool.

A word of caution: The employee survey results should never be used to discipline managers; rather they should be used as a training and educational tool. Managers must embrace the process rather than fear it or use the feedback to retaliate against their employees. It is important for management to familiarize supervisors with the potential effect of survey results on productivity, profitability, and service.

■ MANAGEMENT

Effective management in today's work environment calls for nothing less than a 180° shift from the traditional models and metaphors of the past. Employees are most productive when they are led, not threatened. The amateur manager sees his employees as tools to perform critical functions in the business; the professional manager recognizes that the very success of the business is in the hands of its front-line staff. The front line *is* the bottom line.

Today's successful business leaders reflect a paradox. They are tough as nails and uncompromising about their value systems, but at the same time they care deeply about and respect their employees. They are able to articulate a clear vision of what their operations will look like when they run well, while paying obsessive attention to detail. No element is too small to pursue if it serves to lend the vision more clarity.

Most organizational inflexibility is caused by people who have power and are unwilling to give it up. The professional manager is willing to listen and create an environment in which employees play an active role in the decision-making process and in turn have a stake in the success or failure of the operation. Table 3.1 differentiates the amateur manager from the professional manager.

Today's professional manager is a cheerleader and facilitator, and understands basic human problems. She recognizes the value of the team and encourages participation by the team in the decision process. The professional focus is positive and solution oriented. The professional manager is "hands-on" and looks for

Table 3.1   Characteristics of Amateur and Professional Managers

Amateur	Professional
Police officer	Cheerleader
Enforcer	Facilitator
Judgmental	Understanding
By the book	Flexible
Do it or else	Team builder
Closed-minded	Open-minded
Hypercritical	Supportive, rewarding
Negative focus (what is wrong)	Positive focus (what is right)
Seeks to blame	Seeks solutions
Hands-off	Hands-on
Hire the "right" person, and if they can't do the job, find someone else	Developer of human potential; plans to ensure the success of the staff
Disciplines employees frequently	Uses a systematic approach to ensure their success
Generates fear or anxiety	Builds self-esteem
Reacts	Responds
Poor communicator	Friendly and approachable
Assumes	Ensures
Unclear about standards	Outlines specific expectations
Settles	Asks questions, probes
Waits for problems to arise	Good follow-through
Insecure	Confident

opportunities to develop the strengths of employees, rather than assign blame when things go wrong. The professional manager defines excellence specifically for employees and charts their successes rather than documents their failures. By teaching employees the essential elements that they will need to be successful and outlining the resources and expectations needed to do the job well, the manager is ensuring better performance. The professional manager then becomes a performance developer (Exhibit 3.4).

Psychologists have demonstrated that the power of expectation alone can influence the behavior of others. This phenomenon, called the self-fulfilling prophecy, tells us that if we have high expectations of our employees, they will generally live up to those expectations.

On the other hand, if we expect our employees to perform poorly or give us problems, they probably will.

The job of a manager is to influence subordinates, and some of the most miraculous rescues in the business world have been the result of positive expectations by management, including Lee Iacocca's turnaround of the Chrysler Corporation. Conversely, negative expectations can lead to failure: during the Depression, rumors of financial bankruptcies led to their actual occurrence and the ruin of the country's economy at the New York Stock Exchange, where investors' beliefs

Exhibit 3.4   Fundamentals of Management

1. Frontline staff must be given the authority to make decisions as they relate to customer satisfaction issues.
2. Frontline staff must be encouraged to think and act independently without fear of the consequences of making a bad decision. Create a work environment in which employees motivate themselves.
3. Job content and expectations must be spelled out clearly and reinforced constantly until the employee can understand the philosophy. People work best when expectations are clear, freedoms are spelled out, and consistency is the norm.
4. Managers must have a willingness to understand basic human problems and be sensitive toward all the emotional forces that motivate staff.
5. Managers must act in the role of cheerleader, facilitator, coach, and confidant. They should see themselves as a resource for their employees and look for ways to help them be more effective.
6. Only through constant encouragement and support will the manager be able to build the level of self-confidence in the staff that will let them feel free to serve the customers as if they owned the business themselves.
7. A clear vision of exactly what the business will look like when it is running well must be articulated.
8. Measurable plans must be developed for the execution of the vision based on balancing the needs and interests of the owner with those of the employees and the customers they serve.
9. Managers must build consensus among the staff and create a sense of urgency.
10. Managers should not seek to impress those for whom they work, but those who work for them. Results will always speak for themselves.

about how a stock would perform influenced its value and ultimate performance. Simple human expectation often plays a large part in determining the course of events—*expecting* an event to happen can actually *cause* it to happen. In business, expecting excellence can actually produce it.

A manager's expectations are transmitted using four critical communication factors:

1. **Climate:** Nonverbal messages from the manager or company leadership can exert both encouraging and stifling effects on employee motivation and self-perception.
2. **Feedback:** Managers generally (subconsciously) give more positive reinforcement to employees of whom they have high expectations and negative or very limited feedback to those of whom they have low expectations. We can often see the results of frequent, specific praise contrasted with the results of giving only vague feedback.
3. **Input:** The amount of information given to an employee is crucial. The high-expectation employee receives the resources and a description of the expectations that are needed to do the job well, whereas the low-expectation employee receives little direction or information.
4. **Output:** High-expectation employees are given more opportunities to offer their opinions and more assistance in finding solutions to their problems.

Motivation

Motivation does not just happen because things are going well; it must be planned and managed. Motivated employees are more dependable, self-confident, productive, satisfied, and team oriented. Most important of all, the motivated employee stays in the job longer and ultimately delivers better care to the residents. Motivation is more than being nice to people, complementing them, and creating a friendly work environment. Words of encouragement can stimulate employees to better performance, but never as much as responsibility and the opportunity to accomplish something personally. Motivation is the result of giving employees continuing opportunities to learn more, to test their knowledge, and to gain a sense of achievement and recognition. In short, employees are motivated by responsibility, achievement, recognition, and opportunities for personal growth and advancement.

Sources of dissatisfaction include low pay and benefits, unsatisfactory working conditions, poor supervision, lack of job security, unfair policies and administrative practices, lack of social relationships, and low status. Appropriate financial compensation and benefits are expected, but although bonuses and commissions are effective incentives for some, in general they do little to provide employees a sense of accomplishment and achievement. High performers may become dissatisfied and feel discriminated against as they compare their contributions to those of other less committed employees with similar compensation. Poor working conditions, such as the physical environment or political climate of the workplace, can be a significant source of employee dissatisfaction. Adequate working conditions and user-friendly environmental factors are basic expectations of most employees. Inadequate or incompetent supervision can also be a catalyst for employee dissatisfaction, as well as insecurity about the company or the position. Managers who quote company policy or do not practice service-oriented administration can frustrate and confuse employees looking for answers and reassurance. Employees do not want to be quoted the rulebook; they want to be listened to and respected. Management that treats employees with indifference and operates the community from behind closed doors will create a sense of fear and intimidation. Employees are often looked down upon by more senior level managers, and it is hard to see things eye to eye when you are looking down on someone. Abuse of status and power by management can be divisive, create dissension and break down team spirit.

Employees who are rewarded for performance are more productive, satisfied, and stable. Cash may be important, but cash by itself has no memory—it goes right into the bank or is spent. Today's employees want more from their jobs. They want timely information, opportunities to solve problems and participate in decisions, and assurance that they will be recognized and rewarded for their contributions. Awards and recognition are things they can share with their families; they will remember how they earned them, who sponsored them, and what business goal was met.

Employers should not overlook the many noncash ways to motivate and reward their employees in addition to job-based pay and evaluation systems. Most noncash incentives fall into one or more of the following four categories: merchandise, travel, recognition, and status. Merchandise and travel can fuel performance in the short term, but recognition and status can build an organization. The specific type of reward is less important to the employee than the significance employees place on management's interest in the recognition of employees. The emphasis should be on getting people energized and focused on what it takes to make the operation successful.

Noncash rewards can be as powerful a motivator to increase performance levels as cash. Employee focus groups within retirement communities across the country have confirmed this basic truth about staff motivation and retention. Provided that salary ranges and benefits are competitive, the biggest motivator for employees is to be *appreciated,* recognized, and treated with dignity. Categorically, employees are looking for management to do a better job of training front-line supervisors to manage people and for management to set the right example toward staff from the top. Managers who recognize this teach their supervisors the lessons summarized in Exhibit 3.5.

In his book *1001 Ways to Reward Employees,* management specialist Bob Nelson explains that "employees find personal recognition more motivational than money. . . . Yet it is a rare manager who systematically makes the effort to simply thank employees for a job well done, let alone to do something more innovative to recognize accomplishments."[6] The primary reason why most managers do not more frequently reward and recognize employees is that they lack the time and creativity to come up with ways to do it.

Recognition flows down from the top of an organization, and its source is self-confidence. People feel empowered by recognition; it builds self-esteem and confidence. Managers who look for opportunities to reward and recognize their staffs will themselves be rewarded by employees who take pride in their work and believe that they have a stake in the operation's success. Equipped with this confidence, managers will feel compelled to treat their employees as they are treated by their supervisors. Empowering managers with confidence is like pouring water into a bucket from above. As the bucket fills, confidence tends to overflow down to those waiting employees who also are seeking recognition. As their buckets fill, they become more confident and will start to take on a sense of ownership and assume risk. This confidence in front-line

Exhibit 3.5   Motivating Employees

- Set up a proactive work environment; recognize employees for their strengths and have tolerance for their areas of vulnerability.
- Generate a sense of belonging and team spirit among the group to pull together and accomplish goals.
- Promote the building of relationships with residents and their families.
- Demonstrate that management is "hands-on" and not afraid to roll up its sleeves and participate in the work.
- Talk to employees, ask questions, and *listen.*
- Discourage ego trips and turf building.
- Learn that everyone is responsible for making the operation run well. Managers who say "It's not my job" might as well say "I quit."
- Keep employees informed and involved in the overall operations of the community.
- Build self-esteem among employees and empower them to step into decision-making mode to recognize problems and solve them as they arise. Create an atmosphere that encourages employees to take risks with little fear of retribution when honest mistakes are made.
- Respect employees' intelligence and opinions; seek out their ideas.
- Understand basic human problems and be sensitive to all the emotional forces that motivate people.
- A common thread found among the most successful companies is laughter. Organizations that create a level of urgency mixed with the right amount of humor learn to take themselves only seriously enough to get the job done. Companies that create an atmosphere in which people enjoy their work and each other are far better positioned to be successful than competing firms run by task masters.

employees forms the very foundation for exceptional service to residents. Confidence building is a *continuous* process: when the source runs dry upstream, blame often replaces recognition and mediocrity once again becomes the norm.

Managers must be able to define excellence and communicate to their staff specific expectations designed to create it. Most employees want to do a good job, and the better we can do as managers in showing them what a job looks like when it is well done, the better we equip them to work toward that goal. Walt Disney put it best when he said, "You can dream, create, design and build the number one place in the world, but it takes people to make it happen."[7] If there is not a big difference between what you offer and what your competition offers, there had better be a big difference in the way you treat people.

■■■ WORKERS' COMPENSATION

Workers' compensation is a state-mandated program under which employers are required to pay all the medical bills and a portion of lost wages to workers hurt on the job. Large employers that self-insure pay these claims as a direct expense to their operations; smaller concerns typically purchase insurance, with premiums based in part on their claims experience and job classification.

It is important to check with the Workers' Compensation Rating Bureau to determine the payroll classification for your employees. Slight classification differences can mean big savings on rates. For example, class codes 9052 (Hotel—All other employees, salespersons, and drivers) and 9058 (Hotel—Restaurant employees) both carry a rate per $100 payroll of $4.22, compared to code 8835 (Home health/home care employees), with a significantly higher rate of $4.49. Great care should be taken when selecting a class code, to avoid being classified at a higher rate than necessary.

Experience rating is mandatory in most states for all but the smallest risks. The National Workers' Compensation Council is the primary rating service organization that disseminates workers' compensation experience modifications. The experience rating is a systematic method of modifying your standard premium based on how your actual incurred loss experience compares to the loss experience to be expected of your type of business. The experience modifier is set at 1.00 when your business is established. It is then adjusted up or down depending on your claims experience. A continuous history of high claim frequency can drive the experience modifier up to 1.3, which directly translates to a 30 percent increase in the premiums paid by the employer for the same coverage as his competitor. Conversely, if the claim frequency is less than that of competitors, the experience modifier can drop to less than 1.0, perhaps even 0.80, which means that the employer pays 20 percent less than competitors. In a 100-unit community this can

translate into an annual savings of $6,000 in premiums alone, not to mention time loss, overtime coverage, and excess claims. The experience rating consists of a three-year rolling average, ending one year before the effective date of the policy period. This means that if your claim experience is high, and management implements strategies to lower the claims, the premium will not be reduced for two more years. Therefore it takes a long-term commitment by management to make these programs pay off.

The experience rating plan is designed to give more weight to loss frequency then loss severity. For example, fifteen $3,000 claims would have a much greater impact than one $45,000 claim. Loss experience is split into two components: primary losses and excess losses. Losses of $5,000 or less are considered primary losses and are taken at face value, whereas any loss above this amount is considered an excess loss. These excess loss amounts are further capped by the applicable state's per-claim accident limitation. These larger claims are capped so that they will not have too great an impact on the experience rating. A single large loss may be entirely fortuitous, and it would not be fair to penalize a policyholder three years because of one incident. The reason the formula penalizes loss frequency is that frequent small losses can and often do lead to a severe loss. Loss frequency problems are easily identifiable, and management has more control over loss frequency than loss severity.

Workers' compensation is a manageable expense. The development of a proactive and managed workers' compensation program can save communities thousands of dollars in claims (and premiums) that could otherwise have been spent on employee compensation and other needed areas. The objective of these programs should be to promote safety awareness, reduce injuries, manage the recovery process, and minimize the expense of returning employees to work. Employers who design safety programs to educate their employees and supervisors to create *safety consciousness* will minimize disruption of their operations through time lost from the community and save considerable expense. Safety and loss control must be part of everyday operations, not merely considered when an incident occurs. Employees will generally respond positively to employer programs if they are perceived to be sincere and of value to them, and especially if they are tied to compensation bonuses. Programs must demonstrate management's concern for the welfare of its employees and not be regarded as a way to control costs.

The effective workers' compensation program will be goal oriented and emphasize critical, measurable results, such as days without time-loss injuries. It will include education inservice, wellness programs and community-sponsored fitness events, safety committees, and routine physical plant inspections and be focused on early return through a light-duty program. Incentive safety programs and contests among teams of employees are good ways to heighten safety awareness. The key to the success of any program is employee interest. Contests should be creative, and award thresholds should be within reach and earned at least quarterly to keep the program fresh and on everyone's mind. An awards ceremony can be incorporated into all-employee meetings at which management gives well-deserved recognition to the efforts of winning employees and encourages others to work harder or *smarter* in the coming weeks.

Pre-employment screening can also be an effective tool to ensure that candidates have the physical ability to handle the demands of the position for which they are applying. If the position involves lifting, they should be able to demonstrate ability to do so in previous positions. It is a good idea to contact the state workers' compensation office to review previous claim history. It is illegal to discriminate by not hiring individuals with previous injuries, but knowledge of previous injuries may give the supervisor insight into an individual's need for additional safety training to prevent future injuries.

Some employees have been known to use workers' compensation as a haven for personal problems or the avoidance of income interruption due to job performance issues. All employees should be educated on the *negatives* of workers' compensation. Workers' compensation is a benefit designed to protect those truly injured. Falsification of injury or becoming injured as a result of an unsafe act are simply not worth the time off. Workers' compensation for time-loss cases does not start until the sixth day; therefore employees will need to use up their bank of sick days to guarantee uninterrupted compensation (unless they are severely injured). Also, many are unaware that the compensation rate for workers' compensation is only two-thirds of their normal hourly wage. However, because workers' compensation benefits are not taxed, the typical worker can end up with 80 to 90 percent of previous take-home pay. Finally, if the company suspects a fraudulent claim, it may choose to seek a legal remedy that could ultimately be very expensive to the employee.

Economic trends can also affect the use by workers of workers' compensation. During a recession, workers become fearful that they may be laid off and are more likely to have injuries that prevent them from coming back to work, according to insurance specialists. In effect, going out on workers' compensation becomes a way of guaranteeing a paycheck in hard times. As the economy improves, those fears subside and workers are more willing to return to the job quickly. This relationship is also valid for individual communities that may not be making financial projections: employees begin to become concerned about potential cutbacks by management.

The Workers' Compensation Act of 1991 has established new procedures for filing workers' compensation claims. The important distinction is between time-loss cases and medical-only cases. To qualify for determination as a time-loss case, an injured employee must be incapacitated for a period of five *calendar* days to be eligible for compensation from the sixth day of disability forward. The employee must be incapacitated and unable to earn full wages for twenty-one days to be eligible from the first day of disability. In other words, if the employee is incapacitated for more than five days but less than twenty-one days, he is entitled to benefits for only those days in excess of five days (rules in some states vary).

In about half of the states, the company can specify whom employees will see for occupational care. Employers can identify local physicians with a track record of more conservative treatment and recommend them to injured employees. The object is not only to avoid those doctors who might overprescribe tests and treatments but also to find those interested in returning people to the job.

It is a good idea to have any injured employee initially sent to a clinic with whom management has previously made arrangements. The physician should be provided with a job description for the particular employee and advised whether or not the employer will allow a return to light-duty work. The physician should be willing to contact the employer immediately after seeing the employee to advise on the employee's condition and disability. The cooperation and accessibility of the initial treating physician can position management to influence the case and create an awareness that the employer has a concern for avoiding "indefinite" disability periods. Management should make every attempt to return the employee to work with limitations as soon as possible.

Management should conduct a thorough investigation with witnesses and coworkers to ascertain the circumstances and details of the incident. In some cases, if unsafe practices by the employee caused the accident and resulting injury, the compensation may be reduced by 50 percent. Therefore, any policy or procedural violations should be thoroughly documented.

When workers are hurt, management's communication efforts can have a significant effect on the future course of claims. The community should designate one person as claims coordinator, the liaison to all injured employees. This coordinator can then call homebound employees frequently and make sure they are receiving their checks. The object of this attention is to keep communication channels open and let the employees know that the company misses them and is eager to see them return.

Employees who are returned to light-duty work after an injury will feel useful and valued by their employer. No one likes to be ill or feel disabled, and light-duty work promotes positive emotions that aid the healing process. Light-duty programs also allow people recovering from injuries to stay in touch and feel connected to the routine of working. The program should be managed by someone with sensitivity and an ability to recognize the employee who really does not want to come back to work, for either personal or *personnel* reasons. These employees invariably allege reinjury so that they can collect benefits and stay at home. Once assigned light-duty work, the employee's rehabilitation process should be monitored as closely as if the employee were on temporary disability, and a return-to-work date should be set. The employee, physician, and physical therapist should all be strongly encouraged to meet that return-to-work date. A successful light-duty program requires that the local medical community participate in the company's commitment to the program. Physicians will release patients to light duty if they know that a light-duty program exists and is well managed. Physicians who are aware of a company's light-duty program will be less likely to order three or four days of bed rest for an employee

looking for time off from work. Some companies have started inviting local physicians to tour their property to demonstrate these programs so as to help them make more informed decisions about returning employees to work.

If the employee claims to have been injured in the course of employment and requires medical treatment by a physician but is incapacitated for less than five days, the claim is a medical case only. This means the employee is not eligible for time-loss benefits. Such claims should also be thoroughly investigated, including a check of the accident site, the injured employee's verbal report, and witness verification. Accidents requiring only in-house first aid should be similarly documented, cross-referenced to similar accidents, and reported to the safety committee. They should be reported to the insurer if the incident is itself either very unusual or questionable in terms of its relationship to work.

When the employee is released to work without limitations, this disposition should be put in writing by the physician. The employee's previous position should be offered to him; if it has been filled, then a comparable position should be offered at the same rate of pay (if available). If this offer is refused, the employee should be asked to sign a statement of refusal to accept such employment, or the company should confirm the offer and refusal in writing by mail to the employee.

Clearly, accident prevention is the key to minimizing workers' compensation costs. Educating employees on proper body mechanics and the possible serious injuries they can sustain in their positions can help keep them aware of the risks. To remain effective, however, this training must be done in conjunction with employee-centered, proactive management. Employees should understand the direct benefits to them of a safety program and recognize that absenteeism and workers' compensation costs ultimately hurt everyone.

■ RISK MANAGEMENT

Assisted living community operations are exposed to a wide range of risks. In order to analyze and minimize risks in each aspect of their communities, operators must determine what standards of care apply or should apply and to which they may be held. Assisted living communities are an operational hybrid and differ from other types of businesses for which standards of care have evolved and developed over time. They are similar to other types of housing and service providers for specific populations with special needs and vulnerabilities, such as health care facilities, nursing homes, and group homes for the elderly. They also possess many of the characteristics of the hospitality and residential housing industries.

Standards of performance specific to assisted living may include state regulations and other statutes and regulations, including landlord-tenant, consumer protection, fair housing, and antidiscrimination laws. Other standards to which the assisted living community can be expected to be held will include accepted clinical and professional practices, evolving industry standards, and even representations and promises (oral or written) made in connection with marketing efforts and materials, residency agreements, resident handbooks, service plans, and representations by community employees.

Risk management is as much a mindset as a science. Management must be as committed to implementing and managing risk control policies as it is to marketing the building. The simple fact is that poor risk management will empty a building faster than good marketing will fill it. One widely published incident of resident abuse or molestation can effectively negate thousands of dollars of advertising designed to generate interest in the community and portray a high-quality program.

Effective risk management policies and procedures can easily be developed by working with a loss control professional. Such services are generally available through one's insurance provider, for it is clearly in their best interest that a community minimize risks once they have underwritten a policy covering that community. Most national carriers will have full-time loss control departments specifically created to work with communities to design a risk management program. The goal of any loss control program is to identify risk and then engineer an effective means to reduce or eliminate the chance of loss or exposure.

Loss control programs are designed to mitigate risk by identifying potential strategies to avoid or minimize loss. The following areas are typically covered in a loss control audit:

1. Accident prevention
2. Emergency planning
3. Evacuation procedures
4. Fire prevention and protection
5. Hazardous material
6. Hazardous waste disposal
7. Loss analysis and trends identification
8. OSHA hazard communication
9. Smoke and fire safety programs
10. Vehicle safety

Contracts will often include a section dealing with insurance and or indemnification. Such contracts must be reviewed to consider their overall impact on the risk management program. The review should cover

1. Certificates of insurance
2. General contracts
3. Indemnification
4. Insurance requirements
5. Limits on liability
6. Management agreements
7. Personal care management agreements
8. Procedures and responsibilities
9. Service agreements

Assisted living is very different from other forms of long-term care in the absence of prescriptive regulations. In the skilled nursing environment, regulations have been developed to protect the interests of the patients and ensure that proper and appropriate care is delivered. In many ways, the regulations themselves are specific enough to minimize risks to the patient associated with the delivery of care. This is clearly not the case in assisted living. As residents age in place and as competition drives providers to stretch the definition of assisted living, residents will continue to increase in acuity and expose the community to the associated complications of meeting their ever-increasing health care requirements. These phenomena will inevitably expose the typical assisted living provider to increased risk. It will initially be the responsibility of management to develop procedures to mediate this risk, until legislators succumb to public pressure to regulate assisted living. Regulation is inevitable, and management would be well advised to prepare a comprehensive risk management program proactively as a preventative measure, rather than retrospectively following a serious incident that might have been prevented.

Shared Risk

A defining characteristic of assisted living includes the right of a resident to choose services and negotiate the risk associated with his or her choices. Providers serve both themselves and their residents best when limits on care and risk management are discussed at the onset of residency by negotiating a formalized risk agreement.

Assisted living providers should respect and recognize a resident's right to make individual choices regarding lifestyle, personal actions or behaviors, and the personal service plan. Providers and resident families must recognize that in some cases a resident's decision or action may involve an increased risk of personal harm and may therefore conflict with a provider's responsibility to meet the established standards for assisted living services, care, and supervision. It is here that the concept of informed consent comes into play; such consent can be secured through risk-sharing agreements.

Risk-sharing agreements should be simple and understandable to residents and the employees who serve them. Protocols should be developed by the assisted living community to explain why the decision or action may pose a risk and suggest alternatives for the resident's consideration. Management should encourage a competent resident to discuss his decisions with his family so that the risk associated with those decisions is clearly understood in advance. If after consultation the resident still wishes to pursue an action or refuse service that may involve increased risk of personal harm and conflict with the provider's responsibilities, the provider should

- Describe the action or range of actions subject to negotiation
- Negotiate a "risk agreement" acceptable to the resident that meets all standards for the safety and comfort of the community as well as any applicable statutory and regulatory requirements
- Follow a resident's preferences over his or her family's preference, unless the family has been granted legal powers of decisionmaking
- Record the agreement, the provider's proposed alternatives, and the provider's role, if any, in mitigating the risks in a document signed by the resident and the provider
- Implement any mitigation efforts to which the provider has agreed
- Outline a time frame within which the risk management issue will be addressed with the resident once it has been identified, and a risk agreement developed

- Review the decision documented in the risk agreement with the resident if the resident's mental or physical condition changes substantially from the time when the risk agreement was signed, renegotiating and resigning the agreement when appropriate[8]

A policy statement should be developed by the provider that indicates that risk management agreements are not intended to abridge a resident's rights or to avoid liability for harm caused to a resident by the negligence of the provider. They are simply a format within which to document the resident's decisions regarding his expectations of how the provider will be involved (or the limitations of the provider's involvement) in attending to his personal care needs.

Assisted living providers should consider developing risk-sharing agreements with residents that explain the risks associated with residents' decisions or suggest alternatives that can mitigate those risks. If a resident or family decides to pursue a course of action (or inaction) that may expose them to increased risk, the provider can suggest a risk agreement that details the action or risk and is designed to meet standards for the safety and comfort of the community as well as statutory and regulatory requirements. Such agreements should follow the resident's preferences unless the family has been granted legal authority to act on his behalf.

Typical insurance coverages for retirement housing and assisted living communities are outlined in Exhibit 3.6. Insurance companies can only go so far to provide protection to the community. The manager or owner needs to develop comprehensive protocols and procedures to maximize the effect of the coverage that is in place. No amount of insurance can replace the importance of prevention, operational policies, and staff training.

Most, if not all, hospital professional liability policies (including assisted living) are written as *occurrence policies*. These provide coverage even when the claim is made after the term of the policy period when the incident took place. For example, if someone fell and suffered injuries, and then, a year after the policy term ended, the family chose to file a suit and the company filed a claim, the claim would be covered. This is in sharp contrast to a *claims-made policy,* under which coverage is provided only during the term of the policy. These policies are normally written for special

---

> **Exhibit 3.6   Typical Insurance Coverages**
>
> - Property coverages
>   - → Buildings and personal property
>   - → Loss of business income and rental income
> - Boiler and machinery
> - Crime coverages
>   - → Employee dishonesty
>   - → Forgery and alteration
>   - → Money and securities—inside and outside
> - Commercial general liability
>   (Occurrence form—no deductible)
> - Health care facility professional liability
>   (Occurrence form—no deductible)
> - Employee benefits liability
>   (Claims made form—no deductible)
>
> *Additional Other Coverages*
>
> - Workers' compensation
> - Umbrella liability
> - Business auto policy
>   - → Owned vehicles
>   - → Nonowned, hired car liability
> - Business electronic equipment
> - Employment practices liability
> - Directors and officers liability
> - Fiduciary liability
> - Group health, life, disability, and dental

cases and always require the company to purchase a tail. The tail provides extended coverage beyond the policy term and is normally very expensive, in order to provide the customer with an incentive to renew the policy instead.

Common causes of loss and the underlying concerns they create should be fully understood by all department heads. Slips and falls are the single most common types of loss and typically are the result of a premise hazard. These types of losses can be easily avoided with constant upkeep of the building. If an emergency call system is maintained for the residents, the system must remain fully operational. Such systems are delicate and can fail without notice. The most troublesome risk in facilities where private units have locked doors is the increased chance that residents could fall while alone and go undetected. This could also lead to an invasion of privacy issue when management wants to enter an apartment from which there is no response.

Most people think of abuse or molestation as deliberate acts of violence toward a resident, such as striking or other mistreatment. However, the insurance industry has recently broadened the definition of abuse to include situations of extreme negligence. For example, a male resident in an Alzheimer's unit confined to a wheelchair gained access to the rear loading dock of the facility, which was supposed to be locked. The loading dock was deserted, and the ramp was in the lowered position. The resident went speeding off the ramp and sustained serious injury. The attorney general's office is investigating this incident as a possible abuse case based on the extreme negligence of the facility.

Wandering residents create another exposure for communities that accommodate Alzheimer's residents. There must be a clearly defined agreement with the resident and his family or responsible party so that everyone understands that this resident, unlike the typical assisted living resident, cannot come and go unattended. Otherwise, it is possible that if management attempts to keep the resident on the premises for his own safety, the community could face exposure to a suit for false imprisonment (a personal injury suit).

Most states stress the rights of independence, dignity, and privacy. The community should have permission in the residency agreement or resident handbook to grant permission for entry into a resident's apartment. This is necessary to allow management access for emergency services and response, as well as routine maintenance and the opportunity to show the resident's apartment to prospective tenants once notice to vacate has been given. When the staff is entering for the delivery of daily care or housekeeping, procedures should be established for preapproved scheduled visit times and knocking before keying the door.

Communities that advertise security in their marketing materials must have established procedures in place to guarantee it. In fact, even the implication that 24-hour staffing will ensure a more secure or safe environment may leave the community exposed to lawsuits. Recently, in a retirement community located in Massachusetts, a criminal gained access by leaning on the front door buzzer until someone unknowingly let him in. There was no receptionist on duty in the building. Security staff was employed, but no one was scheduled for this particular shift. An elderly resident who was expecting a visit from the maintenance department had left her door open slightly so that the repairman could come in, and the criminal used this opportunity to rape and burglarize the elderly woman. This horrifying event stresses the importance of enforcing strict security measures at each community. The following suggestions can help to control access to the building:

- All visitors without exception should sign in at a centrally located reception desk.
- A well-organized key control system must be in place to secure second sets of keys to residents' apartments. Each key should be coded to avoid showing the room number and should be kept in a locked area with minimal access.
- The property should be well lit inside and outside to discourage criminals from targeting the community.

Most communities offer transportation services to their residents as one of the basic amenities. It is important to investigate thoroughly all employees who will be providers of this service. Research should be carried out into applicants' personal driving records and criminal histories, if any.

The use of independent contractors is very common in the retirement housing industry and generally increases in frequency with the level of care. Generally, anyone on the premises to provide services creates a potential exposure for the community. If one of the residents is injured or abused by the actions of one of these providers, and the community referred this person to the provider, the community may be involved in the resulting lawsuit. It is a good idea to prepare a waiver of liability that residents can sign to inform them of their obligations when employing private independent contractors.

Management should be able to answer "yes" to every one of the following questions:

- Has management investigated the past performance of all independent contractors to ensure that they are professional and reliable?
- Does management have references or referrals to back up this information?
- Does management maintain files with a current certificate of insurance evidencing the contractors' professional liability insurance?

- Is their professional liability insurance company one of good standing and solvency, with an A. M. Best's rating of A or better?
- Do they carry sufficient limits of insurance (preferably $1 million per occurrence limit)?
- Is the community named as an additional insured on the contractors' policies with respect to their work at the community? The community must take great care to obtain evidence that contractors carry insurance with adequate limits.

Residents will also hire companions or outside contractors such as home health agencies to perform a variety of services in addition to the services they purchase from the community. In fact, some communities do not provide personal care services and contract all such care to outside contractors. This practice can still expose the community to risk from the activities of these "outside contractors." In this case assisted living communities are strongly encouraged to have the resident or responsible party sign a disclosure statement and waiver prior to allowing the contractor to commence delivering any services at the community.

The waiver should certify that the contractor is an independent contractor to the resident, is entering the community solely at the request of the resident to perform services for the resident, and has not in any way contracted with, been solicited by, or agreed to perform any services for the community, or any of their respective partners, employees, officers, directors, affiliates, agents, successors, and assigns. It is also important to acknowledge that the contractor has not represented to the resident that the facility's owners are in any way involved with or in control of the contractor's business, or that the owners have endorsed the contractor or the services to be provided by the contractor to the resident. The owners shall have no control over or charge of or be responsible for any aspect of the services performed by the contractor at the facility. The contractor is validly and properly licensed by any and all applicable regulatory bodies to perform the services for the benefit of the resident. The contractor must certify that the contractor has procured such comprehensive general liability insurance and, if applicable, workmens' compensation and employer's liability insurance that the contractor believes necessary to protect the contractor adequately and that the contractor shall not be covered by any of the owner's insurance.

The contractor should be provided with and acknowledge receipt of the rules and regulations of residence as set forth in the residents' handbook and should comply with such rules and regulations and cause its employees and agents to comply with those rules, including other employees that may work for the contractor within the building.

The agreement should also require that the contractor accept the facility in its "as is" condition and specify that the owners have made no representation or warranty regarding the condition or maintenance of the facility, nor the safety or suitability of the facility for the purposes contemplated by the contractor. In this way, if the contractor becomes injured other than through the negligence of the community, the contractor has limited remedies.

Finally, the contractor should release the owners from and waive any and all claims, damages, fines, penalties, losses, costs, and expenses (including but not limited to attorneys' fees) against the owners or manager that arise from or are in connection with the services performed at the facility. The contractor should also agree to indemnify the owners or manager for any claims relating to the services performed by the contractor or any of its employees or consultants. Such obligations should not be construed to negate, abridge, or reduce other rights or obligations of indemnity that would otherwise exist, whether in contract, at law, or in equity.

Incorporating these acknowledgments into agreements can remind residents of their obligations and responsibility for their own contractors and insulate the community from potential legal risks from contractors not directly hired or controlled by the community.

In most assisted living communities, the in-house operation will want to capture as much of the market for private personal care delivered to the residents as possible. Allowing free access to the residents by outside home health providers seeking to increase their private-pay billable hours will ultimately strip the community of this important profit source and fragment the delivery of good-quality services to the residents. The community management will, of course, be held responsible in the eyes of the families, the state, and the press for any problems (or negligence) associated with the delivery of that care, regardless of who may have been responsible.

Reporting Incidents

Any incident resulting in injury that includes more than the typical slip and fall should be documented and reported to an insurance company. This includes incidents resulting in fractures, dislocations, serious bleeding, mismedication, or any unusual occurrence. It is important to keep to the facts, state only the obvious, and avoid drawing any conclusions. Great care should be taken to exclude any assumptions from the incident report, because they can often be used against management in court. It is important to differentiate between incidents and accidents. All accidents are incidents, but not all incidents are accidents. An incident can be simply an unusual circumstance or behavior up to and including an accident, in which someone may be hurt. A good rule in reporting is that if the incident is worth talking about, it is worth documenting.

The resident record is often the best line of defense in litigation, and it serves as the main communication tool for continuity and evaluation of services. Standards for documenting, handling, and protecting the resident record will help ensure the clarity, validity, and availability of resident information. During litigation, records are scrutinized by plaintiff attorneys for evidence that would support any allegation of tampering, which would render the documentation questionable. Inconsistencies in record keeping can discredit the documentation of the entire resident record. When changes to or entries in this record are made improperly, allegations of a cover-up could create doubt in the minds of jurors. Thus the integrity and preservation of resident records are imperative.

All pertinent records involved in the incident report process should be gathered, analyzed, and locked in a secure area. These records—including the incident report itself and internal investigatory notes and any statements taken from witnesses—are not part of the resident's standard file and should be kept separate. Plaintiff attorneys are not entitled to this information, and it should not be made readily available to them. Any contact with the resident's family or their lawyer must be carefully approached and documented. This is necessary to avoid compromising the defensive posture of the community and its employees. Procedures for receiving and reporting a summons, suit, or subpoena should be clearly defined. This is necessary to avoid penalties for defaults or other legal consequences. If a summons and complaint are forwarded to the community, the date on which these documents are signed for starts a clock ticking that establishes the date by which a response to the allegations must be filed in court or management will face penalties for default. One individual, typically the executive director, should be responsible for notifying insurance carriers, claims management, defense attorneys, workers' compensation authorities, and so on, as well as for the method of notification established.

It is critical for the members of the community to understand their duties as an insured in the handling of incidents at the property. What to report, when to report, and how to report are all important factors in complying with the "Duties of an Insured" clause in the liability insurance contract.

Take *immediate measures* to secure the situation at the time of an incident:

1. Provide any immediate medical care to ensure the safety of those involved.
2. Call all emergency personnel whose services may be required to maintain this safe environment (e.g., police, fire department, EMTs, utility companies, elevator service company).
3. Call the resident or visitor's family to report the occurrence (note the time and record the details of the call).
4. Conduct a thorough internal investigation to ascertain the facts, establish the circumstances, and identify the witnesses to provide a clear understanding of the incident. If the police are conducting an investigation on site, insist that a member of management be present to observe and manage their approach.
5. Call your insurance agent to report the incident.

WHAT TO REPORT. Report any incident resulting in injury and constituting more than the typical slip or fall. This includes incidents resulting in fractures, dislocations, serious bleeding, mismedication, or any unusual occurrence. Anything that you feel is of a serious or unusual nature should be reported to your insurance agent. It is much better to overcommunicate to the insurance company on minor incidents and learn from their reporting guidelines than to fail to report an incident that could potentially "blow up" later.

WHEN TO REPORT. As soon as you have the facts of what happened, report the incident to the insurance com-

pany. Do not wait to hear from an attorney for the victim's family that the problem is worse than you had anticipated. You do not want to create a problem with your insurance carrier by failing to file a timely report. Instead you want your insurer to get involved early, to investigate the facts while they are still fresh in everyone's mind, and to decide with you on how to proceed. Most incidents never become claims, but for the few that do, you definitely want to tap the considerable resources and experience of your carrier in helping you handle them.

HOW TO REPORT. The sample incident report in Exhibit 3.7 will provide all of the relevant information required by most insurance carriers. Most carriers have their own incident forms, so be sure to check with yours first. The more that you can tell your carrier in the report, the easier the investigation process will be. You and your staff will be at the scene at or near the time of the incident. However, many of the details may be lost by the time an insurance claims investigator or adjuster can come out and review the scene. Be factual: only report what you know to be true. Do not bother to theorize about the occurrence, for many times this can lead to the wrong conclusions.

Investigating Incidents

It is critical to any investigation that the integrity of the accident or incident scene be preserved. Much of the tangible evidence that may provide clues that will lead investigators to the proper conclusions will be at the scene. A photograph of the scene of the incident will preserve for future reference the positioning of the furniture, the presence or absence of obstacles, the clothing worn by the resident, the lighting, the presence of housekeeping equipment, or other things that may help investigators determine the cause and contributing factors. A sketch of the scene can also include the position of a fall, or of bedding, clothing, or furniture that may have been involved. It is important to conduct the investigation immediately following the incident, after the victim has been stabilized. Every minute the scene has not been documented allows for disturbances, intentional or unintentional, that may lead investigators to incorrect conclusions. Remember: the first person on the scene is normally a member of community staff, followed by a member of management; whatever material evidence is documented will

---

Exhibit 3.7   **Example of an Incident Report**

Name of community: _____

Address: _____

Date of incident: _____ Time of incident: _____ Date of report: _____

Name of individual: _____ Male/female: _____ Age: _____

Please check: ❑ Resident   ❑ Visitor   ❑ Other

Address (room number for resident; full address for visitor): _____

_____

Entrance date into community: _____

Physical/mental status upon entrance: ❑ Ambulatory ❑ Nonambulatory ❑ Alert ❑ Disoriented

❑ Other (explain) _____

Place incident occurred: _____

Nature and description of incident: _____

_____

Injury sustained? ❑ Yes ❑ No If yes, describe: _____

Hospitalized? ❑ Yes ❑ No If yes, where? _____

Name(s) of witness(es): _____

_____

Resident's family notified of incident: ❑ Yes ❑ No Time _____ Date_____

Family reaction (understanding/supportive versus angry/accusatory): _____

Personal physician notified? ❑ Yes ❑ No Time: _____ Date:_____

Name of physician: _____ Examined by physician? _____

Physician report regarding findings/treatment/change in functional ability:

_____

_____

Final disposition: _____

_____

Report prepared by (signature and date): _____

Personal care director (signature and date): _____

Executive director (signature and date): _____

---

put them in an advantageous position relative to the plaintiff's subsequent investigation.

Prior to conducting the investigation, take a few minutes to develop a list of things that you intend to cover. In this way, the investigator can proceed systematically. For example, the list may include inspecting the scene elements, interviewing other residents and staff, a review of the resident's medications for potential side effects that could cause instability, and a review of her care or service plan and of scheduled interventions immediately preceding the incident.

Having a list prepared in advance will ensure that all major areas are covered, while at the same time allowing the investigator the flexibility to add new things to it as the need arises. There is no substitute for a prompt and thoroughly conducted investigation by management at the time of the occurrence. Even a professional investigator from the insurance company cannot reconstruct the accident accurately several days later.

Listing all the potential witnesses (residents and staff) and collecting all the relevant documents will help narrow the investigation. Reviewing staffing schedules, time sheets, assignment sheets, and visitation records as well as the master logbook will help to determine which staff may be appropriate subjects for interviews.

The interviews should be conducted as soon as possible so that the incident is fresh in everyone's mind and staff do not have the opportunity to discuss the incident with other staff or family members. The longer these interviews are delayed, the lower will be the accuracy of the information collected. Assembly of key documents can help to corroborate testimony. These documents in and of themselves can also generate critical questions and unlock any inconsistencies. Resist the temptation to draw any conclusions until all of the evidence has been systematically evaluated.

Upon completion of the investigation, a written summary of all the interviews and documents reviewed will help to synthesize all of the salient facts. Organize the facts in chronological order or in chart format. This will highlight the chain of events that may have led up to the incident as well as highlight any gaps in the evidence.

Sometimes even the most thorough investigation will remain inconclusive: perhaps a rational explanation can simply not be found. Occasionally pressure from management may even lead the investigator to speculation. Yet it is far better to accept what you do not and cannot know than to make something up. It is important to remember that investigations are aimed at *fact finding*, not *fault finding*. People will be more likely to share accurate information with you if they trust that you are not out to blame them or retaliate against them. In addition, misinformation that is later proven false can subject the entire investigation to criticism and actually improve the opposition's case.

Before summarizing the findings in written form, it is essential to consider the purpose of this report and who will be its audience. Prior to the setting down findings in detail, an outline should be prepared to document the investigation process; use the list described above as a guide. The investigation report should lead the reader to conclude that the investigation was impartial and focused on the facts, and it should of course ultimately support any conclusions reached. The more impartial the report, the better it will serve to clarify the conclusions. The report should demonstrate how the causes of the incident were discovered as well as underline the logic of the findings. A thoroughly pre-

pared report can help not only to protect and limit management's liability, but also to build credibility. The report can also be used to develop action plans and safety recommendations to prevent recurrences.

Frequently a community will receive its first indication that a claim or suit is contemplated when the family of a resident (or its attorney) requests a copy of the resident's file. Simply responding to this request without requiring the proper authorization papers will compromise the confidentiality and integrity of the file. When this type of "fishing expedition" occurs, the insurance carrier and local defense counsel should be notified. There should be an incident report already on file pertaining to the family's inquiry. The insurer will then direct its adjuster or company-assigned defense counsel to handle the requests of the plaintiff's attorney. Information released will be strictly limited to that required to fulfill the purpose stated on the authorization. Authorizations specifying "any and all information" or other such broadly inclusive statements are generally not honored by defense counsel. They understand that release of information that is not essential to the stated purpose of the request is specifically prohibited and will do everything to protect your community from release of confidential information.

NOTES

1. *Wall Street Journal* (Sept. 13, 1995), 1.
2. R. Half, *Robert Half on Hiring* (New York: Crown and New American Library, 1986).
3. For a free color catalog featuring hundreds of preformatted papers and cards, write or call Paper Direct, 100 Plaza Drive, Seacus, NJ 07094-3606, (800) A-PAPERS.
4. *Retirement Housing Business Report* may be obtained from CD Publications, 8204 Fenton Stret, Silver Spring, MD 20910, (301) 588-6380.
5. NASLI (National Association for Senior Living Industries), 184 Duke of Gloucester Street, Annapolis, MD 21401-2523, (410) 263-0991. In conjunction with Lewis Consulting International, Inc., NASLI conducts an annual compensation analysis nationwide. Information is collected and analyzed on senior industry community-based staff compensation, sales compensation, and executive compensation packages. The surveys can be ordered together or separately through NASLI's bookstore at the address listed here.
6. B. Nelson, *1001 Ways to Reward Employees* (New York: Workman, 1994), xi.
7. *The Disney Keys to Service Excellence.* Disney University Professional Development Programs (Lake Buena Vista, Fla.: The Walt Disney Company, 1995), 4.
8. *Mass-Alfa Quality Guidelines: Risk Management in Assisted Living* (Woburn, Mass., 1997), 12.

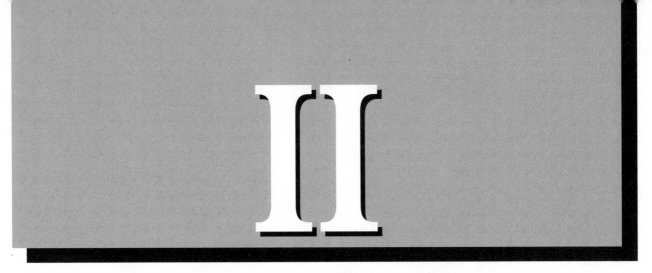

Resident Services

Concierge and Reception

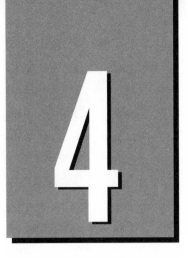

The concierge position is one of the most important within the community. Not only is this the hub of activity and communication to the residents, but the concierge is normally the first contact for community guests and inquiries. All too often the sales staff has invested as many as ten phone contacts in a prospect, finally convincing her to come in for a tour, only to have their valuable prospect ignored or kept waiting in the lobby. It is very rare, indeed, that prospects are impressed enough with the "sticks and bricks" to confirm the sale. Most successful salespeople understand that they are selling relationships and solutions, and that takes the personal touch.

It is important to get off to a good start, especially with the typical, reluctant prospect who may be looking for an excuse to delay what is at the moment the biggest decision in his life. It is critical that all guests and visitors be greeted with a warm smile, a cheerful and friendly attitude, and an air of professionalism and confidence that will make them feel welcome and reassured that the community will be able to deliver on the quality it projects.

The primary responsibility of the concierge is public relations, both internal and external. The individuals operating the front desk should be hospitality-oriented professionals who can perform multiple tasks simultaneously and thrive in a fast-paced and challenging environment. The concierge is the one person in the community who has daily contact with the residents, either in person or on the telephone. In addition, the concierge is usually the first person to whom a resident will turn with a problem, request, complaint, or question. It is essential that the concierge provide prompt, courteous, high-quality service at each resident encounter. Happy and satisfied residents are a key marketing ingredient and contribute to good referrals. The concierge must create and maintain an atmosphere of warmth, personal interest, and positive emphasis as well as a calm environment in the lobby, over the telephone, and through written communication—despite the daily chaos of this highly "charged" position. The successful concierge possesses a high degree of patience and understanding of the senior population. The way people behave toward you is usually dictated by the way you behave toward them. Behavior is not something we are born with; it is not a constant, like gender or the color of one's eyes, but a variable, like a hat one wears. It is a performance that the employee chooses to put on. The professional concierge can choose behavior to suit every encounter he has with the public, and this behavior should be a cloak for all the concierge's personal problems, prejudices, and feelings. In short, reception staff should not feel as though they are at work and should treat visitors as if they are visiting their own home. They should be primed always to be in *decision-making mode* to solve problems and manage the traffic at the front desk.

There are several essential functions of the concierge or reception desk. Not only are these employees positioned to greet visitors and perform a "switchboard" function for the community, they are also the conduit between the residents and the various department heads for communication of their needs and the community's policies. In addition, the front desk often serves as a monitor of the emergency call system and can even monitor building security and document incidents. Many operators also use night shift reception staff to perform administrative support services, including typing for department heads, light accounting such as summarizing meal credits, or special projects that can be done on a portable computer or by hand. They can also assist the marketing department with the collation of direct mail pieces, flyers, or other time-consuming projects that normally distract salespeople from otherwise valuable selling time. Because of the importance of the concierge position to the overall success of the community, guest and telephone protocol are discussed here in detail.

▪▬▬▬ HANDLING INQUIRIES AND GUEST PROTOCOL

Every person entering the lobby should be greeted immediately by the receptionist. Whenever possible, this greeting should be verbal: "Good morning, Mr. Smith." When speaking on the telephone and unable to speak to a guest in the lobby, the receptionist should acknowledge the visitor with another form of greeting. The best way to do this is with eye contact and a smile, nod, or wave. Every visitor should know that the receptionist is aware that he has entered the lobby and will be with him as soon as possible. If the person entering the lobby is not a regular visitor, it is even more important to speak to him immediately, as he will most likely be looking for information and assistance. At times it may be necessary to put a caller on hold so that the concierge can greet a visitor immediately.

During the first few seconds of the interchange, the visitor should be given the name of the receptionist and have been asked for his. It is important that the receptionist learn the proper name and pronunciation; if necessary, ask the visitor to repeat it. The first-time visitor is often ill at ease and in need of reassurance. After learning his name, it is helpful to *use it* in conversation in order to put him at ease.

After determining the visitor's needs, the receptionist should tell him who will be contacted to assist him. To do this effectively, the concierge staff must have a thorough understanding of all administrative and marketing personnel—who they are and exactly what each person is responsible for. Be sure to put the visitor in contact with the correct staff member; do not give him the runaround! If the visitor will be kept waiting, be sure to make him comfortable. Ask if he would like to have a seat while you contact the person who will be helping with his request. Offer refreshments if possible.

After making the visitor comfortable, contact the appropriate staff member and advise her of the visitor's name and the nature of the visit. Be sure to find out exactly how long the visitor should be kept waiting. If the staff member is going to be delayed for more than 10 minutes, contact a backup staff person to help the visitor. Advise the visitor of the anticipated waiting time and then monitor the situation. During the time the visitor is waiting, engage him in light conversation or give him something to read or a photo album to browse through.

When the appropriate staff member arrives, make the proper introductions using the visitor's and staff member's names. Also, provide any necessary background information to the parties involved. Advise the staff member of any questions or pertinent information mentioned in conversation with the visitor. Remember to give the visitor a parting acknowledgement: "Have a good afternoon, Mr. Smith."

I once visited a retirement community and, while waiting for a tour by the sales director, noticed a small sign behind the reception desk that said "OUR REPUTATION IS IN YOUR HANDS," an obvious reminder to the reception staff of the importance of their part in creating a positive impression. This is as important over the telephone as it is in person. It is usually easy to tell how a person's day is going by the way in which he answers the phone. The telephone is often the first encounter with many prospects, and just as people size each other up in person within the first few seconds of meeting, so it goes with the telephone, only on a more critical level. They do not know (nor do they need to know) that you're having a bad day or that the telephone is lighting up like a Christmas tree. All they have to go on is the tone of your voice and the attention they receive.

Each phone call may be a potential sale. Although each person who calls may not be eligible for your community, he may have a family member or friend who is. The caller may be a center of influence for the larger community or an area business owner, either of whom can be critical to the success of your community.

Advertising, marketing, outreach, and print media are all very expensive. The money and time spent to make each sale is far too great to be negated by a cranky person at your end of the phone line. Everyone involved with the community, staff and residents alike, is a potential salesperson. Be equipped with the proper information about the services and amenities your community offers; understand the concept; be helpful and patient while offering this information. You never know who's on the other end of the phone. It could be anyone, from the president of the company or a potential resident to a wrong number. It doesn't matter; each caller should be treated with the same polite manner.

Special consideration should be given to persons inquiring about job openings. The job search process is at best intimidating, humbling, and a bit scary. The applicant is normally forced to step outside his comfort zone and go through the motions with a statistically very slim chance of landing the job as a result of the visit. Good management recognizes this often stressful situation, takes measures to make job applicants feel welcome, and indeed makes them feel that they would want to work in the community. While there are normally far more applicants for any given position than openings (if management treats its current employees as well as it does its customers), you want to send the applicant away feeling that this would be a great place to work so that he will refer friends, and even relatives, to your door. It is just good business to make everyone feel special.

Attitude is hard to disguise, but is much easier done in person; visual image can be very deceiving. Unfortunately we cannot pull off such a deception over the phone. In order to compensate for this, put on a smile each time you answer the phone. Proper phone etiquette is expected; poor phone etiquette is remembered.

Today's marketplace creates the need for all of us to deal with the competition: marketing, selling, consumer demands, and advertising. This demands that each employee recognize herself as a salesperson respon-

sible for the image of the project. The concierge should provide only basic information in response to inquiries; requests for more detailed information should be directed to the sales staff. This will lessen the possibility of incorrect or outdated information being given out. Sales staff are trained to prequalify these call-ins over the phone and are better equipped to create a sense of urgency for a visit.

The following tips can facilitate a positive first impression by telephone. Always answer the telephone by the third ring; this lets the caller know you are anxious to help them. SMILE as you speak: the caller can *hear* a smile! Finish your words and sentences in more formal language than casual conversation. Unless you are speaking to a friend, use formal address: "Thank you, Mrs. Jones. I'll put you through as soon as she is off the line." Ask permission to put the caller on hold. If more than one line is ringing, answer by saying the community's name and asking "Would you hold, please?" When you get back to the line on hold, say, "Thank you for holding. This is [your name], may I help you?" *Do not leave the caller on hold for longer than 30 seconds* without checking back. Make sure a transfer call is completed and reaches the proper person, if the phone system allows. If you are not able to connect the caller with the appropriate staff member because she is unavailable at the time, ask if you may assist the caller or if she would like you to take a message and have the staff member return the call. Always be sure the caller understands what the outcome or action of her call will be.

Always use a message form that produces a carbon copy of the message. Be sure to note legibly *all* pertinent information, so that the staff member will be completely informed and prepared when he returns the call. Document name, time, date, return telephone number, reason for call, and action necessary. As soon as possible, deliver all messages or notify staff members that there are messages at the desk for them. Deliver any uncollected messages left at the end of the shift.

We usually visit various businesses with preconceived expectations about how we will be treated. If we are treated better than we expect, we are pleasantly surprised and register the first impression as quality. The key is to make people feel special, and the only way to do so is to exceed a visitor's expectations. The best way to do this is to think of how *you* expect to be treated when you enter a senior living community, then treat your own visitors just a little bit better. First-time visitors will be impressed with the building; with each successive visit the concierge must look for ways to keep these visitors impressed. The little extra personal touches are remembered, simply because most people do not bother with them.

■■■■■ STAFFING

Staffing a concierge or reception desk depends on the level of care provided at the project, the property configuration, the emergency response system, and the number and expectations of the residents. Normally the reception desk is staffed around the clock (24 hours/day, 7 days/week—4.2 full-time employees [FTE]). However, in assisted living communities, the front desk is usually staffed 16 hours per day (7 AM–7 PM), with night calls forwarded to the nursing station. In some larger communities (over 300 units), a second person may be necessary during the busy afternoon/evening shift to assist residents and their guests. This second person can work from 3:00 PM to 11:00 PM and also serve as the *manager on duty* to avoid the need for a night maintenance person. This *manager on duty* or *night manager* should be trained in the essential elements of emergency maintenance and elevator operations. They should also be certified in cardiopulmonary resuscitation (CPR) and trained in how to handle resident emergency calls. In addition, the night manager should respond to and assist in emergency situations, monitor evening activities and programs, and respond to resident needs. There are a number of ways to provide coverage for the concierge during breaks, lunch, and bathroom visits. Never leave the desk uncovered—without exception, the most vocal resident or family will have an "emergency" just at the precise time that the front desk staff ran to get a coffee warm-up. The night shift is the best time to run the community laundry operation; not only is there an ample supply of hot water and less distraction, but the staff can also be cross-trained to cover the front desk during breaks and even staff absences. During the day, break coverage can be handled by administrative or activity staff.

It is a good idea to cross-train several key employees on the finer points of operating the front desk. Normally the office manager or resident relations director supervises this function. In smaller operations, the office manager should actually be scheduled to take one shift per week on the desk to maintain contact with the residents, understand the workload of the employees, and monitor the overall communication flow of the building. This can save up to $3,000 per year in staffing costs while demonstrating to the residents and other employees management's commitment to creating a team environment by sharing the workload.

■■■■■ RESOURCES

As the concierge desk is "communication central," a well-organized resource file will help to position the staff to be knowledgeable and competent. The file should include directions to and from the property, airport, local restaurants, sports facilities, and downtown by way of local, recognizable arteries, along with copies of a city map that can be handed out. Reviews of local restaurants sorted by cuisine type may also be useful to residents and their guests. Most better hotels will have a computer-based description and review of major restaurants that produces a printout that can be copied and kept on file for distribution to your guests. In addition, it is helpful to have a telephone directory that lists the numbers of the local pharmacies and grocery stores that deliver, along with numbers for cab companies, city tour operators, major city attractions such as the museum and aquarium, hospitals and nursing homes, emergency numbers, and so on. It is also a good idea to keep a copy of the week's entertainment listings from the local newspaper, which include movies, theater, concerts, opera, and the symphony. Some communities also keep jogging maps and information on other local attractions within walking distance of the property. Local bus schedules and the location of the nearest stop can help ease pressure on the transportation department. The concierge desk should also maintain a small amount of change to sell stamps to residents. The stamp supply can be replenished by the driver between runs. The fund should not be used for resident postage due or COD deliveries, and the cash balance should be reconciled against a daily count of stamps sold. Stamps can also be purchased by mail using Postal Service order forms.

■■■■■ DELIVERIES

The residents must be told that they should notify the concierge or reception staff of expected deliveries so that they may assist if possible. If the resident is home when a delivery arrives, she will be notified and the package can be brought to her apartment by the delivery person. If she is not at home, the concierge will accept the package and notify the resident when she returns. All deliveries should be entered into the logbook. The community should not accept furniture or other large deliveries.

If the resident plans to be away and cannot accept a large delivery, the concierge can have a staff member let delivery persons into the resident's apartment *only* with advance written permission. The staff member should remain in the apartment with the delivery person until the delivery is completed. The concierge should not accept COD packages or grocery deliveries in the resident's absence.

For residents' convenience, local pharmacies, dry cleaners, grocery stores, and various eateries provide delivery services. These telephone numbers should be made available at the concierge desk and through the resident relations office. The resident should notify the concierge to expect the delivery and notify the resident when it arrives. It is the resident's responsibility to pay the delivery person for all items delivered. Checks may be held at the front desk, but the concierge should not be permitted to hold any cash for delivery payments or for any other purpose. Delivery persons should not be permitted to transact business on the premises unless authorized by the management at the resident's request. The concierge should not be permitted to hold residents' incoming or outgoing dry cleaning at the desk, in order to avoid accusations if articles become lost.

Resist the temptation to provide bell services such as parcel delivery or grocery assistance on request. These items can either be delivered to the resident's room by the delivery person or stored in a convenient location near the front desk to be delivered to the resident's apartment at the end of breaks or by the drivers at the end of their shift. The concierge should not accept perishables or valuables, as the community may be held responsible for any losses. Some communities provide small wheeled carts or wagons for residents to transport their packages and groceries to their rooms themselves. Residents have been known to run businesses out of their apartments, with continuous parcel deliveries to the front desk. Shipping companies will usually refuse to deliver the items to residents' apartments, and storage and handling of such deliveries may become burdensome. Arrangements should then be

made with the residents to deliver the parcels for a small fee. It is always a good idea to encourage as much independence in the residents as possible, even if they complain about it. The exercise is good for them and helps offset additional staffing costs. If residents are unable to ambulate for these purposes, another level of care may be more appropriate, unless of course their condition is temporary.

The higher the level of care, the more night staff the community will employ. Rarely does one find night reception staffing in assisted living or skilled nursing facilities; this function is normally performed by transferring the phones to the nurses' station. One assisted living community transferred its phones to an answering service that could page the night aides if necessary. Where the emergency call enunciator is located on the assisted living floor, or can be tied into the paging system, one can eliminate the need for a nurse to sit at the desk at night (if allowed by regulations). Other systems can be adapted to send an emergency alert by computerized voice through a two-way radio held by the night shift employees.

SECURITY

Security is an increasingly important issue for property owners and managers, not only because crime is on the rise in many areas but also because, according to data compiled by a Massachusetts security analysis firm, apartment owners and managers are increasingly being held responsible for crimes occurring on their properties. Forty-three percent of all reported suits were brought in Texas, New York, California, and Florida. Lawsuits against property owners primarily involve rape, robbery, and assault and battery. Average jury verdict and settlement amounts are increasing and cover a wide range. Just over 78 percent of all cases receive awards of less than $1 million; however, some have been as high as $3 million. A number of recent legal developments have made it easier for plaintiffs both to sue and to succeed with their claims.[1] As seniors age they experience a heightened sense of vulnerability that is manifested in their call for additional security measures and (usually) more staff.

Operators must be extremely cautious not to advertise *security* in their marketing materials unless they plan to have trained personnel on staff or contract out regular patrols of the hallways and grounds. "Security" should not be confused with a 24-hour concierge, an emergency response system, the use of security cameras, or simply a building that is locked at night. It must be made very clear to the residents and their families that, although you attempt to screen visitors and guests, the property does not employ security staff (unless it does). Even if the property *has* a security service or security staff, they are usually unarmed and are instructed to contact local law enforcement officials at the first sign of trouble.

It is advisable to conduct thorough multistate background checks on any candidates who are being considered for security positions. Local law enforcement agencies have advised us that the security profession often attracts individuals who have been previously deemed inappropriate for public service employment and who are therefore looking to the private sector for work in an *enforcement* capacity. Many of these individuals are also ardent firearm enthusiasts, which could present additional complications. Recently the security chief of a luxury hotel on the east coast entered the property through the employee entrance just after midnight and shot and killed one of his employees, ending a long-standing squabble between the two; he later turned the gun on himself. This incident illustrates the fact that, whereas operators may be exposed to risk without a security staff, they may also be inviting trouble with one. An excellent solution to the problem may involve the local police department. Some communities take advantage of their significant political influence in city and county governments and persuade the chief of police to schedule several daily visits by uniformed officers who cruise the hallways, or at least the grounds, on a regular patrol. Although this scheme may not provide much of a deterrent, it does help ease the residents' fears. At the very least, operators can encourage the local patrol officers to stop by daily for coffee and fresh muffins.

Staffing

Proper staffing of a security department depends on a number of factors. Assuming the operator has determined that security is necessary, the size of the force can range from a night watchman (10 hours/day, 7 days/week—1.75 FTE) to 24-hour security at a guard station (24 hours/day, 7 days/week—4.2 FTE) plus night patrols around the property (1.75 FTE) depending on its size, its configuration, and crime statistics in the neighborhood. Additional temporary

security staff may be necessary from time to time to protect residents and staff from potential workplace violence or to guard new construction projects or additions. Twenty-four-hour security staffed with qualified, experienced employees, along with benefits, insurance, communication, and supplies, can easily add more than $100,000 per year to the operating budget. Like most types of services, once implemented this one is not easily withdrawn from the residents.

Normally, the use of security cameras positioned to cover the parking areas, loading dock, and employee entrance and monitored by the concierge will provide adequate routine coverage. Over the years, in my experience operating some 63 communities across the country, the worst problems have involved some stolen or damaged cars in the parking lot, one disgruntled employee who had to be physically removed from the property, and one drive-by shooting. All these incidents were effectively handled by the local authorities to the satisfaction of the residents, and two cars were even stolen while my security guard was on duty checking room flags! I did experience an armed robbery of my contract valet parking attendant, but the entire event was successfully recorded on camera and the police apprehended the perpetrator sometime later without incident. In fact, the residents never knew of the incident and surely would have found out from facility-employed security staff.

In certain circumstances, some security employees can be used for housekeeping duties in the common areas and the lobby, as can the night concierge. It is important to inform these job applicants that their duties may include some of these services and inquire if they would be comfortable performing them. Depending on the facility, these duties might include carpet cleaning, changing light bulbs, polishing brass and furniture, updating information boards, or other duties. In addition to performing their regular patrols, some operators use night security staff to perform the "I'm OK" door flag program.

"I'm OK"

A number of systems are employed by retirement communities to check on the daily status of each resident. The type of system varies by the size of the community. Both electronic and manual systems are available, and each works quite well for its intended use. The door flag system is one of the best. Stated simply, each apartment door frame is fitted with a small oval-shaped clear Plexiglas tag about three inches long with a hole drilled at one end attached near the top of the door. The tag is loosely attached to the frame so that it rotates freely around the hole. When the tag is rotated up against the door and the door opens, the tag will drop to the down position. Equipped with a resident roster of all occupied apartments, the security guard is then able to determine if the resident has opened his door, if marketing, housekeeping, or maintenance has visited a vacant apartment, or other entry has been made. The occupied apartments with flags still in the up position will then be checked out, usually by 10:00 the next morning. All flags are then reset each night.

Electronic systems such as Marlok™ that use electronically programmed keys can track each time a door is keyed to open. Specifically coded keys can be issued to the resident, housekeeping staff, maintenance crew, or whoever has a need to enter the apartment. The system can be programmed to search all daily entries and exits made by the residents on all occupied apartments and print out a list each morning of "no activity" doors for the morning concierge to call to check up on residents. This system is also effective for determining who entered an apartment in case something is declared missing; it can also be hardwired to the emergency response system. The key readers in each lock do fail regularly and require trained personnel to replace or override manually. In addition, as with any electronic system, they can be very vulnerable to power surges and spikes. There are also battery-operated card reader lock systems that are capable of memory, but unfortunately the batteries all seem to fail at once and their replacement can be both expensive and very inconvenient for residents who may find themselves locked out. Another useful daily check-in now being installed in newer communities features a green flashing lighted button, adjacent to the pull cord in the bedroom, that the resident will simply push upon arising each morning. A central computer will then print out a report listing the apartments that have not checked in, so they can be called by the concierge staff. The system can also be tied into the resident and outside doors, or can be disabled at the resident's request. Other systems using a button by the resident's phone that is tied to lights on a central board at the front desk are equally effective.

Manual systems can be used for any size population but are best suited to communities under 200 units. The most effective manual system should account for residents at the time when they are out of their apartments for meals. A resident roster can be printed each day and posted at the entrance to the dining room, where residents can check off their names as they enter or leave, or residents can be checked off by the dining room manager or hostess. The roster first goes to the concierge to be updated to account for people who are out of town or at the hospital, then is passed to the dining room staff to verify either room service or the residents' presence in the dining room. After the evening meal, the evening concierge calls those residents who are unaccounted for. All residents should be checked daily. Residents are encouraged to call the concierge if they will not be coming down for a meal.

LOGBOOKS

There should be several different logbooks kept at the concierge desk. They should be hardbound books with sequentially numbered pages so that a continuous, unalterable log can be kept. A log of all entries and exits through the lobby can be very useful in reconstructing events; tracking residents, staff, and deliveries; noting comments made by residents or changes in their behavior; and recording emergency pull-cord activation and daily traffic through the lobby. This enables the supervisor to track resident patterns, staff workload, and follow-up on resident questions and incidents. The work order log and system is also helpful for maintenance to track and prioritize requests while ensuring that the concierge is the one central location to record both staff and resident service requests (see Chapter 12 for more on the work order system). The activity sign-up log will ensure that residents document their reservations for group tours and trips on the community bus for outings, shopping trips, religious trips, and the mall run. Another essential log is the transportation appointment request book. This enables residents to schedule their transportation requests by automobile into the available time slots on a first-come, first-served basis. The concierge should be aware of all daily activities and any scheduled changes with full information on upcoming events. Finally, the reservation book for the guest apartments should also be maintained by the concierge.

■■■■■ GUEST SUITES AND OVERNIGHT GUESTS

Most communities have furnished guest suites that are available for use by resident guests on a short-term and first-come, first-served basis. During their stay, guests may have access to meals in the dining room at the current meal rates. The resident host is normally held responsible for his guests' behavior and all charges incurred by them. There is usually a charge per night for the use of guest suites that is competitive with the going rate at local hotels; most operators normally include continental breakfast. There should be a list of charges at the concierge desk or in the resident relations office for the resident to check. Normally, residents like to treat their guests, and this can be done discreetly by appearing on the next month's bill through the normal billing cycle. There should be no payment or cash accepted for meals in the dining room. If guests insist on settling their accounts themselves, this can be done in the form of a check to the property accountant when they check out. Residents are normally allowed a certain number of meals per month that are included in their monthly fees. Those residents who do not use all these meals will want to apply these meal credits to their guests. This should be strongly discouraged. A resident guest meal that costs $6–$8.00 to produce and serve can be sold to a guest for $10–$15.00. Operators will not adjust their purchasing or staffing if residents miss a few meals; the same overhead applies whether they are there or not. The fact that there is some economy of scale to mass-producing meals and other services allows for the profitability in the operations. Furthermore, when residents are away for an extended period (more than a week), they should receive a meal credit only for the food costs.

Reservations should be made for the guest suite and for each meal by contacting the concierge and the dining room. Children are permitted in the guest suite only when accompanied by an adult. Even adult children can be a problem. A situation once developed in which the daughter of a resident felt strongly that she should be able to use the facility during her mother's extensive travels. She felt that she should be entitled not only to use her mother's apartment and eat her meals, but also to enjoy use of the common areas. House rules can be established for overnight guests and companions to clarify expectations and limit the use of common-area amenities to residents only. This way the privacy of the residents' extended living areas can be respected. Most insurance policies will cover accidents that befall both residents and their guests, but these do little to appease angry residents who feel that their facilities are being abused and their home has been invaded.

Check-in time for guest suites should be after 1:00 PM and check-out by 11:00 AM to allow housekeeping time to tidy the apartment and the kitchen time to deliver the arrival amenities such as cookies or a fruit bowl. Amenities are usually a very inexpensive way to charm residents' guests and ultimately impress your residents. Nothing impresses people more than having their guests think that they are receiving special treatment because of a resident's influence.

There should be a fee for all telephone calls placed from guest suites. Long-distance charges should then be billed to the resident when the monthly telephone bill arrives.

The resident relations department, along with the housekeeping supervisor, should develop a standardized list of expendables for the guest rooms and apartments. The list should include bath linens and amenities, bed linens and pillows, clock radio, notepads, telephone instructions, room service menu, coat and skirt hangers, kitchen equipment including place settings and flatware, glasses, coffee maker, pots and pans, tea kettle, water pitcher, knives, paper goods, arrival amenity, television set with remote, ash trays, and so forth. This is a partial list intended to illustrate the need for an organized approach to ensuring that guests have all the essentials needed to make their visit comfortable. It is also a good idea to include an information packet that includes a welcome letter, floor plan of the building, menu, and brochure. In most states the operation of the guest suites falls under the jurisdiction of the Inn Keepers Act, and a copy of this, along with the emergency exit path and directions, must be posted in a conspicuous location, usually on the back of the door.

Residents should be encouraged to invite friends or relatives to be guests in their apartment. For security purposes, they need to notify the concierge when guests are staying with them. Overnight guests must sign in at the concierge desk on arrival. A person living in a resident apartment for more than thirty days should automatically be considered a second occupant and should be charged as such on the next month's statement. Be cautious not to allow residents to permit relatives to stay with them for any extended period; once they move in while they are "between jobs," they are very difficult to extricate without permanently affecting your long-term relationship with the resident. Most resident agreements and the Americans with Disabilities Act allow operators to maintain the age requirement exclusion for these types of properties. Some communities charge a "companion fee" for a resident's private duty aide who spends 18 hours or more per day at the property.

ANSWERING THE EMERGENCY CALL SYSTEM

Each time a resident's pull cord or call light is activated, staff should consider the situation an emergency. Residents must be instructed on orientation to the community and their apartment that the pull cords are for use in a medical emergency and are not to be pulled for room service, for maintenance requests, or because their housekeeper is late or they cannot find their glasses. They also need to be instructed on the emergency procedure that will follow and the importance of filling out an emergency information card that can be used by the paramedics. The emergency information card can be attached to their refrigerator and should include at a minimum such important medical data as preexisting conditions, a list of current medications, any allergies, hospital and religious preferences, name and emergency number of their personal physician, medical insurance information (including their Medicare number, if they are eligible), names of relatives to be contacted, the existence of a living will, or other pertinent instructions and information. Two copies of this emergency information should be maintained at the concierge desk and updated periodically. Computerized, state-of-the-art emergency call systems now include a feature whereby emergency information can be input into the system and pulled up on the screen during an emergency. The information can be printed and sent with the paramedics to the hospital.

Residents' call lights need to be answered promptly, for the resident may be alone and in an emergency situation, such as having fallen or experiencing chest pain, a heart attack, difficulty in breathing, or some other life-threatening situation. The resident's apartment should immediately be called to determine the nature and urgency of the request and to reassure the resident that help is immediately on the way. The concierge phone system must have a separate trunk set-up to deal with emergencies, just in case all the rollover lines are busy. The community operations manual should detail the appropriate procedure along with the emergency numbers to call. The paramedics should be met at the entrance nearest to the resident's apartment and escorted there. The resident should not be left unattended until help arrives. The concierge is best able to coordinate emergency response from her station at the concierge desk and should call other trained community personnel to wait with the resident until emergency crews arrive. If the facility's smoke alarm system activates the alarm, a back-up call should be placed to the fire department. Most alarm systems are connected directly to the fire dispatcher but have been known to fail.

ADVANCE DIRECTIVES

Every individual has the authority to determine her own medical treatment, including the right to execute advance directives related to health care proxy and cardiopulmonary resuscitation. A health care proxy is a legally recognized document that allows an individual to appoint someone as an agent to make medical treatment decisions on his behalf. Many people complete a health care proxy as a way of ensuring that their values and wishes regarding medical care are followed by health care providers should they lose the ability to decide. This enables health care providers to rely on the proxy agent's decisions without fear of liability.

Patients may also arrange with their physicians for Do Not Resuscitate (DNR) orders, a doctor's order directing that the individual not be resuscitated in the event of cardiac or respiratory arrest. The retirement community may choose to assist in the storage and dissemination of DNR information, including positive identification of residents through photo documentation or bracelets.

Operators must decide in advance if it will be their policy to perform CPR routinely on their residents or to determine if their physician-documented DNR order is on file. (With the passage of the Patient Self-Determination Act of 1990, residents can arrange for advance directives that legally prohibit the use of life-sustaining care for the terminally ill.) A copy of a resident's living will can go to the hospital with the ambulance driver. It is usually best to let the hospital handle the appropriate administration of the living will. In most cases the law will protect employees from liability arising out of providing CPR on a resident against his wishes. For assisted living and skilled nursing communities, state regulations require resuscitation attempts unless it can be determined that the patient has been dead for some time. Normally, in most operations CPR should be initiated on any resident, staff member, or visitor who experiences an acute cessation of respiration, pulse, and consciousness. Optimally, the facility staff should be trained to provide an efficient, safe, and professionally calm environment during such an incident and to enable an advanced life support team of paramedics to function efficiently within the facility.

When a resident, employee, or visitor is found unconscious and does not respond to shake-and-shout, the staff member who finds the victim immediately alerts the nearest supervisor or other person in charge. The supervisor will assess the victim and begin CPR (if appropriate) according to the *American Red Cross Guidelines*. The concierge or attending staff will call 911 and ask for the advanced life support team. The concierge can also place a call to the resident's physician to notify her of the patient's condition and receive orders. The executive director or alternate should then be notified as soon as possible. Be sure to protect the rights of residents with regard to privacy during transfer and discharge. Many times a resident will be somewhat embarrassed by all the attention and will refuse transport and downplay her condition. When in doubt, transport or allow the paramedics to make that decision. When paramedics arrive, the incident is turned over to them and the staff should document the events in the resident's medical record, or fill out an incident report with a copy being placed in the resident's file. If a resident refuses medical attention or transport to a hospital, he should be asked to sign the incident report, noting such refusal.

The patient's attending physician and other responsible persons should be notified by the supervisor

---

Exhibit 4.1   Guidelines for DNR Orders

■ Development of a residence policy statement regarding DNR orders that is compliant with current law and recognizes a resident's right to choose the treatment course in case of cardiac arrest, including a system to communicate DNR orders to emergency medical services (EMS) personnel.

■ Communication of this right to the resident, legal guardian, or health care agent as a part of the service plan discussion.

■ Proactive communication and education of local EMS regarding this policy of the residence in advance regarding DNR orders.

"Advance Directives in Assisted Living, Health Care Proxies, and DNR Orders," Massachusetts Assisted Living Federation of America Quality Guidelines, August 26, 1997, p. 2.

---

on duty of any accident involving the patient or other significant change in the patient's physical, mental, or emotional status. At the resident's request, his physician can obtain and complete a DNR Order Verification Form and bracelet. This provides a mechanism for emergency medical personnel arriving at the scene to determine the resident's wishes. A new program, "Comfort Care DNR Verification," has been developed by the Massachusetts Department of Public Health Office of Emergency Medical Services, in consultation with local physician groups. The resident can wear the bracelet and keep the form available in her apartment. This way, the responsibility is on the resident to communicate advance directives, rather than on management to sort out the information during an emergency.[2]

NOTES
1. Liability Consultants Inc., "Major Developments in Premises Security Liability." The report is available directly from the firm by calling (508) 872-5222.
2. Free brochures are available by calling the Massachusetts Office of Emergency Medical Services at (617) 753-8300.

Resident Relations

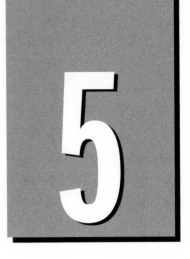

Residents can be a challenge. Not only are we financially dependent on them, but for many senior living professionals they are the source of both anxiety and job satisfaction. As managers of senior living communities, we are uniquely positioned to make a difference in the quality of people's lives. Many need-driven seniors inquire at a senior living community looking for solutions. It can be a very difficult time for people who may have been living independently to take this first step toward declaring their own "dependence." The transition into a community lifestyle can be traumatic, and seniors deal with this trauma in a variety of ways. Normally they begin the process in denial, then exhibit anger and hostility, followed by bargaining and ultimately acceptance. It is much like a bereavement process. In fact, they may be experiencing one of the most disruptive losses of all—their home, and with it a good piece of their independence. For many, this loss can touch their very identity, an identity that may have been developing for the past 75 years.

Although most residents will accept and adapt to their new environment after a few months, others will find it more difficult. As people age, they become more resistant to change, but the aging process itself demands change, much of which catches them unprepared. No one ever plans to lose a spouse, or have a hip replaced, or face difficulty with simple tasks such as preparing meals. For some, these constant changes in lifestyle can be a struggle.

Fortunately, those who have a difficult time adjusting represent the minority and are easily identified. But employees and other residents sometimes label them "chronic complainers" or "difficult residents." It is important for employees to recognize that it is not these people who are "bad," only their behavior. There is normally a cause for behavioral problems, such as stress, medical problems or physiological imbalance, anger at the loss of a spouse, family or financial problems, or simply rejection of the normal aging process. Some people choose to internalize these problems, whereas others will outwardly criticize and exhibit hostility to the world around them.

HANDLING COMPLAINTS

A complaint is not always a criticism, and indeed it is not always a simple matter to identify the real problem behind a complaint. Residents may be experiencing difficulty adjusting to the community, a difficulty that may be complicated by feelings of rejection and guilt.

Today's residents may have grown up during the Depression and may have become conditioned to austerity. When first introduced to a modern senior living community, many react negatively to a lifestyle that they may personally consider "lavish." It is the dream of many to pass on their life savings to their heirs, and many find it very difficult to spend this money on themselves. Therefore, they may be concerned about how their hard-earned money is used by management to deliver resident services and may feel that they do not deserve this lifestyle. For most, at the very least, it is a significant departure from the frugal lifestyle they may have been living in their own home or apartment.

Family members also experience guilt about influencing their mother or father to move into a senior living community. After all, these are the people who raised them and provided for their every need as children. Many are forced by busy careers, geographical isolation, and other family commitments to seek professional help in dealing with their aging parents. Unfortunately, senior living communities are still viewed by the uninformed majority as "homes." This view may lead families to feelings of having abandoned their parents. Residents recognize this, and many will play on the guilt that their children may be experiencing, consciously or subconsciously. Residents are much harder on their families than they ever are on management. For example, residents' families are normally the first to hear of their problems and complaints. They usually preface their complaints with, "I told you this wasn't right for me" and expect family members to take a personal interest in their problems. This behavior normally occurs more frequently among residents who recently moved into the community than among more established tenants. Residents may complain more early in their residency because of loneliness and feelings of isolation. Complaints to families will normally decrease with time as residents adjust to their new environment and make new friends. Most complaints directed at management from family members are in response to their parents' complaints to them. It is important to discuss these issues with family members and to remind them that their parents may be experiencing difficulty adjusting to their new lifestyle and that their barrage of complaints may be a manifestation of other, broader issues. Remind family members that everyone must support the resident and be patient.

Many times management will be the last to hear residents' complaints. Normally the cycle starts with their families; next to be told are other residents, then line staff, and ultimately management. Residents may feel somewhat captive in the senior living community and may withhold their concerns for fear of either retribution or being labeled as "troublemakers." In addi-

tion, they may not have the confidence that management will treat their concerns confidentially—or respond at all. They will in fact confide their complaints to all sorts of people while asking each of them to protect their anonymity. Family members who may relay their parents' complaints to management normally do so without their knowledge or approval. Family members should be reminded that management will do everything reasonable to resolve their parents' issues discreetly. However, they should encourage their parents to be proactive and report their concerns to management first in specific terms so that specific solutions can be developed. When a resident says, "I told them about it and they never do anything," it could also mean that his request may have already been denied or that granting it would be inconsistent with community policy. Residents will always seek "special" treatment or try to differentiate their situations from those of other residents. Any success in convincing management to "bend" the rules for their personal needs can be considered a triumph to be flaunted before other residents. Management should take great care to ensure that all residents are treated fairly and equally.

It is important to distinguish residents who may be upset from those who may be difficult. When a reasonable person gets upset she may have momentary lapses of unreasonableness, but she is basically rational and reasonable. But difficult people have a psychological need to get attention by disruptive and negative means. They are chronically hard to communicate with and may have lived their entire life this way. It is almost as if they live in a constant storm, moving around in a vortex of anxiety from one place to the next. They seek satisfaction through validation and solicit the support of others. When management, staff, or even fellow residents are pulled into their storm, these other individuals are at risk of losing their perspective as they become caught up in the turmoil. When we lose our perspective, we also lose our objectivity and become part of the problem rather than part of the solution. Storms may come and go, but difficult people tend to hang around, and if it isn't one thing, it will soon be another. If this behavior continues, residents and staff alike will begin to exhibit creative avoidance, which can further isolate the difficult resident and make matters worse. He may soon find himself sitting alone in the dining room or with new residents, until they also become weary of the negativity. We all need to recognize that there are some people who will be unreasonable no matter what you do. Normally they will compose only about 1 percent of the resident population. In extreme cases, some communities may temporarily refuse service to difficult residents in the main dining room, delivering their meals to their apartments instead. Other residents have the right to quiet enjoyment of the community's common areas, and this alternative can be very effective in isolating disruptive behavior problems while protecting the atmosphere for the other residents. This strategy normally also has a moderating effect on the difficult resident's behavior, as isolation can be somewhat embarrassing.

The business of operating senior living communities is unique in that our customers are to a large extent a captive audience. They can't just go away or be appeased with an amenity or free meal. We need to satisfy them permanently or clearly communicate the limits of what can or cannot be done for them. If you are firm and confident in your interaction with a resident, she will respect you more than if your response is ambiguous. If management has a reputation for quick, courteous responses to complaints, residents will be more apt to begin their conversations with you rationally. When they scream or yell, it is often because that is what another resident had to do to get results. How current resident concerns are handled will set the stage for how future residents may behave toward management. Word of mouth spreads like wildfire through a community, especially if it involves gossip or the actions of management. Studies have shown that

- For every resident who bothers to complain, there are 24 silent, unhappy residents. Yet if residents do complain and the complaint is resolved quickly, 90 percent will recommend you to their friends.
- The average "wronged" resident will tell 8 to 16 people, each of whom may tell 5 others. In a tight social circle such as a senior community, word can spread fast.
- On average it can cost as much as five times more to attract a new resident as it takes to keep an old one happy.

Encourage your residents to complain. The act of complaining can open communication lines, dispel rumors, and build resident satisfaction and referrals. Retailer Marshall Field aptly summarized the impor-

tance of constructive complaints when he said, "Those who complain teach me how I may please others so that more will come. Only those hurt me who are displeased but do not complain. They refuse me permission to correct my errors and improve my service."[1] In 1979 and again in 1986, Technical Assistance Research Programs Institute of Washington, D.C. (TARP) conducted landmark studies of the handling of consumer complaints in America. TARP found that one in four customers of the average American organization is upset enough to consider taking her business elsewhere. Yet only 5 percent will actually register a complaint; the other 95 percent would rather switch than fight. According to TARP, consumers overwhelmingly believe that "complaining won't do any good; no one wants to hear about my problem." The TARP report goes on to conclude that this pessimism is well founded: more than 40 percent of the consumers were unhappy with the action taken to resolve their complaints.

Residents can become upset for a variety of reasons. As mentioned earlier, sometimes the real source of their problems is difficult to isolate, whereas at other times it may be clear and justified. Either way, in working to resolve their problems it helps to understand what may set them off. Residents may become upset because

- They have an expectation that may not have been met. You or someone in the organization promised them something that was not delivered or has changed. They may have made a wrong assumption about what the community's lifestyle would do for them. It is critical that sales representatives avoid making promises that do not reflect operational reality. *Never overpromise and underdeliver.*
- They may already be upset at someone or something else that may be beyond your control. They may feel tired, sick, stressed, frustrated, or abandoned. They may feel like victims, as personal power or influence in their lives seems to erode with age.
- Sometimes residents will use any excuse to prove they are right, whether or not they are. A resident may have a chip on his shoulder or hold deeply rooted prejudices.
- Someone on the staff may have been rude, indifferent, or discourteous to them. They may have been told one thing by one staff member and something else by another. They may have acted on something they were told by a staff member that was

wrong. They may have been embarrassed about doing something incorrectly or have had their integrity or honesty questioned.

■ *They may have a real and valid complaint.*

Annoyances that a person usually tolerates become intolerable when that individual is upset. Although you cannot control another person's behavior, you can adjust *your* behavior to avoid escalating hers. Don't react—respond to difficult situations. A good example of this is when your doctor tells you your body is *reacting* to medication; this has a very negative connotation. However, if she reports that you are *responding* to the medicine, it's good news. We *react* when our immediate instincts take charge; we *respond* when we listen, consider the alternatives, and develop a workable solution to a difficult situation.

Upset residents will be looking for a variety of responses from you. They will want to be taken seriously and treated with respect. They will not respond well to condescension or arrogance. They will expect immediate action. They do not want you to "look into it" but to do something *right now.* They may want compensation or restitution, someone to pay. This might include expectations of a reprimand or disciplinary action against a staff member up to and including termination. Inform the resident that corrective action will be taken, in order to reassure him that you understand the seriousness of his concern. Sometimes the resident just wants to know that his complaint will somehow make a difference and that some action has been or will be taken, so that no one else will have this problem again. Most of all, residents want attention and to be listened to. If they feel neglected or ignored, they will go to great lengths to make their points. Great care must be taken not to patronize an errant resident, as she may already feel vulnerable in her new environment. It is important to focus not only on what the resident is saying, but on how she is saying it. The resident may not *say* she's angry, but her voice conveys it loud and clear. Listen carefully for emotions as well as facts.

Residents will occasionally confront management publicly. It is very important to validate the residents' concerns and separate them from the group in order to maintain control. Resident meetings can get out of hand quickly when residents successfully maneuver management into a defensive posture. It is like the dog

and the mail carrier: if the carrier shows fear, the dog will give chase. The residents will also grab hold of your leg and hold on. Come to resident meetings with an agenda and stick to it. There should always be something special on the agenda, such as announcing the employee of the quarter or offering some resident recognition, to add a positive note to the meeting (you might want to save this for last). It is always well received if you ask residents for ideas. If things begin to get off track, schedule the topic for another meeting to allow yourself time to research the situation and ask key residents for support for your position.

Residents can quickly discern whether or not you are paying attention to them. If they were mildly agitated before, your inattention can push them to anger. Upset residents may call you names, curse, or say other unpleasant things about you, your coworkers, or your organization. Avoid letting them "push your buttons." Otherwise you may lose your objectivity, and you must remain in control if you are going to find a solution to the situation. Repeat or paraphrase what you understand the resident to have said. Sometimes hearing you say it makes it sound worse than the resident believes it really is, and he will frequently back down a bit. At the very least he will know you are really listening to him.

Handling resident complaints involves much the same process employed by salespeople to overcome objections. Residents want to be heard and empathized with. Tell them you understand how they could *feel* that way. Validate their concerns by admitting that others have *felt* the same way. Finally, offer an explanation that has been acceptable to others: "What they have *found* is that two separate dining times can create a more intimate setting and better service." In this way your explanation will help clarify matters so that they understand more fully. The *feel, felt, found* technique acknowledges residents' feelings, substantiates the importance of their concerns, and offers solutions based on experience. Always remember to be consistent in your responses. Consistency of response will be tested by the residents, and consistency equals credibility. Treating favorite residents differently from the general population will be transparent to most residents and staff; it is never worth the short-term benefits. Sometimes the hardest thing for the manager to do is to say no and mean it. It is much easier to give in to a resident's demands to get him off your back, but you may pay for it later. It is usually better to say no to a resident's request if you are not sure it is possible to comply. This will buy you some time, perhaps to resolve the problem in the resident's favor and surprise her. If you merely say you will "look into it," there is no closure. You are accepting the responsibility to follow up personally and run the risk of rejection if you are unable to deliver.

Residents who are not satisfied, or become frustrated with management's inability to resolve their concerns reasonably, will seek validation through other residents. In extreme cases, such situations can deteriorate into conflict. When lines of communication break down, residents will seek other alternatives to make their points. They may attempt to organize other residents by circulating a petition, seek legal advice, or even report their complaint to an ombudsman or to state regulatory authorities who may be required by law to investigate personally. People who hire attorneys to do their talking for them either have a close relative who will do it for free or are truly desperate. Although some extreme circumstances may end up in court, 90 percent of all litigation is normally settled out of court. Large sums of money and energy can be spent because someone was unwilling to listen to a problem.

Resident petitions can set a dangerous precedent when management is ultimately forced to give in. It is within a resident's rights to circulate a petition, but management should make every attempt to resolve a resident's concerns before a petition gains momentum. Some residents may even be intimidated into signing a petition by other more influential residents. It is appropriate to speak to the person(s) responsible for circulating the petition if other residents complain about being pestered to sign it. However, management should never give the impression that it is afraid of a petition or is attempting to derail it. Simply address the issue and state your case or policy proactively, or call the residents together and make a presentation on the subject. Most residents understand business practices and are reasonable. Corporate management responsible for multiple sites must be careful not to accept the role of arbitrator, or it may compromise the executive director's authority to manage the community. Whenever possible, the decision of the executive director should be viewed as final.

Proactively manage your residents' expectations and opinions. Recognize their contributions through volunteer appreciation socials, resident appreciation and newcomers' dinners, pictures and features in the community newsletter and other marketing materials, a "hall of fame" for recognizing resident council service, and pictures of successful events on bulletin boards and easel displays. Share pertinent information with residents through flyers and memos about community affairs, accomplishments of the owner(s), formal responses to important issues, and good news about marketing accomplishments or details on the new-resident referral program. A suggestion box should be set up and referred to at all meetings and informally when residents complain. Tell them that if they want action, they should document their specific concerns along with signed suggestions on how things could be improved, so management can follow up. Management should then respond to all suggestions by documenting the suggestion along with the appropriate response in a report distributed monthly to the resident council president. In this way, as resident concerns are identified, specific solutions can be offered by management to derail residents' criticism that "nothing ever happens if you complain." The resident council can refer to previous suggestion box responses from management on issues that may resurface. Don't be afraid to say, "I don't know" or "I don't have the answer right now." Tell them, "That's a good question. I'll find an answer for you and get back to you tomorrow." Don't be afraid to share problems, and *never* cover anything up. Residents should be encouraged to recognize the value of positive reinforcement as well.

The extent to which residents use the suggestion box as a communication tool will depend solely on how management responds to it. One of the world's largest and most successful food stores is Stew Leonard's Dairy in Norwalk, Connecticut; sales are approaching $100 million a year. Sales volume per square foot is about ten times the level of conventional grocery stores. The Food Marketing Institute figures that $100 million in annual sales is about normal for a *ten-store* supermarket chain. Profits are $250 per square foot, according to *Boardroom Reports*. Obviously, the Leonard family are onto something here. The secret of their success revolves around their obsession with customer service. Near the front door is a suggestion box where customers are encouraged to share their comments, suggestions, and complaints. Each morning the contents of the box are emptied out and typed up on as many sheets of paper as it takes (100 suggestions and comments a day is the average). By 10:00 A.M. the comment sheets have been photocopied, distributed to all department managers, and posted and left on tables in the employee break areas, so that everyone knows how well they are doing in the eyes of their most important managers—their customers. It doesn't end there. Within 24 hours, someone on the store's management team—often someone named Leonard—has followed up with a phone call to thank the customer for his or her comments, explore the details of the suggestion, or discuss ways to resolve the problem. Within 48 hours, there's a letter in the mail to follow up yet again. Customers who take the initiative at Stew Leonard's find out quickly how highly their input is valued.

People tend to avoid conflict because it is a stress producer. Real problems don't just go away. Managers who avoid dealing with issues as they arise run the risk of their escalation. Left unchecked, they can ultimately become expensive and require massive amounts of unproductive time to resolve.

Finally, it is natural to feel attacked personally when a resident is actually upset at the organization, a policy, one of your coworkers—or even himself. He is lashing out at whatever is near, in this case you. More often than not, his misfortune was not caused by you; remind yourself of this. If a resident says "You screwed up my order," he probably means "My order didn't arrive in a reasonable amount of time and you people are unorganized in the kitchen. Whoever is responsible for this is in big trouble and *you* are going to hear about it." Of course, sometimes the mistake may have been your fault. We all make mistakes. Experience teaches us to recognize them when we make them again! It will often disarm residents if you admit that it was your fault and apologize. Exhibits 5.1 and 5.2 offer suggestions on handling complaints and adopting a responsive approach to others.

■■■ RESIDENT ADVISORY COUNCILS

No business can ever be successful without the support of its customers. Residents can be your greatest ally and your worst nightmare. Residents are paying large sums of money for the services they receive; it is only reasonable that they should expect some voice in how the services are delivered. Many communities have found the resident council to be the best way to

---

| **Exhibit 5.1** | **Handling Complaints: A Step-by-Step Response** |

- Disarm the resident with a calm response.
- Isolate him from other residents or guests.
- Verbally cushion the resident's behavior.
- Use the *feel, felt, found* approach.
- Apologize for the situation.
- Assure the resident that you want to help.
- Probe to identify the *specific* problem, not just the symptoms. Pin the resident down on sweeping accusations.
- Paraphrase the resident's concerns to clarify your understanding.
- Find something in the resident's remarks with which you can agree.
- Avoid being defensive and trying to make excuses.
- Show the resident that you value this information and appreciate her courage in bringing it to your attention.
- Inquire as to how she would like you to respond or specifically resolve her concern.
- Explain available options; offer choices.
- Summarize actions to be taken—yours and hers. She may be part of the solution.
- Thank the resident for bringing the matter to your attention.
- *Follow up!*

| **Exhibit 5.2** | **Response Tactics** |

- Listen carefully and clarify before you respond.
- Engage the resident. Face him and look him in the eye.
- Adopt an open, not defensive, body posture; show your concern.
- Avoid being condescending or impatient.
- Never argue or interrupt; let him get it all out. The resident may be just blowing off steam.
- Be sincere and show empathy.
- Eliminate distractions.
- Use a pleasant tone of voice.
- Be solution oriented.
- Don't take things personally.

give the residents that voice while controlling special interest groups. Residents should be placed *in an advisory role only* and not be expected to participate in the management of the community. After all, part of what they are paying the management company for through their rent or monthly service fee is professional supervision. Normally resident councils will accept as much authority as is formally or informally delegated to them by management. You do not want your residents managing your community for you, as such a situation will only complicate management's efforts to control costs and increase revenues. This should be clearly understood by new and existing resident council members.

Resident councils by definition should serve to represent the interests of the *entire* resident body. The selection of the resident council should involve a democratic process based on display of the candidates' objectivity and interest in representing the resident body as a whole. The election process should not be a popularity contest, and great care should be taken to advise residents to screen potential candidates to avoid potential conflicts of interest. They should never be perceived as a "rubber stamp" committee that only sings management's praises. It is important for the resident council to understand the importance of a balance between the objectives of the owner(s) and the expectations of the employees and the residents they serve. The operation will run best when everyone's needs are addressed.

The resident council should be made up of no fewer than six residents. Some communities will elect a president and a secretary plus a representative from each floor, building, or wing. Management should set up procedures for electing resident council members, establish initial bylaws, and recommend standing rules of procedure. Although community needs may differ, the following suggestions will facilitate the creation and clarify the role of a proactive resident advisory council.

Electing Resident Council Members

The council should limit the term for residents who serve on the council to a period of two years. Council members should not be allowed to run for immediate reelection, in order to limit the development of special interest groups. To ensure objective representation, terms should be staggered. Each year the council

should have a minimum of two to three new members, depending on the size of the council. A nominating and elections committee should be formed to prepare a slate of two candidates for each vacancy on the council. In addition, residents not on the committee may nominate any number of additional candidates with additional petitions signed by 12 other residents. The committee should verify that each nominee has indicated a willingness to serve. The names of the candidates should be placed on the ballot in alphabetical order.

The committee should establish an annual schedule to begin the process and announce the slate of candidates. Before the election, an all-resident meeting should be held to introduce the candidates. The election should be by means of sealed ballot, and those candidates receiving the greatest number of votes will become new members of the council. Ballots for the election should be placed in residents' mailboxes on a specified date. For a ballot to be counted, it must be placed in a sealed envelope and inserted into the ballot box on the receptionist's desk by a specified date, normally one week following distribution. The ballots are then counted at a meeting of the nominating and elections committee. In case of a tie, a runoff election should be held using the same procedures as in the first election. When the candidates elected to the council have been determined, the remaining candidates should be listed in order of the number of votes received and used to fill unexpected vacancies on the council. If any council member is unable to complete a term of service, the council should name as a successor the person who received the greatest number of votes on the list remaining from the last election. The winners of the election should be published without reference to the actual count.

Bylaws of the Resident Advisory Council

The bylaws should establish the name of the organization, normally the "Resident Advisory Council of [your community]." They should also establish its purpose: to bring to the attention of the management any concerns and questions brought forth by the residents and to act in an *advisory* capacity to the management on behalf of the residents. The bylaws should specify the number of members, their overlapping terms, and the policy for replacement of members who are unable to complete their terms. Three unexcused absences should result in a letter, giving the dates of the absences and advising the member that she will be dropped from the council. Absences should be considered excused when the president is notified in a timely manner before the meeting. The president of the resident advisory council should be elected for a term of only one year and can be renominated only after a one-year break in service. The officers of the council should be defined and confirmed by an affirmative vote by a majority of all council members.

The bylaws should establish the duties of the officers.

DUTIES OF THE PRESIDENT

- Preside at all council meetings
- Develop an agenda for monthly meetings
- Report to all resident meetings on the work of the council
- Appoint, with council consultation, chairpersons and members of standing and other committees
- Preside as chairperson of the nominating and elections committee
- Serve as ex officio member of all other committees
- In the absence of the secretary, appoint a secretary pro tem

DUTIES OF THE SECRETARY

- Record in the official minutes actions taken at council meetings and distribute copies to council members and management
- Act as custodian of council minutes and related notices, communications, and reports
- Act as custodian of the official documents of the council, including the bylaws and rules of procedures
- In the absence of the president, call the meeting to order and preside over the election of a president pro tem

Meetings should be held monthly unless otherwise provided for by the council. A majority of all council members should constitute a quorum. Special meetings can be called with advance notice by the president, at the request of management, or by three members of the council. Written notice should be given stating the business to be conducted, and only such business should be taken up as is stated in the meeting call. Each member is entitled to one vote, and any member may abstain from voting. Motions are passed by a majority vote of those members present and vot-

ing at the meeting. Meetings should be called to order by the president or, in her absence, by the secretary. An agenda should include introduction of guests; reading, correction, and approval of minutes of the previous meeting; reports of the president, secretary, and committees; unfinished business; and new business. *Riddick's Revised Rules of Procedure* can be used to govern council proceedings unless otherwise provided in the bylaws and the standing rules of procedures.

There should be two standing committees: the nominating and elections committee and the employee appreciation fund committee. Other ad hoc committees may be created to address specific issues that may come up from time to time. Some communities establish committees for each department, but the council may expect each committee to report on its activities every month. There is in fact peer pressure to find things to report on, even when the department may be running smoothly. The department head may at times feel scrutinized by residents who may be looking for problems where none exist. Limit the number of ad hoc committees whereever possible.

■ Employee Appreciation Fund

Management in senior living communities usually discourages employees from accepting tips and in fact may have a policy expressly prohibiting the practice. This is necessary in order to discourage employees from favoring some residents. In addition, the potential distribution of these tips would unfairly favor dining room and housekeeping employees. And of course it takes the combined efforts of all employees to bring the service package to life. An employee appreciation fund is normally established by the resident council to provide a vehicle for the distribution of gratuities to all employees. Residents will normally ask management for guidance in determining eligibility in order to ensure fairness.

Although the community can certainly assist residents in administering this fund, it must be clear that this is an undertaking of the residents and is not sponsored by the community. This distinction is important because the Internal Revenue Service (IRS) and the state department of revenue are likely to view any disbursements by the community to employees as compensation requiring the necessary withholding and employer matching taxes. A separate non–interest-bearing account can be established as the employee appreciation fund. The account can be opened using the name and social security number of the executive director as the primary contact. Because this is a non–interest-bearing account, there are no income tax implications or reporting requirements for the account. Residents can then make gifts payable by check to the account. A general notice can be given to the residents outlining the purpose of the fund, giving the contribution deadline date, and describing the basis on which amounts will be distributed, in terms of both eligible employees and the basic allocation method. The money can then be withdrawn and distributed to the eligible employees in cash.

Department heads should not participate in this distribution if they are otherwise compensated by bonus or other performance incentives. The executive director should never participate in this distribution, and only sales staff who are not paid commissions as part of their compensation should be included. Ultimately, it should be left to the residents to decide who are appropriate participants, but it is in the best interest of the residents to recognize those employees who directly serve them. Normally the resident council will collect the funds annually for distribution two weeks prior to year-end holidays. Some communities collect twice a year, with a summer collection as well. Other communities have established a "Christmas club": contributions are made monthly to the fund and then distributed at year end. This is helpful for residents on a budget or those living in a high-cost environment such as an assisted living facility, where it may be difficult to come up with the money at a time of the year when they are buying gifts for relatives.

To ensure fairness, the collected funds should be distributed to the employees based on total hours worked. For example, the amount collected should be divided by the total hours worked during the past 12 months for all eligible employees. To calculate the dollar distribution multiply the per-hour figure by the total hours worked for each employee (to a maximum of 2,080 for a full-time employee). For those employees who work less than full time, their share is then fairly prorated based on their total hours worked. Most communities will require the employee to be employed actively at the time of distribution and for at least three months before being eligible. Normally the resident council will aim to collect $365, or a dollar per day for the preceding year from each resident; other communities may choose a more modest contribution, such as $10 per month. Although some residents may not be able to afford this level of contribution (resident contributions will average about $150 for most communities), all gifts are appreciated by the employees. In one large, affluent continuing care retirement community, the fund accumulated in excess of $140,000; when divided among the 200 employees, this resulted in a distribution of up to $700 per person—a nice holiday bonus. I have even heard of a distribution per employee of $1,200. Normally the funds are distributed in sealed and labeled envelopes in cash. Employees should be reminded by management that this distribution is considered tip income and should be reported to the IRS. Management should be prepared for some employee resignations after fund distribution, as employees planning to leave will wait for this bonus before announcing their departure.

RESIDENTS ON BOARDS

The subject of the participation of residents on governing boards can be a very sensitive one; their voting status can complicate matters even further. Residents will nearly always request representation on governing boards. In some states, resident representation on boards of continuing care retirement communities (CCRCs) is required by law. In addition, there is considerable support among some legislators for giving residents voting status on boards. In a recent survey of directors and officers of Florida CCRCs underwritten and initiated by FORCE Financial Group (an investment banking firm specializing in the financing of CCRC projects), 20 percent of the boards were found to have one or more residents as voting members: 12 percent elect one resident to the board, and 8 percent elect more than one resident to the board. An additional 30 percent of the boards have nonvoting resident members, and 26 percent of boards open their meetings fully or partially to resident attendance. Only 24 percent of the boards do not promote resident attendance or participation.[2] Governing boards of CCRCs are realizing the value of resident participation for the success and acceptance of their policy initiatives. Residents who participate on boards without voting rights will be viewed as "token" representatives by other residents. This can even create animosity between resident representatives and the residents they are elected to represent, for having responsibility without authority can place the resident board representatives in an awkward position. Residents will insist that they be represented by vote to establish formally their position on critical issues, even though they may be ultimately outvoted. This can in turn lead to demands for equal representation. The danger of this situation comes when a conflict of interest arises on initiatives, such as increases in monthly service fees, that may not be well received by the general population but that may be necessary to ensure the financial stability of the project. Nevertheless, boards are increasingly recognizing the rich resources of skill and experience among their residents, which can be tapped to facilitate the problem-solving and long-term planning processes.

■■■■■ RESIDENT SATISFACTION

There are many ways to quantify the residents' support of the management of the community. As with any business, word-of-mouth endorsements by your customers are your best advertisement. Residents will define quality as simply the difference between what they expect and what they get. If their expectations are exceeded (or even just met), they will represent your community as a quality operation. Conversely, if you are unable to meet their expectations, or fail to deliver on your promises, they will not recommend your community to friends and can even become hostile.

New residents will often walk into senior living communities with negative expectations. Those with little prior exposure to these communities will expect them to be restrictive, cold, and institutional. It is important for staff to be trained to recognize the forces that shape resident expectations. Some communities even go so far as to provide sensitivity training in gerontology to equip employees at all levels to understand the aging process and to develop a sensitivity toward the emotional forces at work in their residents.

Exceeding expectations is often simply a matter of doing little things properly. Communities that ensure that all employees are service oriented and empower them to handle small problems for residents as they arise will often exceed the residents' expectations.

The average length of stay in a CCRC is about 12.5 years. During this time the average resident paying a modest $2,000 in monthly service fees represents an asset to the community of approximately $300,000, not including his entrance fee. For an independent living community whose average resident will stay 5.5 years, the same monthly fee represents a $132,000 asset. In this light, the value of rewarding the employee's initiative on the resident's behalf becomes crystal clear to management. To estimate the average length of stay, first calculate the number of move-outs for the year divided by the average number of occupied units to calculate the percentage turnover. Then divide this number into 1 for the average stay in years. In the preceding example, an 18 percent annual turnover will result in an average length of stay of 5.5 years for independent living (8% turnover for the CCRC example).

The characteristics that define high-quality service are personal attention, dependability, consistency, promptness, and employee competence. It is not as critical for residents to always get what they asked for as it is for them to receive a prompt, courteous, and competent response. Boardrooms and executive offices are full of senior managers who are all for signing service proclamations and making speeches reminding "those people down in the trenches" how important residents are, but who cannot seem to find the time to tackle the problem of improving resident satisfaction. Resident satisfaction does not happen simply because you have a beautiful building complemented by a high-quality service package. In fact, the nicer the property, the greater the residents' expectation for service. I have often walked into a luxurious community only to be ignored by the receptionist. The combined effect leaves one with the impression that "something just isn't quite right." Resident satisfaction is an attitude that absolutely requires the commitment by employees at all levels to make the dream a reality. It is the personal touch that brings the whole package to life. Resident satisfaction mirrors employee relations. Developing effective and proactive human resource practices builds an essential foundation for supporting your resident service package (see Chapter 3 for more on developing employees into resident relations assets). If managers want to improve the level of resident satisfaction in their operation, they must first start by looking at the way their employees are treated. Contented employees are better equipped to serve the residents with a positive and cheerful attitude. Conversely, happy residents are easier to take care of and are less demanding, which creates a positive work environment.

A critical component of the service cycle (Figure 5.1) is employee turnover. Long-term employees

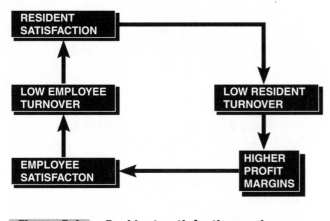

Figure 5.1   Resident satisfaction cycle

Source: Adapted from Leonard A. Schlesinger and James L. Heskett, *Breaking the Cycle of Failure in Services* (New York: Free Press, 1993)

become very aware of the personal needs of the residents. For example, even though Mrs. Cameron orders ice cream for dessert every night, Rose, her server, knows that she is lactose intolerant and serves her low-fat frozen yogurt as a substitute. Housekeeper Micaela knows that she must be extremely careful with the seashell collection of Mr. Crane's deceased wife. This knowledge of the personal needs of the residents cannot be easily replaced when long-term employees become dissatisfied and seek employment elsewhere. When they walk out the door, they take with them your high level of resident satisfaction, which is often rooted in their personal knowledge of the preferences of the residents. The well-intentioned new replacement will, of course, serve Mrs. Cameron ice cream as she requests, thereby causing her extreme discomfort and dissatisfaction. Management must place a premium on the importance of keeping its employees in their jobs and communicate to them their value to the entire operation.

Resident satisfaction is the result of a dynamic, not a static, encounter. The resident evaluates both the process and the outcome and values both. For example, residents will accept a marginal food product temporarily if they receive consistently good service, and vice versa. However perception of a poor product cannot be overcome by a good relationship with the residents—at least not for long. Nor will a good product overcome poor treatment. Fail at both and the residents will become part of the problem by turning off the tap on referrals. The mandate is clear: to create a high level of resident satisfaction necessary to earn resident

endorsements, management must understand and even shape the residents' expectations.

Resident Opinion Surveys

Resident opinion surveys have long been the bellwether of resident satisfaction. The goal of any resident survey is to maximize the response to achieve statistically valid results, to identify any problem areas, and to quantify the residents' response to your management of the service package. Resident surveys can take on many shapes, from a leisure interest survey on admission to specific food preference surveys, exit interviews, marketing perception surveys, and resident satisfaction surveys. I limit the discussion here to resident satisfaction, as the other survey tools are discussed in detail in other chapters. Among the most important factors in conducting a meaningful survey are frequency, design, distribution and collection, interpretation of results, and follow-up.

FREQUENCY

Most communities conduct an annual resident satisfaction survey; however, residents will also respond to a biannual survey if they perceive that there are some problems that need management's attention. Communities who inundate their residents with survey requests may place a burden on the residents, who will become very reluctant to respond. In the end, those who do return the surveys may represent only a small minority of chronic complainers, rather than the views of the resident population as a whole. If management demonstrates that it is acting on resident feedback, residents will be more tolerant than if the survey process simply becomes a routine event or a token attempt by management to convince residents that it is customer oriented and that their opinion "really matters." If the survey results reveal a high level of dissatisfaction in a given department, then an abbreviated follow-up survey of that department may be useful after steps have been taken to correct the problem.

DESIGN

When designing your survey instrument, first decide on what you hope to learn from your residents. Surveys tell management what residents perceive to be the real values of the community. They should be designed to measure the percent satisfaction and dissatisfaction with the community's services and amenities—essentially how well the promise was fulfilled by the delivery. Surveys should also measure how well an organization is functioning internally in terms of how the various departments and functions service each other. Survey instruments will evolve over the life of the community. At first, management may want to issue a more comprehensive survey that evaluates residents' experiences from their initial visit with marketing to their orientation, responsiveness of staff, dining room service, food quality and quantity, frequency and variety of activity programs, condition and cleanliness of apartments and common areas, landscaping and curb appeal of the property, transportation frequency, and communication by, fairness of, and confidence in management. It is also a good idea to ask the residents if they think the staff are treated fairly and are happy in their work. Normally if employees are not happy the residents are among the first to know. Finally, ask the residents if they would be willing to recommend the community to their friends, and if not, why not. In order to guarantee a good return of surveys from the residents, the survey size should be limited. Most residents will fill out a two- or three-page survey; however, if the survey exceeds five pages, your response rate may drop to less than 50 percent.

After the community has reached stabilized occupancy and the expectations of the residents have taken shape, a more abbreviated survey may be appropriate. Ask residents to rate the overall performance of each department as *excellent, good, fair,* or *poor.* The favorable responses can be tabulated from the *excellent* and *good* responses, and the unfavorable opinions from the *fair* and *poor* responses.

The process of designing questions for the survey is a great opportunity to manage the residents' expectations. For example, a question that asks the resident to check the appropriate ending for the statement "The food is delivered promptly to my table: *always, seldom,* or *never*" can imply that it is management's goal always to have food delivered promptly—a standard that may not be realistic, or even expected in fine restaurants among leisurely diners. Rather if it is worded "My meals are normally delivered to my table within a reasonable period of time: yes or no," the statement implies that residents may expect routine operational problems that can delay their meals occasionally, but this is not considered normal. Great care should be taken not to set management up for failure by design-

ing questions that attempt to define a perfect world. It may be financially prohibitive *always* to deliver residents their meals promptly. Aim for realistic targets when designing questions.

DISTRIBUTION AND COLLECTION

Surveys should be professionally copied (at a copy or reprint shop) in double-sided format to make them appear shorter. Be sure to typeset the survey in large print so that it is not a burden for your visually impaired residents to read. The distribution and collection of the survey should be proactively managed to assure an acceptable response. Residents who are dissatisfied and claim to speak on behalf of all the residents will be the first to respond. Others who may feel that everything is fine will normally not bother to fill out and send in the survey unless specifically requested to do so. Although it is important to identify areas of dissatisfaction, surveys with a low response rate can be quite negative. These results may not be representative of the resident opinions as a whole and can at times be very discouraging and adversely affect employee morale. For the survey to be objective, it must represent the opinions of the resident majority. An aggressively managed survey process can yield up to an 80 percent response rate with results that can motivate employees; if the process is left to chance, a 40 percent response is not uncommon. Two surveys should be distributed to apartments that are double occupied to ensure that all residents have the opportunity to comment. Spouses often have differing opinions on community services, and communities that distribute only one survey per apartment run the risk of alienating one spouse or both from participating in the process. It should be emphasized that everyone's opinion is valued.

Management should call a general meeting of the residents to go over the survey instrument and explain the importance of everyone's participation. When asked for our evaluation of something, most of us tap into our short-term memory, and the results of a successful resident event or recent fee increase may positively or negatively influence the results. Distribute the surveys during a neutral time of year when there is not much happening that could lend subjectivity to the questionnaire. It should be stressed that the survey is intended to summarize the residents' opinions over the last year (or whatever period of time has elapsed since the last survey), and residents should be cautioned not simply to evaluate their most recent encounter with each department. Furthermore, residents should be asked to be certain that their surveys objectively represent their personal opinions and not what they may have heard from other residents. Management should also conduct individual floor meetings and select resident wing or floor captains to be responsible for collecting the completed surveys from the residents in their sections. The surveys should be returned in sealed envelopes to the resident floor captains, who are equipped with a check-off list.

Finally, the survey should be reviewed with employees prior to distribution (especially the housekeeping staff) to ensure that they have a good understanding of the survey and its importance. Some communities offer incentives to residents to complete the survey, from a free guest meal to "I've been heard" stickers or buttons. Surveys should be tabulated off-site, either at a corporate headquarters or by a consultant, if for no other reason than to guarantee the participants' complete anonymity and confidentiality. If there is a high rate of negative responses to questions dealing with the degree of openness and trust in management, this same lack of trust will carry through to the sur-

vey data. On the other hand, if there is a high level of resident confidence in and endorsement of on-site management, the residents will want to tell the world about it.

The survey should be distributed along with a cover memo to explain its purpose and its importance to management. The cover memo in Exhibit 5.3 provides an example.

INTERPRETATION OF RESULTS

As mentioned earlier, the response rate to the survey will establish its validity. Response rates of 60 percent or less, while providing some useful information, will do little to offset criticism of a department. Response rates greater than 75 percent truly represent a majority and are statistically valid. The percent response to each question should be tabulated as *excellent, good, fair, or poor,* or whatever the evaluation criteria might be. Try to make the questions consistent from one survey to the next to allow for comparisons that can help identify trends. Changes in resident response from favorable to unfavorable or vice versa may occur for a variety of reasons, including but not limited to survey response percentage, changes in staffing, proactive

---

Exhibit 5.3   Sample Cover Memo for Resident Survey

Dear Resident:

Your happiness and satisfaction are critical to us. I hope that every day our staff is doing everything they can to make your move to our community a rewarding experience. We invite you to take a moment to review how well we are meeting your needs, and we also welcome suggestions for improvement.

Please complete the following questionnaire, seal it in the attached envelope, and return it to your resident representative. Your comments and observations are critical to us and will help shape our services and amenities. In addition, we will be using your responses in part to evaluate our staff at your community. So even if you feel everything is fine, please write "fine" on your survey and send it in so your opinion can be properly recognized. If the survey is difficult for you to read, or if you have a question, ask your housekeeper or any management representative.

We also would like to take this opportunity to thank you for the many referrals you have given us; clearly a fully occupied community is in everyone's best interest.

Thank you for taking the time to share your impressions with us.

Very truly yours,

Benjamin W. Pearce
Senior Vice President of Operations

versus reactive resident council leadership, differences in resident perception of value following a significant monthly fee increase, or a legitimate decline in service or product quality. Resident surveys often directly reflect the popularity of a department head. Department heads who are responsive and well liked by the residents consistently score higher on surveys of this type. However, poor service cannot be overcome by a good relationship with the residents, at least not for long.

The survey results should be tabulated in a spreadsheet format so that an overall score can be determined. An unfavorable change in the residents' opinion of any department that exceeds 10 percent could indicate a problem to be addressed. Management should expect at least a 90 percent overall endorsement when combining the favorable responses. More important, management should carefully evaluate the differences, both positive and negative, from one survey to the next to determine if progress has been made in correcting resident perceptions of previously identified areas of vulnerability. Management should not settle for anything less than 90 percent of the residents indicating a willingness to recommend the community to their friends, for resident endorsements are the cheapest and most effective form of advertising. Communities that routinely receive fewer than 25 percent of their new leads from resident referrals may have serious service issues to address.

Managers of multiple properties can rate their resident satisfaction results comparatively using a Quality Index (QI) system, which indexes individual service area ratings against companywide service ratings. This method enables the company to use the QI to rank the performance of each community against a common norm. It is similar to that used to calculate the consumer price index. All QI scores are based on combined favorable responses: *excellent* plus *good,* or *yes* percentages for the yes/no questions on the survey. For example:

Housekeeping— All communities		Housekeeping— Community A	
Excellent	43.3%	Excellent	47.2%
Good	48.2%	Good	50.9%
TOTAL	91.5%	TOTAL	98.1%

Index score
for Community A = (98.1% / 91.5%) × 100 = 107.2

The average of all *excellent/good* responses is set at a baseline of 100, and the QI scores are measured against this baseline. In this case, the score of 107.2 indicates a level of resident satisfaction with housekeeping in Community A that is considerably above average levels for other operated communities. In general, scores above 100 indicate acceptable performance, whereas scores below 100 show a need for attention. The farther above or below 100, the higher or lower the relative level of resident satisfaction. The long-term objective for the company is to decrease the spread of QI service ratings around the score of 100 for all communities. Using this system, corporate operations managers can easily identify and prioritize problem areas in their portfolios.

FOLLOW-UP

Residents must be convinced that management will act on the results of the survey, or they will not respond in numbers. In addition, if management fails to demonstrate a response to the survey, it may damage its own credibility in the eyes of the residents and their families. Any combined *excellent/good* or *yes* response level less than 85 percent, or any increase in combined unfavorable *fair/poor* or *no* response level greater than 10 percent, should automatically trigger a plan of correction, which should be formulated by the department head and her direct supervisor within 30 days of the tabulation of the survey. This should not be an exercise that simply identifies existing problems with general recommendations that are "ongoing." Department heads should call all their employees together to brainstorm, so that they all can be part of the solution. Plans of correction should describe the area in need of improvement in specific terms, detail a solution, assign a responsible party, and target a completion date. In asking residents for their opinions, you must also earn their confidence that the information they provide will be acted on. Some communities are very reluctant to publish the results of their surveys, citing fears that some specific departmental results may add fuel to arguments by special interest groups and affect employee morale. A survey of any nature will raise the expectations of the population served. When residents give their valuable input, it is with the clear expectation that management fully intends to respond positively, quickly, and thoroughly to the issues and concerns raised. If management is unwilling to commit itself to feeding back survey results to the participants, and to addressing the survey findings as quickly as possible, it is better not to do the survey at all. Conversely, positive results from a resident survey can severely damage the credibility of chronic complainers by providing documentation of the endorsement of the service package by the majority of the residents. Resident survey results can quickly derail the negativity and influence of a vocal minority.

Resident survey results should never be used to discipline a manager, to find an excuse for discharging someone, or to coerce someone into a behavioral change. To do so will cause employees to fear the process rather than receive it as a useful management tool. It is important for management to familiarize supervisors with the impacts of the survey results and to coach them on their potential effect on productivity, profitability, and service. It is up to management to motivate employees to want to deliver good service and equip them to do so, not threaten them if they do not.

Remember: residents define quality as the difference between what they expect and what is consistently delivered to them. With an overall rating of 90 percent satisfaction, management is obviously exceeding their expectations. This level of endorsement is even more impressive when the community can earn the residents' satisfaction while completing its fiscal year under budget in expenses. At this point, the staff's ability to balance these often conflicting objectives consistently is clearly a reflection of their professionalism and commitment to building real value in their operation.

■ RESIDENT HANDBOOKS

A well-written, concise, and thorough resident handbook is instrumental to the operational translation of the service package. In many cases, the resident handbook is also an integral component of the residency agreement and is often considered a legal document. The purpose of the resident handbook is to outline in detail operational procedures for the residents as well as basic information about the community. The handbook provides an opportunity to manage the residents' expectations about the services and amenities the community has to offer. It should include at least the following components: a welcome letter, a list of important telephone numbers, a description of services, general community policies and procedures (including policies regarding use of public areas), emergency and safety information (including security procedures), rules and regulations, other useful information, and a community map and floor plan.

WELCOME LETTER. Written as an introduction to the community by the executive director, the welcome letter should be warm and friendly. It should set the stage by explaining that the community is exemplified by residents who care about each other and actively pursue lives of growth and fulfillment, and that the community is designed to enhance their lifestyle by providing services that promote greater individual well-being. The welcome letter should also define the purpose of the handbook: to provide some basic information about the community's operations and services and the management's expectations of the residents. It should discuss the importance of resident feedback and outline the procedures for offering comments. Finally, it should state the open door policy of the management staff, all of whom are personally committed to balancing the needs and interests of the owner(s) with those of the residents and employees.

IMPORTANT TELEPHONE NUMBERS. Included here should be emergency numbers for police, fire department, ambulance, hospitals, and pharmacies. Telephone numbers for the front desk, executive offices, dining room, marketing department, beauty shop, bank, and other businesses should also be included. Some communities also publish a resident directory that is included in the resident handbook.

SERVICES. A short description of each service should be offered, outlining what residents may expect and what is included in or ancillary to their monthly service fee. Residents have a tendency to coerce management into stretching services. By outlining the limits of each service in advance, management can refer resident inquires back to the community policies as outlined in the resident handbook, allowing for a baseline interpretation of the policies and establishing a consistent response for all employees.

POLICIES AND PROCEDURES. Operational policies and procedures that directly affect the residents, such as those governing apartment changes, billing, deliveries, privately employed personnel, parking, pets, smoking, and tipping, can be detailed in this section. Included here are the routine expectations that management has of the residents and their guests. Describe how residents can maximize the benefits of the services provided and do their part to ensure that things run smoothly in the community.

PUBLIC AREAS. Management should place emphasis on the importance of having common areas where residents can socialize with others and enjoy special activities. The residents should consider these areas as extensions of their apartments and an integral part of their home. Make it clear that these areas are used by all residents and that family members and guests have use of the common areas and amenities only when accompanied by residents. Describe the intent and use of each room along with any associated rules or restrictions. Don't be afraid to ask the residents to maintain the common areas and to leave them as they found them so that all residents may enjoy the amenities of each room.

EMERGENCY AND SAFETY INFORMATION. Provide a detailed description of procedures to be followed in the event of an emergency, along with a description of the community's fire alarm and emergency call system. Each resident should be provided with an evacuation route map to the emergency exit nearest his apartment. It is also a good idea to explain how the fire alarm and sprinkler systems work and to specify the location of the nearest alarm station and fire extinguisher. Inform residents that they will be required to participate in monthly fire drills and evacuation practices. Give specific instructions for procedures to follow in the unlikely event of a fire, along with the fire department emergency number (it may not be 911). Explain the medical emergency procedure and provide the number of an ambulance service, if appropriate.

The procedure for contacting the police department should also be included, along with a description of the community's security measures, key control policies, and visitor access procedures. If the community has an established program to check on each resident daily, such as an "I'm OK" program, it should also detailed here.

RULES AND REGULATIONS. Detailed here should be rules concerning use of residents' apartments, parking, use of the grounds, storage, apartment modifications, locks and keys, and conduct of guests, as well as other liabilities and responsibilities of tenants.

■■■■■ MEDICAL CHALLENGES

According to the Bible, mankind is given threescore years and ten (70 years) within which to grow our spirit on this earth. Modern gerontologists are much more optimistic, estimating life expectancy for an infant boy born in the 1990s to be 71.8 years and for a girl, 78.6 years. The average entry age of seniors in CCRCs today is about 78 years; for congregate communities, about 81.5 years; and for assisted living communities, 82.5 years. Residents who are 80 years old today have significantly exceeded their life expectancy at birth in the 1910s of 50.2 years for men and 53.7 years for women. More than 25 years have been added to the life expectancy of infants in the United States since 1900, largely owing to our improving ability to combat infectious diseases.

As stewards of the elderly living in senior communities, we cannot escape our obligation to assist our residents in facing the inevitable medical challenges that will shape their lives. At this point in their lives, many seniors who inquire about retirement living options may be interested in a supportive living environment where they can have access to care that will enable them to continue to function independently as they grow older. Seniors who continue to live in their home after the loss of their spouses tend to focus on all the things that they cannot do anymore—their limitations. This attitude can lead to chronic depression and despair. The power of the mind to heal the body has been well established in medicine; conversely, seniors who become lonely and depressed can in fact shorten their lives. We are social creatures; we flourish when we are around other people with similar interests and when we have purpose. Time and again I have seen residents, who had moved into senior communities chronically depressed or with extensive medical complications, out on the dance floor after six months of companionship and activity. Herein lies the primary motivator for many employees, who are uniquely empowered to give residents back their lives by bringing out the best in them through others.

In his book *How and Why We Age,* gerontologist Leonard Hayflick differentiates between life expectancy and active, healthy, or functional life expectancy.[3]

Active life expectancy ends when a person's health declines to a point at which she loses independence in matters of daily living and must depend on others for some form of care. Most Americans over the age of 65 are healthy and live normal, productive lives, but with increasing age, health generally deteriorates and the need for care increases. In one study it was found that 45 percent of those over the age of 85 needed help with one or more basic activities of daily life. The quality and longevity of the resident's life can be measurably improved through companionship and preventive care.

Mark Twain said, "Age is a thing of mind over matter—if you don't mind it, it don't matter." For many old people "it don't matter," and apathy or denial of age-related health complications can lead to serious consequences. The best thing that seniors can do to optimize their healthy years is to understand and identify potential common problems while they are still treatable. Residents should be encouraged to contact their primary care physicians to establish a course of preventive checkups and screenings. These can be designed based on health, medical, and family history. The following tests and procedures are based on guidelines recommended by the American Heart Association and the American Cancer Association.

- Immunizations: Flu shots can be helpful to avoid complications brought on by common viruses.
- History: Health history should be taken every two and a half years after age 61 and annually after age 75 for healthy individuals.
- Mammogram: A mammogram is an X ray of the breast that searches for indicators of cancer too small to locate manually. This test is recommended once between the ages of 35 and 40 to get a baseline and then every two years until age 50. Thereafter, an annual test is recommended.
- Stool slide tests: This is an analysis of the stool to search for hidden traces of blood, the appearance of which could signal cancer or some other disorder in the digestive tract. Tests are recommended annually for everyone over 50.
- Urinalysis: The urine is a veritable road map of the workings of many vital organs. This test is recommended annually.
- Blood tests: Blood tests should be taken every two and a half years.

- Pelvic examinations: All healthy women over the age of 40 should have a pelvic exam annually.
- Electrocardiogram (EKG): The American Heart Association recommends a baseline EKG at ages 20, 40, and 60.
- Physical examinations: The American Heart Association recommends an annual physical after the age of 75. The American Cancer Society recommends an annual screening for cancer after the age of 40, especially for cancer of the thyroid, testicles, prostate, ovaries, lymph nodes, and skin.

Many operators also establish proactive programs to identify potential health problems in their resident populations. During weekly meetings of department heads, the agenda should include changes in resident status that have been noticed by the employees during the course of the week. Employees of key departments such as housekeeping should be trained to recognize health changes in their residents and to report them promptly to their supervisors. They should be made aware that residents will have a propensity to conceal their health problems for fear of being asked to transfer to a more supportive environment. Many health problems, when detected early, can be managed by a physician, enabling residents to continue to function independently and live in greater comfort. At the first sign of a change in health status, a resident should be approached for a consultation by the executive director. In extreme cases, it may be appropriate to notify the resident's family members or physician immediately. It is advisable to initiate contact with the family at the first sign of changes in the resident's health status to establish a dialogue concerning physical, physiological, or gerontological issues, keeping them informed and soliciting their support. Working with the family or their support network in turn facilitates cooperation by the resident in dealing with age-related challenges. It may be appropriate to schedule quarterly or semiannual meetings with the family and key department heads to monitor the status of some residents. Never wait until a resident's condition becomes unmanageable before involving the family or physician. These meetings can be a valuable source of information on the level of the resident or the family's satisfaction, health and dietary concerns, and affordability issues. No one likes surprises, particularly if one is forced into a confrontation with a loved one who may be in denial. As with any problem-solving exercise, issues are best dealt with as they arise, with attempts to build consensus early on among all interested parties.

For people over 65, the top three causes of death are heart disease, cancer, and cerebrovascular disease (stroke); they represent the cause of death in about 75 percent of all those who die after age 65. Thus it may be helpful for managers to understand these afflictions and learn to recognize the symptoms of these and other common disorders of the elderly, including incontinence, Alzheimer's disease, and substance abuse.

Heart Disease and Stroke

Cardiovascular disease is the leading cause of death in the United States and other developed countries. Atherosclerosis, a thickening and hardening of the walls of the coronary arteries, is the most common form of heart disease. This condition begins early in life and may in later years result in a heart attack (myocardial infarction), angina, or a stroke (cerebrovascular accident). Symptoms include pain in the chest, shoulder, or jaw lasting more than two minutes. Vomiting and sweating frequently accompany the pain. Patients may also experience a sudden state of confusion or change in mental status, or simply feel breathless. Some people experience small heart attacks that are symptomless and show up only on EKGs. Heart disease can often be prevented with a simple change in diet to reduce cholesterol combined with a regular exercise routine. The American Heart Association has a wealth of educational materials that are easily accessible.[4]

Risk factors of stroke include hypertension, heart disease (including coronary artery disease), previous stroke, smoking, obesity, high cholesterol levels, consumption of large amounts of coffee, cancer, or infection. The incidence of stroke is directly correlated with blood pressure throughout its range: higher blood pressure can force small blood clots to the brain or heart, causing a stroke. Up to 50 percent of all strokes occur in patients with a history of previous strokes or transient ischemic attacks (so-called mini-strokes).

Cancer

Cancer is an insidious disease that can present itself as a tumor (as with colon and breast cancer), as a skin lesion, or as a condition of the blood (such as leukemia). It can be fatal, but in many cases can be cured with early detection. Some gerontologists believe that the increased incidence of cancer with age is the result of an immune system less capable of detecting and destroying cancer cells in the elderly. The "Seven Danger Signals of Cancer" as developed by the American Cancer Society[5] are as follows: (1) a change in bowel or bladder habits; (2) a sore that does not heal; (3) unusual bleeding or discharge; (4) a thickening or lump in the breast or elsewhere; (5) indigestion or difficulty in swallowing; (6) an obvious change in a wart or mole; or (7) a nagging cough or hoarseness.

Treatments for cancer include chemotherapy, radiation, and surgery. Dr. Bernie Siegel's *Love, Medicine and Miracles* explains how the patient's mental state and attitude can significantly influence the progression of the disease.[6] The American Cancer Society hotline is (800) 4-CANCER.

Incontinence

Incontinence is the involuntary loss of control over the elimination of urine, stool, or both. This loss of control can range from a slight leakage, in the case of stress incontinence triggered by a sneeze, to a total loss of control. There are four main causes of the condition: urological (medical problems in the genitourinary tract), neurological (medical problems with the nervous system or brain), psychological (depression, nervousness), and pharmacological (adverse reaction to a medication or medications). Eighty percent of all incontinence is manageable; in extreme cases surgery or catheterization may be necessary. The national organization that serves the needs of incontinent people is Help for Incontinent People (HIP), and their telephone number is (803) 585-8789. Incontinence can be a very embarrassing condition for many residents, and problems that arise must be dealt with promptly by management. Many incontinence problems are caused by something as simple as a urinary tract infection, an overreaction to pain medication, or even lactose intolerance that develops unexpectedly. Teach your employees to look at an incontinence problem as an opportunity to learn more about this unpredictable condition and to be solution oriented. Take the time to find out the cause; often the problem is temporary and quite treatable. Explain to the resident that in many cases the condition is treatable and one should seek a doctor's advice. Follow up with a call to the physician to determine the cause of the problem and to express your concern for the resident's well-being. Adult sanitary products, such as Attends or Depends, can allow residents considerable freedom to move about the community. The housekeeping staff are normally the first to become aware of a potential problem and should be questioned routinely during weekly staff briefings to identify changes in a resident's status.

Alzheimer's Disease

Until recently public awareness of Alzheimer's disease was limited, and there was still a widespread belief that senility was always associated with old age. Scientists now know that the loss of mental capacity during the aging process is not inevitable. Not all older people become senile; however, short-term memory does decline with age. The main complaint of most older people with respect to the aging process is changes in their cognitive ability. The risk of developing Alzheimer's disease increases with advancing age, and after age 65, the percentage of people who suffer from it doubles with every decade of life.[7] The disease, first discovered by German neurologist Alois Alzheimer in 1906, is a debilitating and ultimately fatal illness that destroys mental functions, including memory, speech, comprehension, and awareness. The disease was formerly difficult to diagnose and was positively confirmed only by removing the brain during autopsy, revealing the characteristic nerve tangles and protein deposits (plaques) in the brain. Scientists have now discovered a definitive method to diagnose Alzheimer's using an extremely weak solution of tropicamide, the same drug used by eye doctors in regular exams. Researchers found that in Alzheimer's patients pupils dilated by about 13 percent, versus 4 percent in healthy elderly patients. Gerontologists' estimates that 47 percent of all Americans are afflicted with the disease by the age of 85 may need to be revised as a result of this new discovery.

Alzheimer's normally begins with memory deficit problems or difficulty in performing routine tasks. As the disease progresses, victims can undergo severe personality changes and experience confusion; ultimately the individual can no longer care for himself. At this point, 24-hour supervision becomes necessary, with ultimate transfer to a special care facility. In the early stages of the disease, residents can adjust their lifestyles by making notes to supplement memory loss and establishing routines for taking their medications and locating keys, glasses, dentures, and other

important items. "There are many behaviors which are common to the Alzheimer's victim. Some of these are paranoia, agitation, pacing, fidgeting, verbal abuse, and wandering. While each of these behaviors may be common to the Alzheimer's victim, it is important to realize that they may be manifest in different ways in different patients."[8]

Most important, management and staff must be patient with residents and teach them and their families to accept help. The following suggestions have been offered by Emma Shulman and Gertrude Steinberg.

- Do not ask the patient to do things he cannot do, or try to reason with him or use logic.
- Alzheimer's victims can startle easily; always approach the patient from the front and communicate face to face.
- Exercise the patient frequently and use range-of-motion exercises. Avoid excessive stimuli, such as crowds or loud noises.
- The caregiver should know the patient best or ask a family member about the patient's habits.

"It is normal for the caregiver to react to an Alzheimer's victim by feeling helpless, angry, fearful, upset, or bewildered. The caregiver must always remember they are in control and their reactions will either calm the resident or create bigger problems. It is important to realize that the resident may not be fully aware of his actions and the problem behavior may not necessarily have any meaning. It is critical for the caregiver to react with warmth and tenderness."[9]

The only drug approved by the Food and Drug Administration for the treatment of Alzheimer's disease, tacrine, is manufactured by Warner-Lambert and marketed under the name of Cognex. The drug comes with the disclaimer "Cognex is not a cure for Alzheimer's disease. Even in those people who are at first helped by Cognex, the drug's positive effects are likely to lessen as the disease itself gets worse." Another promising drug that is currently in the trial stage is called Galantamine. A variety of evidence suggests that degeneration of cholinergic neurons may contribute to the cognitive impairments experienced by Alzheimer's victims. These impairments can be slowed or reversed by administration of acetylcholinesterase inhibitors.[10] Galantamine is a reversible cholinesterase inhibitor that can be isolated from a number of different plant sources, including daffodil bulbs, and initial studies indicate that Galantamine can improve learning and memory performance. The current clinical trials and research are being sponsored by the Janssen Research Foundation in Titusville, New Jersey.

Be cautious about labeling. The term "senility" is not a medical diagnosis but has come to be used somewhat indiscriminately to cover a variety of symptoms and behaviors, including forgetfulness, confusion, lack of responsiveness, and depression. Many of these symptoms can be brought on by reversible causes, such as malnutrition, anxiety, alcoholism, or adverse reaction to multiple medications.[11] The Alzheimer's Disease and Related Disorders Association (ADRDA) is available to assist families and victims with educational materials and advice for the victim and caregiver alike.[12]

■ Substance Abuse

Too often we equate the problems of alcoholism and chemical dependency with America's youth. The reality is that these problems can occur in populations of any age or economic background. Alcohol dependency among elderly people living in retirement communities is a growing concern. The number of elderly persons who abuse alcohol in the United States is estimated at 4 million. Community-based cross-sectional studies generally define two patterns of use: abstention and daily use. In a review of these studies, abstention ranged from 31 to 58 percent, and daily drinking ranged from 10 to 22 percent in samples of older patients. The most consistent findings of cross-sectional and longitudinal studies are quite revealing[13]:

■ Elderly men drink larger amounts of alcohol and drink more often than elderly women.

■ No definitive relationship exists between ethnic origin and alcohol use.

■ Lower-income elderly persons consume less alcohol than those at higher income levels.

■ Abstainers tend to remain abstinent; alcohol consumption by light drinkers tends to remain stable with age.

■ About one-third to one-half of elderly alcohol abusers experience the onset of problem drinking late in life.

■ Elderly people generally respond better to treatment and stay with treatment programs longer than do younger people.

Alcohol tolerance decreases significantly with age. This lower tolerance is attributed to a combination of factors. As the body ages, there is a reduction in lean body mass and a decrease in the percent of body water, which results in higher blood alcohol concentrations for a given amount of alcohol. In addition, there can be a decrease in the oxidation or metabolism of some medications and alcohol due to a decrease in blood flow and functioning of the liver. Alcohol affects some organ systems in the body preferentially. The nervous, cardiovascular, and gastrointestinal systems all have reduced functional reserves in the elderly, and consequently the elderly alcohol abuser may be at a higher risk of developing clinical illnesses of these organ systems.[14]

A strong correlation also exists between alcohol abuse and depression in the elderly alcohol abuser. Alcohol induces depression by direct action on the central nervous system. The elderly may further self-medicate this depression with more alcohol. When alcohol abuse and depression coincide, the resident is at greater risk for suicide.

Symptoms of alcohol abuse are often misinterpreted as dementia. In the elderly, alcohol abuse and dementia may be difficult to differentiate because frequently the symptom in both of these disorders is a slow, progressive loss of memory. Some common symptoms that may indicate alcohol abuse include a history of repeated falls, forgetfulness, depression, gastritis, confusion, hypertension, and malnutrition. Alcohol abuse can often be precipitated by stress factors, such as the death of a spouse or significant other; recent diagnosis of a significant illness; a significant downward economic shift; retirement; significant loss of memory, vision, or hearing; or social isolation.[15] The combination of severe stresses associated with these conditions with the use of prescription and nonprescription drugs can have potentially disastrous results.

With early detection and treatment, many late-onset abusers can be put back on track. The treatment of alcohol abuse and chemical dependency goes through three stages: denial breach, detoxification, and rehabilitation. The breaching of denial is more easily accomplished in the elderly than in younger populations. Detoxification is also easier to carry out in the elderly, because they do not need to drink as much as the young to experience the same effects. Disulfiram

(Antabuse) is a drug used to maintain sobriety while a person undergoes treatment. If taken as prescribed, it produces highly unpleasant symptoms—including pounding of the heart, nausea, vomiting, and shortness of breath—whenever a person drinks. Many physicians are reluctant to recommend this medication to older alcoholics for fear that their coexisting medical problems might increase the risk associated with the drug. Alcohol rehabilitation programs focus primarily on education, outreach to the family, group counseling aimed at helping improve alcohol-free day-to-day functioning, vocational training, and attendance at Alcoholics Anonymous (AA) meetings. The programs are usually offered as a two- to four-week inpatient or outpatient session, which is almost always followed by six to twelve months of continuing therapy at decreasing intensity. Interestingly, approximately one-third of all AA members are over age 50.

The National Institute on Aging publishes a *Resource Directory for Older People,* an excellent summary of the many active senior advocacy groups operating in this country.[16] The directory lists the various resources in alphabetical order along with short descriptions of their services. The toll-free publication number is (800) 222-2225.

◼◼ MEDICATIONS

The incidence of chronic disease conditions and other health-related complications increases with age. The conditions that occur in the older adult can range from minor to severe and result in varying degrees of inconvenience or disability. Prescription medications, nonprescription medications, and non-drug items are all used to resolve or manage these problems; many disease states are managed by one or more prescription or nonprescription medications to combat concurrent problems. Nonprescription medications account for approximately one-third of all expenditures for medications by the elderly because they are generally less expensive and more easily accessible.

A significant problem in the elderly is the potential psychological and physical hazards associated with the array of medications they may be taking. Some residents have been known to share their medications with other residents who have complained of similar symptoms. Many residents will be routinely taking as many as six or eight nonprescription medications in addition to those prescribed by their physicians. Although most pharmacies screen prescription requests for incompatibility, many do not, and doctors may be unaware of the use of nonprescription drugs.[17] (See also the section on "Polypharmacy" in Chapter 17.) Some residents will, in fact, change physicians if they do not like their doctor's diagnosis or prescription. In one case, an elderly resident who was exhibiting inappropriate behavior in the community was ultimately found to be taking some 44 different medications from three separate pharmacies! Upon medical evaluation by the community's medical director, several of the medications were found to be chemically incompatible, with harmful side effects, including violent mood swings. The following medications can be a "red flag" for current and future health complications.

BARBITURATES (Nembutal, phenobarbital, seconal). These medications may be used to manage convulsive disorders. They are no longer used with great frequency, but some older people still have doctors who prescribe these drugs for sleep. Serious problems with dependency and their continued use may lead to behavior that can be disruptive. These medications can contribute to morning "hangover" effects that leave the resident feeling "dopey" and can lead to falls.

ANTIDEPRESSANTS—SEVERE DEPRESSION (Marplan, Nardil, Parnate). These medications are typically used for cases of severe depression when other agents have not been effective and are more prevalent among the "young elderly." Residents with severe depression may pose management challenges and have difficulty assimilating into the community. If not monitored carefully and taken correctly, these drugs can have serious hypertensive side effects. Residents on these drugs will have many dietary restrictions as a result of serious food-drug interactions. Lithium bicarbonate is used to moderate peaks and valleys for manic depressive states.

ANTIDEPRESSANTS—MODERATE DEPRESSION (Desyrel, Elavil, Norpramin, Prozac, Sinequan). These medications are typically used for cases of moderate depression and may also help the anxiety that accompanies depressed states. It may be useful to determine the resident's behavior before the medication was started to anticipate behaviors that may be disruptive if the resident becomes noncompliant with the drug regimen.

TRANQUILIZERS—MAJOR (Haldol, Mellaril, Navane, Prolixin, Stelazine, Thorazine). These medications are used to treat psychoses and severe anxiety and for sedation. Behavior problems, such as confusion, delirium, short-term memory problems, and disorientation, may occur. Neuromuscular side effects can contribute to falls and are common in elderly patients who use these drugs.

TRANQUILIZERS—MINOR (Ativan, Buspare, Librium, Serax, Tranxene, Valium). These medications are given for moderate anxiety and nervousness. Prolonged use may cause dependency, confusion, and impaired attention.

ANTICONVULSANTS (Clonopin, Depakene, Diamox, Dilantin, phenobarbital, Tegretol). These medications are given for seizure disorders. Noncompliance may trigger seizures, resulting in falls and other accidents.

CEREBRAL VASODILATOR (Hydergine). This medication is given for confusion arising from dementia. It is usually started early in the condition, when the confusion may not be as obvious. Disruptive behavior may arise as the condition progresses.

SPASMOLYTICS (Daricon, Ditropan, Urispas). These medications are given to control urinary incontinence. The drugs decrease spasms in the bladder and increase its ability to hold urine. Side effects include severe memory impairment, blurred vision, and constipation. It may be important to determine if the resident is psychologically stable and independent of the use of other external control measures.

This is by no means a complete list, but it does provide an effective illustration of the potential side effects of many medications commonly used by older adults. In addition to the *Physician's Desk Reference*,[18] there is an excellent reference book entitled *Worst Pills, Best Pills*. This book, published by the Public Citizen Health Research Group, explains the risks and benefits of 287 of the drugs most commonly used by older adults; it is intended to reduce the amount of drug-induced disease and increase the likelihood of benefiting from appropriate drug therapy.[19]

■■■■ WELLNESS PROGRAMS

It is a good idea to set up a wellness clinic where residents can go to have their vital signs and weights checked on a regular basis by a qualified registered nurse or licensed practical nurse. During weekly or bimonthly sessions, the nurse can quickly identify potential health risks and provide counseling. Sessions such as these also help the resident become more comfortable with the natural aging process. If a manager suspects that a health problem may be arising for a resident, she can consult with the nurse and perhaps recommend, through the resident's personal physician, that an evaluation be conducted (with the resident's permission). A resident who is in denial or refuses to cooperate with an evaluation leaves management with limited options. It is important to emphasize the issue of safety and outline to the resident and his family the risks involved in continued residency. Physicians are normally trusted and respected by the elderly and can play an important role in influencing the reluctant resident. Management may request that the family or physician attempt to influence the resident; request that the resident or family employ the services of a licensed home health agency; request transfer to a more appropriate level of care; or give the resident notice to vacate per the conditions of his residency agreement. In extreme cases, management may wish to notify the local or state department of adult protective services to report an inappropriate and dangerous condition. The Fair Housing Amendments Act of 1988 allows residents to remain in their apartments as long as they can afford to finance their additional care requirements. Most residents will agree to management's recommendations if they are properly prepared in advance to understand their options. For residents living in licensed communities, regulations are quite clear on the limits to the level of care that can be provided in each setting. Some residents may qualify for home health services provided under Part B Medicare (see Chapter 18).

There is no evidence to support the theory that exercise will promote longevity. However, exercise combined with a healthy diet will significantly reduce or even eliminate the occurrence of cardiovascular disease. Seniors who regularly exercise will generally feel better and remain stronger than their sedentary counterparts. Residents who are healthier are normally easier to deal with and better balanced emotionally. Encourage residents to exercise regularly by setting up walking programs and water or low-impact aerobics. Gerontologists agree that the people who generally live the longest are those who are physically, mentally, and emotionally active.

Proactively manage the perceptions of your residents and prospects concerning the use of supportive devices; do not allow them to set your admission standards. Not all people who use wheelchairs are unhealthy; the law clearly protects their rights to be treated equally, and rightfully so. The same principle applies to walkers. Explain to prospects that walkers are simply a supportive device to enable people who may be experiencing problems with their mobility to get back on their feet. Point out that the device does not define the person but is simply a tool designed to allow independence, not promote dependence. It should be management's philosophy to encourage residents to use supportive devices as a rehabilitation tool with the ultimate goal of abandoning the devices as they recover. Seniors do not like to be confronted with supportive devices because of their association with the stereotypical nursing home resident. Do not allow your residents to become blinded by this misperception.

Many communities will be approached by residents with requests to allow the use of motorized carts. Many of these carts are capable of speeds of up to 12 miles per hour and will be driven by people who would not normally qualify for a driver's license. Although the courts have not ruled specifically against the use of these carts within retirement communities, they are sensitive to the safety hazards they may pose to deaf, blind, and other disabled residents. In addition, these carts can cause considerable damage to building fixtures and furnishings when operated using the typical "bump and go" method. Carts parked in the corridors can also pose a significant obstruction to evacuation in case of an emergency. Operators who do allow the use of these carts within the walls of their communities are well advised to establish reasonable restrictions by imposing speed limits, requiring the use of an audible device while going around corners and backing up, and prohibiting elevator use during the evening meal "rush hour." For those communities that have outdoor pathways and grounds, caution residents that these carts may become unstable on hillsides and are prone to tipping over. (This happened to a resident in a cart playing ball with her dog: as she went to retrieve the ball from near a lake, the cart overturned, pinning her underwater. Fortunately for her, an alert maintenance man managed to free her and pull her to safety in time.)

NOTES

1. R. L. Desatnick, *Managing to Keep the Customer* (San Francisco: Jossey-Bass, 1987).
2. FORCE Financial Group, 111 Riverside Avenue, Suite 320, Jacksonville, FL 32202.
3. L. Hayflick, *How and Why We Age* (New York: Ballantine Books, 1994).
4. The American Heart Association can be reached at (214) 373-6300.
5. Reprinted by permission of the American Cancer Society.
6. B. S. Siegel, *Love, Medicine and Miracles: Lessons Learned about Self-Healing from a Surgeon's Experience with Exceptional Patients* (New York: HarperCollins, 1990).
7. National Institute on Aging, National Institutes of Health, "Progress Report on Alzheimer's Disease" (Silver Spring, Md.: NIA/NIH, 1995).
8. N. M. Willingham, "Understanding Alzheimer's," *Spectrum* 5(11) (Nov. 1991): 30.
9. "Progress Report on Alzheimer's Disease," p. 2.
10. J. E. Sweeney, C. F. Hohmann, T. H. Moran, and J. T. Coyle, "A Long-Acting Cholinesterase Inhibitor Reverses Spatial Memory Deficits," *Pharmacology and Behaviour* 31 (1988): 141–47.
11. R. N. Butler, *Why Survive? Being Old in America* (New York: Harper & Row, 1975).
12. The Alzheimer's Disease and Related Disorders Association can be reached at (800) 621-0379. The Alzheimer's Disease Education and Referral Center provides excellent resource materials; call (800) 438-4380 or visit their Web site at http://www.alzheimers.org/adear.
13. J. G. Liberto, D. W. Oslin, and P. E. Ruskin, "Alcoholism in Older Persons: A Review of the Literature," *Hospital and Community Psychiatry* 43(10) (Oct. 1992): 975.
14. R. Jain and J. McGinness, "Neuropsychiatric Aspects of Alcohol Abuse in the Elderly," *Geriatric Medicine Today* 9(7) (July 1990): 60.
15. Ibid., p. 62.
16. *Resource Directory for Older People* (Bethesda, Md.: National Institute on Aging, 1993).
17. W. Simonson, *Medications and the Elderly: A Guide for Promoting Proper Use* (Rockville, Md.: Aspen, 1984).
18. *Physician's Desk Reference,* published annually by Medical Economics Data.
19. S. M. Wolfe, L. Fugate, E. P. Hulstrand, et al. *Worst Pills, Best Pills* (Washington, D.C.: Public Citizen Health Research Group, 1988).

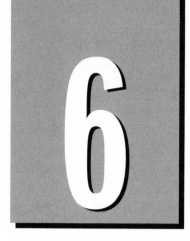

6 Transportation

The transportation department is the residents' conduit to the outside world. For those who no longer have the ability to drive, the scheduled bus and car transportation represents their only means to do their grocery shopping, visit their physician, run errands, and take other routine trips. Occasionally, family members can augment this function, but operators should not count on them for relief.

There are a number of important considerations when organizing a transportation department. First and foremost should be the determination of the extent of transportation that will be included in the monthly service fee and what level of additional services should be billed to residents. Residents will expect routine transportation for shopping, health care needs, visits to the grocery store, attending religious services, and going on tours or trips. Much of this transportation can be handled in groups on the community's bus or vans. A typical schedule might include a run to doctors' offices on Mondays, a visit to downtown on Tuesday, an outing on Wednesday, a run to the grocery store on Thursday, routine servicing on Friday, use on Saturday for lunch out, and religious services on Sunday. This information is best disseminated to the residents using a *Schedule of Transportation Services* that lists the normal transportation schedule and states transportation policies and any additional charges.

It may be best to designate specific drop-off and pick-up points along with their corresponding scheduled times. This policy serves two purposes: it motivates the residents to be at the pick-up point at the appointed time or run the risk of having to take a cab back to the property; and it allows the driver to refuse special requests for alternate drop-off locations that are out of the way and may jeopardize making the pick-up appointment. In addition, between drop-off and pick-up times, the driver can return to the property and perform other duties such as delivering parcels to residents' apartments or doing routine maintenance on the vehicle. There is a good argument against the driver remaining with the residents: under some circumstances, the community could be held responsible and perhaps liable for anything that may happen to a resident while he is under the driver's supervision. It is better to leave the residents alone to do their business and let them exercise their independence.

EQUIPMENT

When determining the type of vehicle to purchase, the comfort of the passengers should be the first concern. Larger van manufacturers can custom build a van to meet the needs of a special population. Seats should be firm with proper lumbar support. Resist the temptation to include armrests, as residents will catch their bags and parcels on them. Residents will frequently complain about the ride and comfort of the van. Larger 26-passenger vans that have three axles and adjustable air suspension are much more comfortable than two-axle vans. In addition, the larger van may be easier to equip with a storage area for groceries and wheelchair accommodations. Seniors are very sensitive to temperature extremes, so be sure to consult the manufacturer on the appropriate climate control devices as well as the size of motor that will be necessary to support this equipment. Other considerations when considering the purchase of a new van should include an analysis of the intended usage and any potential physical barriers. The distances traveled routinely to and from the community, terrain, street width, parking availability, overhead clearance for the front entrance, and service availability will all be very important factors in making the final decision.

The Americans with Disabilities Act may require operators to make the "reasonable accommodation" of a wheelchair lift for communities with disabled residents. Although this may be an expensive option, it can also provide the residents a great convenience. For safety reasons, the driver should always accompany the resident on the lift as it is being raised or lowered. Never leave a resident alone on the lift platform, as the vehicle may not be completely level and, if the resident were to release the wheelchair brakes, she could possibly roll off the platform to the ground. It is also not advisable to transport residents in Amigo or motorized carts in the van. The wheelchair tie-downs are not designed to handle the weight of these heavy carts, and they could possibly break loose in an accident, with potentially serious consequences to the other passengers. There are two basic locations in which to install the wheelchair lift—rear-load and front- or side-load. The rear-load location is very convenient for the driver and allows the ambulatory residents to self-load from the front while the driver assists other residents with the lift platform at the back. The lift can also be used to transport heavy materials and supplies when it is not being used to carry residents. The front- or side-load configuration also has advantages. First and foremost, disabled residents can sit up front and communicate with the driver and fellow passengers, rather than feel like second-class citizens forced "to the back of the bus" because of their disability. In addition, when the wheelchair areas are vacant, the tie-downs normally are recessed and residents can store their groceries and parcels in this location rather than being forced to wrestle them back to their seats, a situation that limits the occupancy of the van because of the lack of suitable storage space.

In addition to multipassenger vans, larger communities also have a luxury sedan to provide more customized transportation needs. At the start of a new community's operations, it may be possible to structure the transportation program such that the sedan is used solely for transportation services that are billed to the residents. Not only does this arrangement generate additional revenue for the project, it also discourages the overbooking of the vehicle. For existing operations, it is best to set up a *free zone* around the property, usually five to six miles. Trips beyond this zone can be charged by the trip, or preferably by the hour. Drivers should be discouraged from waiting for the resident at an appointment; if it is possible to wait, the resident should be charged for the wait time as well. Drivers must be directed to hold to their schedules and not get into the habit of accommodating special requests—one resident's special request could result in another's inconvenience. There are few things that residents dislike more than being delayed at a pick-up spot or missing an appointment, especially if the problem is caused by another resident.

██████ MANAGEMENT

When opening a new project it is advisable to provide only limited automobile service. As the community fills, residents who were among the first to move in may have become spoiled by having a car to themselves and will find it intolerable to be forced to share the sedan with newcomers. As the community fills, residents can be informed that, should more than one resident be going out in the same direction or within the same time period, they may be asked to carpool and will be riding with a fellow resident or residents. Carpooling should be at the discretion of management.

For best results, the residents should be advised to schedule their transportation needs as much in advance as possible, to allow the drivers some flexibility in scheduling. At times, situations arise in which residents may have last-minute needs for transportation. Unfortunately, the driver may not be able to accommodate them owing to previously booked appointments. To place a request for transportation, residents should contact the concierge. They should be prepared to give the following information: the date and time of their appointment; the name and address of the doctor or dentist (including suite number, if applicable) or destination, and the telephone number; and their name and telephone number. The concierge will relay the transportation request to the driver, who will then call the resident (or put a note in her in-house mail slot) to confirm the availability of transportation at that time. It is important to advise the resident that leaving a transportation request with the concierge is not sufficient—it must be confirmed by the driver, preferably on the same day it was received. To ensure fairness, transportation requests should not be accepted more than thirty days in advance. It is also advisable for residents to reconfirm appointments with their doctors' offices the day before. Should their plans change, they should leave a message for the driver with the concierge. When the appointments are completed, residents should call the concierge and ask to be picked up by the driver. In some cases, residents may have to wait at their destination before they can be picked up.

To avoid costly overtime, be sure to set up a quitting time each day that dictates when the driver must return the vehicle to the community, such as no later than 5:00 P.M. each day. Therefore, if residents schedule a doctor's appointment late in the day and the driver will not be able to pick them up and return to the community by 5:00 P.M., they must be prepared to arrange for their own return transportation. If residents wish the driver to pick them up after 5:00 P.M., and the driver is able to do so, an additional charge should be billed.

Except for scheduled group trips, planned by the program director, driver service should be scheduled each day of the week depending on the extent of the department's budget. It is rarely necessary to schedule transportation eight hours per day, seven days per week, unless it can be billed to the residents. Many communities limit transportation services to six days a week with the seventh day reserved for servicing the vehicle. The amount of scheduled service will, of course, depend on the community's size and budget. Abbreviated schedules can be offered during holidays and inclement weather.

It is vital to ensure that all vehicles be maintained in safe working order and have all the appropriate safety equipment on board, including distress signals, a fire extinguisher, and a first aid kit. They should be managed as a fleet, with regularly scheduled routine maintenance performed on a tickler basis based on mileage and hours of service. Although major vehicle servicing may require the services of professionals, the lead

driver should be responsible for routine maintenance in accordance with the vehicles' owner manuals. Services such as topping off fluid levels, changing the oil and wiper blades, checking tire pressure, doing paint touch-ups, and replacing burned-out lights and fuses can easily be scheduled and handled by the driver. Yet, even with the best preventive maintenance program in place, community vehicles have a habit of breaking down at the most inconvenient time. I well remember being called at the corporate office in the Midwest by a resident on the car phone of our stalled vehicle on the George Washington Bridge in New York City, during a summer heat wave, to be offered explicit advice on vehicle maintenance procedures—five years later, I still had not heard the end of it. As most community vehicles are conspicuously marked with the project's name and logo, they are a public reflection of the property's standards, and it is important that they be cleaned and washed weekly. In addition, any scratches and scrapes, however minor, should be repaired immediately, to keep the vehicle looking new. A daily checklist, such as those used by car rental agencies to document deficiencies in appearance or performance, should also be developed.

All transportation employees' driving records and licenses should be verified at least annually in written form with the state, in accordance with Occupational Safety and Health Act (1970) rules, and a copy of each employee's license should be kept on file. All drivers should know how to handle an accident or emergency situation; these can occur with surprising regularity. Proper reporting procedures should be kept with each vehicle at all times, along with insurance records and the vehicle's registration.

Resist a resident's preference to be transported to the hospital in the community's vehicle. The driver cannot perform emergency care in the event of a sudden change in the resident's condition. A subsequent inquiry may find the community negligent or guilty of exercising poor judgment in making the transfer decision, even if it was made at the resident's request. Personal staff vehicles should never be used to transport residents. The community's insurance may not provide coverage in the event of an accident, and there is no guarantee as to the mechanical soundness of the employee's vehicle.

Residents should always be assisted into and out of all vehicles and given assistance with their parcels when required. Always park and lock the vehicle when assisting residents into the doctor's office or other areas; I once had a sedan stolen (along with an entire trunkload of dining room linen returning from an outside laundry contractor) on such an occasion. The driver left the car at the curb with the keys in the ignition and the motor running. Fortunately, insurance companies will, in may cases, even insure you against your own stupidity.

The driver should schedule some time after the grocery and shopping runs to deliver residents' packages to their rooms. In addition, during slow times the driver should be available to assist the activity department in the set-up and take-down of events and special functions.

▇▇▇▇ STAFFING

Staffing the department will obviously depend on the resident population. To protect against absenteeism and to maximize flexibility, several other employees should be licensed and trained to operate the vehicles, including the activity director and other management personnel. In addition, it is a good idea to have one or two on-call drivers on the payroll to fill in as needed. Except for prearranged group trips, planned by the program director, driver service should be available on a scheduled basis. Exhibit 6.1 is an example of a transportation schedule for a 200-unit community that offers service hours to accommodate most residents' needs.

This translates to about 18 minutes per week per resident for 200 units. The amount and type of transportation services will depend to a large extent on the profile of the residents. The more active the population, the more transportation they will require; however, properties that have a high proportion of assisted living residents may find it necessary to make more frequent runs to doctors' offices. Once residents transfer

to skilled nursing, the services are mostly self-contained and doctors visit them. A good rule of thumb is to schedule about 15–20 minutes of transportation time per week per unit, or more if there are a large number of double occupants or a high percentage of frail residents who may require frequent doctor's visits. Some economies of scale may be achieved in larger communities. For a 150-unit community, to provide minimum transportation service seven days a week will require 1.4 FTE (full-time employees) or 56 hours, which translates to about 22 minutes per unit per week. A 225-unit project that requires the same transportation schedule translates to 15 hours per resident per week, and such a program is still within acceptable limits. Supplemental transportation can be scheduled using the community sedan on a charge-per-trip basis.

▇▇▇▇ OTHER TRANSPORTATION RESOURCES

Most communities will provide supplemental transportation services free or for a modest fee using a van service specializing in the transportation of seniors or those with handicaps. Many taxi services offer senior discounts. In larger cities, the local bus transportation agency usually offers special services for seniors as well.

Section 16 of the Urban Mass Transportation Act of 1964 as amended outlines a program that provides assistance in meeting the transportation needs of the elderly or physically challenged persons where public transportation services are unavailable, insufficient, or inappropriate. Three categories of applicants are eligible for Section 16 funds: (1) private nonprofit organizations, determined by the secretary of the treasury to be organizations described by 26 U.S.C. Section 501(c) as exempt from taxation or that have been determined by state law to be nonprofit; (2) public bodies that certify to the state department of transportation that no nonprofit corporations or associations are readily available in the area to provide the service; and

---

Exhibit 6.1	**Typical Transportation Schedule**		
Monday through Friday from	8:30 A.M. to 5:00 P.M.	—8.5 hours/day 5 days/week	= 42.5 hours
Friday nights	from 7:00 P.M. to 11:00 P.M.	—4 hours/day 1 day/week	= 4 hours
Saturday	from 10:00 A.M. to 5:00 P.M.	—7 hours/day 1 day/week	= 7 hours
Sunday	from 9:00 A.M. to 5:00 P.M.	—8 hours/day 1 day/week	= 8 hours
		Total hours/week	= 61.5 or 1.54 FTE

(3) public bodies approved by the state to coordinate services for elderly persons and persons with disabilities. These funds may be used to acquire transportation vehicles for these purposes. However, vehicles acquired by private nonprofit agencies may be leased to private for-profit entities where services could not otherwise be provided and where such arrangements result in more efficient and effective services for elderly or disabled persons. For-profit organizations can, in fact, coordinate their transportation needs with those of nonprofit agencies receiving these grant monies; this possibility should be investigated in communities where transportation constraints have become an issue with the residents. Interested parties should contact their state department of transportation to obtain more details and the names of plan participants.

Activities and Enrichment

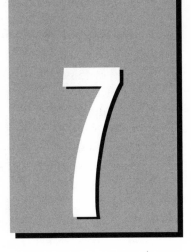

For many seniors, seeking information about an "independent" retirement community is in fact the first step toward declaring their own *dependence*. Many inquiries and subsequent admissions to retirement communities are triggered by events in the lives of the seniors involved. Seniors tend to investigate lifestyle changes as a result of some type of loss in their lives: loss of a spouse, of driving ability, or of ability to care for themselves without help. It is human nature to mourn these losses and through this process reevaluate one's life. One tends to compare actual accomplishments and position in life to one's mental image of what one expected to be like at this stage. At forty, when one comes to the conclusion that one's life is not meeting expectations, there is ample time to adjust priorities and get back on track. At eighty, however, the opportunities for change become more limited. John Barrymore Sr. once said, "A man is never old till regrets take the place of dreams." Research into the attitudes and behavior of seniors suggests that anxieties related to future adverse health conditions are less important than fears about the loss of opportunities to be what they wanted to be.[1] Old age is the time in life when one's physical world may be perceived as continually shrinking. Many face this time and the bereavement process alone as they reevaluate their lives and are confronted with their own mortality. There is a tendency among seniors to focus on their limitations and all of the obstacles that aging presents. When sad-

ness turns to depression, they are headed for trouble.

Much of the stress of this process becomes internalized, and thus seniors may be very vulnerable to depression. Ample research demonstrates the mind's capacity to influence a person's health, both positively and negatively. If left unchecked, depression and despair can inhibit recovery from illness and lead to hopelessness and premature death. Researcher Ken Wells, in the landmark Rand study at the University of California, Los Angeles, found that 50 percent of all depressed people are over 65. Wells studied depressed versus nondepressed people and found that depressed elderly patients used four times the amount of health care dollars used by nondepressed seniors and had a 58 percent greater mortality rate within the first year of admittance to a skilled nursing facility than their nondepressed counterparts.[2] For example, depressed people tend to lack motivation to get up and move about. This inactivity makes them susceptible to urinary tract infections and pneumonia, which if left untreated can lead to kidney failure and death.

Reluctant admission to a retirement community is for many seniors yet another reminder of their inability to live at home independently. Americans of this age group, who struggled through the depression years to achieve the American dream of home ownership, derive much of their identity from their living environment. It is indeed a challenge to give up a home in which one has lived for many years, to learn to identify with one's new retirement "home," and to function in a communal environment.

For a community's enrichment and activity program to be effective, it must be sensitive to the emotional forces that motivate people in this age group. The program must be designed to redirect their focus away from their limitations and toward productive educational and social activities with a positive emphasis that will enhance the quality of life.

Today's senior apartments are full of activity. Residents are attending college courses, playing golf, traveling, and remaining active in service organizations in the community. Variety and respect for individual preference are key elements in a successful recreational activities program. Leisure interests are lifelong habits that each person develops. These interests continue into later life, even after one has entered a retirement community.

A community's life enrichment or activity/recreation director is instrumental in maintaining the satisfaction of residents. The activity department should provide residents the opportunity to maintain a balanced and involved leisure lifestyle. To achieve this, the program should include activities that provide potential for growth, educational opportunities, physical activity and exercise, social programs, creative expression, and travel networks. In addition, the activity department may be a bridge to the community via intergenerational programs with children, fund-raising, and the formation of active residents' councils. The list is endless and may be highly individualized based on the leisure interest survey conducted at move-in and the creativity of the program director.

Each retirement community should have its own activity identity—what residents like to do and like to see: what's important to them. This personality becomes the community and is reflected in the appearance of the newsletter, the calendar, and even the holiday decor in common areas. The same holds true for assisted living communities and skilled nursing homes.

With the OBRA (Omnibus Budget Reconciliation Act) guidelines, HCFA (Health Care Financing Administration), and in some cases JCAHO (Joint Commission on Accreditation for Hospitals Organization) and CARF (Certification Administration for Rehabilitation Facilities), the recreational activity programs of skilled nursing units are being scruti-

nized more than ever. This trend can be expected to proceed down the continuum of care as regulators look to assisted living communities as a more cost-effective setting in which to deliver care. The old standby of the "4 Bs"—birthdays, Bible, bridge, and bingo—as the basis for programming activities falls short in this heavily regulated part of the continuing care retirement community industry. For this reason, the position of activity director must be filled by a qualified recreation professional.

▪ STAFFING

For continuing care retirement communities (CCRC), it is best to hire an activity director who is a certified therapeutic recreation specialist (CTRS). This professional not only has a bachelor's degree in recreation administration and activity programming for special populations, but is also nationally certified by the National Council for Therapeutic Recreation Certification (NCTRC). Communities with assisted living facilities and skilled nursing services may eliminate the need for outside activity consultants at substantial savings. Regulations concerning activity consulting vary from state to state; however, many states have specifically named therapeutic recreation specialists as qualified candidates for the position of activity director. The CTRS is trained to perform activity assessments, programming, planning, documentation, evaluation, and supervision for the elderly and special populations. This level of sophistication adds depth to an enrichment program while meeting the needs of active, independent residents as well as those of the frail elderly who may be aging in place or are in higher levels of care. In the CCRC setting, the independent apartments are not currently regulated, but the skilled nursing component is. Operators would be well advised to consider hiring a professional activity director with a clinical background and knowledge of documentation and activity adaptations. The successful director will have a high energy level and an empathy for the elderly.

Activity assistants can be individuals with high school diplomas or graduates of 36-hour activity therapy courses and who have some experience or interest in working with the elderly. More mature individuals who may have aging parents of their own are usually better equipped to connect with seniors. However, people of any age with the right attitude, solid communication skills, and sincerity can earn the trust and respect of the residents.

There are currently no industry guidelines for staffing ratios across all levels of care. The appropriate staffing complement for each community must be customized according to internal factors such as the residents' profile, the extent of programming offered in the service package, the number of volunteers, the interests of the residents, and the nature of the activities. External factors that may influence staffing include regulatory requirements, the extent of programming offered by local competitors, the geographic location of the community, its proximity to entertainment sources, and transportation. For skilled nursing, the staff-to-resident ratio should be no less than 1:50. Therefore, a 99-bed home would have one activity assistant and one director. The assistant may work Sunday to Thursday or Tuesday to Saturday, or rotate weekends off to provide activity programming seven days a week. A typical schedule also includes two late nights per week to provide for evening programs. The staffing in retirement centers is adjusted downward. The activity director may work alone or with one assistant and may have access to a van driver for community outings. Many smaller communities with staffing constraints have effectively used volunteers or entertainers and have offered courses and seminars to supplement evening and weekend programming. Table 7.1 lists full-time equivalents by resident population and is offered as a general guideline.

Staff should be responsible for maintaining certification, and the activity director must keep records of all in-services provided to activity assistants, aides, and nursing home staff where applicable. All certificates pertaining to employees' credentials must be on file in personnel records or with the human resources director at the property for review by regulators. Based on the hiring package, the CCRC may reimburse some tuition and continuing education toward the certification of its employees, particularly if the certification is a regulatory requirement.

VOLUNTEER PROGRAMS

Typically, the activity director also performs the function of the volunteer services coordinator. This double role is not always ideal, as the activity director's time may be at a premium. Recruiting a volunteer to act as volunteer coordinator is a good alternative; many residents have the leadership skills and management experience needed to coordinate volunteer services. Volunteers can provide activity programs, teach courses, assist with large functions, provide one-on-one activities to assisted living and skilled nursing facility residents; some may even work in the business office or provide musical entertainment.

The process of recruiting volunteers should start with the leisure interest survey given to residents at move-in time. In the survey, a resident may be asked if he is interested in working in any number of areas or if he has a talent to share with his neighbors. If the response is a positive one, the resident is asked to fill out an application as would an employee; then, after receiving a thorough orientation, the volunteer is scheduled according to specific job descriptions provided by the activity director. In this way the activity director and the volunteer clearly establish their mutual expectations. The more structure provided the volunteer, the better the outcome of the relationship and the less chance of misunderstanding regarding each other's role.

Networking the neighborhood is another way to recruit volunteers. Place announcements in church bulletins, contact local high schools for community service students, call university recreation and leisure departments, gerontology and psychology departments, and schools of social service. Many programs require internships; the student intern is a wonderful asset for providing additional staff at little cost. Students can be offered a per diem, a vacant apartment, meals for each day worked, or even a bus pass as possible incentives in return for a full-time employee. Many communities hire temporary interns after graduation

Table 7.1	Activity Staffing Analysis (full-time employees)		
Number of residents	Independent living facility (1:150)	Assisted care living facility (1:100)	Skilled nursing facility (1:50)
< 50	0.5	1.0	1.0
51–100	1.0	1.0	2.0
101–150	1.25	1.25–1.5	3.0
151–200	1.5	1.5–2.0	4.0
201–250	1.75	2.0–2.5	5.0
251–300	2.0	2.5–3.0	6.0
301–350	2.25	3.0–3.5	7.0

as these entry level employees are already trained and familiar with the community's operations and residents. If the activity director is a CTRS, she can act as a preceptor to many university therapy programs. These may include, but are not limited to, therapeutic recreation, gerontology, occupational therapy, and psychology student interns.

In 1991 Marriott Senior Living Services and the United States Administration on Aging conducted a senior volunteer study in conjunction with ICR Survey Research Group of Media, Pennsylvania, that included 962 telephone interviews with respondents 60 years of age or older. The landmark study served to confirm a tremendous pent-up demand among the elderly for opportunities to volunteer. The following highlights of the survey portray a spirit of volunteerism that is largely untapped by community operators.

■ More than 41 percent (5.5 million) of the 37.7 million Americans 60 years of age and older performed some form of volunteer work in the past year. The 65 to 69 and 70 to 74 age groups had the greatest percentage of volunteers, 46 and 45 percent, respectively. Seniors over the age of 80 had the smallest percentage of volunteers, 27 percent.

■ Fourteen million older Americans (37.4%) are potential volunteers who are or may be willing to volunteer if asked.

■ Among current volunteers, 25.6 percent indicated they would have preferred to volunteer more time if asked.

■ Eighty-three percent of seniors said they performed volunteer services in order to help others, and 56 percent did it to feel more useful or productive. Slightly more than half of those asked (52%) felt they volunteered to fulfill a moral responsibility, and nearly one-third volunteered because they felt volunteering was a social obligation. One of every four seniors volunteered as a way of finding companionship, and only 5 percent volunteered to alleviate feelings of guilt.

■ Most seniors (57%) volunteered their services to church or religious organizations, followed by social service agencies (32%), civic or cultural organizations (25%), schools or institutions (22%), and health-related organizations such as the American Red Cross or the Alzheimer's Association (16%). Less than 10 percent indicated that they donate time to a political party or campaign.[3]

The senior volunteer study states that among potential volunteers, retirement communities replaced social service organizations as the second most preferred type of organization for which to volunteer. This could perhaps in part be attributed to seniors' curiosity about their own senior living options.

A well-organized community outreach program designed to promote volunteerism within your community can help to dispel the myths and fears among seniors about senior living. As volunteers become accustomed to the senior living community and make friends there, they begin to realize its inherent value and the benefits that may apply to their own lifestyle needs. Clearly, operators who recognize the marketing potential of this form of community outreach may realize that the benefits of these programs stretch well beyond the intended value to their resident population.

■ MANAGEMENT

Organizing an efficient activity department begins with clearly written policies and procedures. Policy and procedure manuals are OBRA and HCFA requirements. The policy and procedure manuals of the activity department should be on file in the executive director's office as well as in the activity office for review by surveyors. Activity staff should review the manual annually and update its contents. Policy and procedure manuals should also be included in the new-employee orientation process to ensure that activity standards are consistently taught. The policy and procedure manual should generally include the following items.

■ A philosophy or mission statement concerning the life enrichment or recreation services of the community.

■ Clearly stated objectives for providing services to residents.

■ Organization of the department including detailed responsibilities of all personnel.

■ Staffing and personnel policies including: employee orientation in-servicing, job descriptions, staff meeting outlines, volunteer and student intern programs.

■ Scheduling of activities and programs and staffing.

■ Documentation policies for activities including skilled nursing facility initial assessments, resident leisure interest survey, patient care plans such as minimum data sets (MDS), progress notes, and frequency and participation records.

- Program descriptions outlining in-house activities including program protocol information for each group provided by the activity department. All outings should have an outing policy and emergency van procedures. For communities with Alzheimer's residents, an escort policy for safety must be in place.

- Communication procedures such as monthly calendars and newsletters with the frequency of their distribution, along with guidelines concerning when and where to post them and distribution by mail, bulletin boards, and decorations as essential communication tools.

- A quality assurance plan to evaluate participation in programs and the effectiveness of the activity department in meeting the needs of residents, including some form of resident satisfaction criteria.

SUPPLIES

Many companies provide mail order arts and crafts items, decorations, and computer software.[4] Mail ordering may seem appealing at first because of the time constraints in a busy activity department, but it is wise to establish local accounts with stores in the neighborhood to take advantage of sales and specials. Also, with any mail order supply house, there is the *hidden* cost of shipping that offsets the convenience. The use of local vendors can also reduce receiving and administrative paperwork and create a sense of community among local businesses toward the property. Local accounts may include video stores, stationery shops, and arts and crafts stores; even the company that delivers oxygen to the resident in unit 216 may be able to deliver a helium tank for activities, marketing, special events, and to cheer up ill residents. It never hurts to ask, and it can save considerable expense. Traditionally activity budgets are small in retirement communities, and the seasoned, shrewd director becomes skilled at making every dollar count.

Control of inventory in the activity department is the most effective way to contain costs. How many times have executive directors heard that a tape recorder is missing or that "we can't find the Christmas decorations" when hundreds of dollars were spent on these items during previous budget years? Activity directors need to keep an organized inventory of all equipment, supplies, and decorations in storage or in the activity office. All materials must be checked out by staff and returned to a designated location. Time is lost when items cannot be found, and the last thing in excess in a successful activity department is time. A simple clipboard with a list for signing out items will suffice. An organized inventory list should be devised according to the needs of the community and based on resident interests.

In addition to an inventory of supplies and equipment, all sales receipts should be copied and attached to or placed on file with warranty information and instruction manuals. It is a good practice to record all serial numbers of equipment inside the front cover of the instruction manual of expensive equipment to facilitate identification in the event that they are lost or stolen.

Most communities provide food and beverage supplies from in-house kitchens. The activity budget should include a line item for food and beverage charges, so that these are not included in the kitchen's average-cost-per-meal calculations for the resident population. A separate budget amount for this purpose will create an atmosphere of cooperation with the chef who will not be penalized in his food costs when sponsoring resident events. Most chefs can acquire everything from birthday cakes to nonalcoholic beer. The activity director should fill out a special function request form well in advance of the proposed event to allow the kitchen some lead time to work the request into their daily production planning. Waiting until the last minute to request cookies or fruit plates will only create resentment among the kitchen staff and could degenerate into conflict.[5] Depending on the community's accounting procedure, the activity director should be notified by the kitchen or property accountant of the amount of food and beverage charges that will be allocated to her budget. Careful planning of events by the activity director should include keeping a running tally on all charges against the budget. This practice will earmark dollars in anticipation of an upcoming major event. It is always better to be ahead of your budget and manage your limited resources in anticipation of needs than to try to catch up by skimping elsewhere.

RESOURCES

Every activity department can benefit from subscribing to a variety of publications. Maintaining a library of activity reference sources in the activity office can provide new ideas when you are at a loss. Newspapers list community events, and the activity director should contact the senior editor of the local paper to receive lists of upcoming programs. The Chamber of Commerce is also an excellent resource. Most communities maintain membership in this organization and should make use of this important connection to the outside community for programming ideas. Service organizations may also be encouraged to hold their meetings in retirement community public areas. These meetings normally involve lunch service that can be arranged at a small profit through the community's food and beverage department. Be sure to involve the residents' council in this decision; after all, you are inviting guests into their home. Also be aware that parking may impose some limitations. Designate specific areas where service organizations may park, so as not to inconvenience residents and their guests or marketing prospects. Residents may become agitated when their parking spaces are taken while they are out, particularly if they are being charged extra for their use. Local churches may hold services or Bible study open to residents, or even initiated by residents. These events can be important resources for activity ideas and also have marketing advantages.

Schools are excellent and inexpensive resources as well. Local elementary or middle schools can be outlets for residents' volunteer interests and may also provide some fascinating intergenerational potential. In one community in Colorado, residents and high school drama students joined forces during the summer months to produce a play that earned statewide recognition. Not only did it provide a creative outlet for interested residents, it also served to bridge the generation gap with the youngsters. The resulting press coverage in the local newspaper and on television made great progress toward dispelling the myth about a retirement community being an "old folks home" (and didn't hurt the marketing efforts either). Another successful school program that made the news involved a class project to document early life in the local community. Junior high school students interviewed residents who had lived in the surrounding community most of their lives. The residents were asked to share their impressions about how the town had changed over the years. The activity director and the schoolteacher had the completed reports edited and then archived them at the local library. In

a skilled nursing home in Washington state, a lonely but highly educated patient, who was unfortunately confined to her bed by rheumatoid arthritis, was recruited by the local special education director of the elementary school to record books on audiotape for developmentally challenged students. This activity gave the patient a new purpose in life and allowed her to make a contribution, while adding significantly to the audio library of the local school system. Residents can also attend community college courses or act as mentors or tutors of students in some circumstances. The opportunities are unlimited for someone with a bit of creativity.

The activity director should be an active member of the local activity director association or, if she is a CTRS, be a member of the local chapter of the American Therapeutic Recreation Association (ATRA). These organizations provide continuing education opportunities, programming information, networking resources, and legislative updates pertaining to standards for activity therapy in higher levels of care. Active memberships in these organizations will help the activity director avoid the isolation that leads to stagnation, the last thing an effective activity department needs.

The activity profession is extremely demanding, both emotionally and physically. Not only are the activity director and staff expected to keep the community decorated to reflect every season and holiday, but also to rearrange furniture for programs, arrange food service, set up functions, create signage and information boards, and physically assist with the residents' mobility and transfers. From an emotional standpoint, the position is very service oriented. All day long, the activity staff gives residents the emotional support and encouragement needed to help them through the challenges of the aging process, expecting little in return. This constant giving requires a very strong individual who can meet the expectations of the residents and management without becoming drained. Management must recognize the enormous strain involved in meeting the demands of the job and encourage the activity staff to become involved in organizations in which they can share their frustrations and victories with peers. These organizations can provide a much-needed balance for the director and staff, allowing them to maintain their positive attitude, energy level, and creativity. Exhibit 7.1 provides an orientation checklist of the complexities of this critical position.

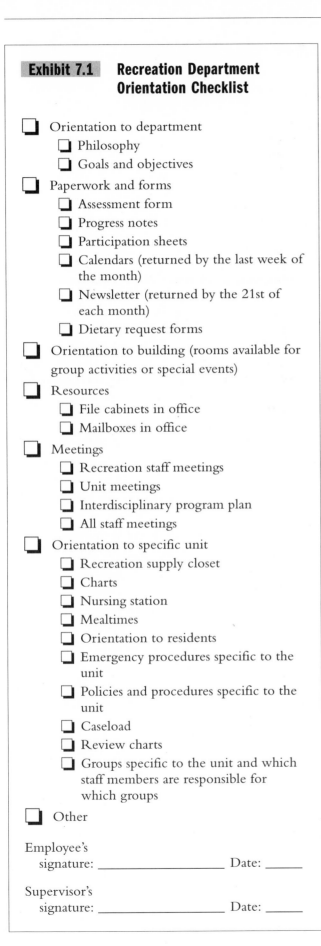

Exhibit 7.1 **Recreation Department Orientation Checklist**

- ☐ Orientation to department
  - ☐ Philosophy
  - ☐ Goals and objectives
- ☐ Paperwork and forms
  - ☐ Assessment form
  - ☐ Progress notes
  - ☐ Participation sheets
  - ☐ Calendars (returned by the last week of the month)
  - ☐ Newsletter (returned by the 21st of each month)
  - ☐ Dietary request forms
- ☐ Orientation to building (rooms available for group activities or special events)
- ☐ Resources
  - ☐ File cabinets in office
  - ☐ Mailboxes in office
- ☐ Meetings
  - ☐ Recreation staff meetings
  - ☐ Unit meetings
  - ☐ Interdisciplinary program plan
  - ☐ All staff meetings
- ☐ Orientation to specific unit
  - ☐ Recreation supply closet
  - ☐ Charts
  - ☐ Nursing station
  - ☐ Mealtimes
  - ☐ Orientation to residents
  - ☐ Emergency procedures specific to the unit
  - ☐ Policies and procedures specific to the unit
  - ☐ Caseload
  - ☐ Review charts
  - ☐ Groups specific to the unit and which staff members are responsible for which groups
- ☐ Other

Employee's
signature: _____ Date: _____

Supervisor's
signature: _____ Date: _____

RECREATIONAL ACTIVITIES

Recreational activities involve two areas of concern to the operator of a retirement community: in-house programs and community programs. Each area includes both shared-cost and community-provided activities.

In-House Programs

Residents of either a retirement center or a skilled nursing facility should have completed an initial assessment upon placement or a leisure interest survey at move-in. These tools indicate which in-house programs should be available to residents. The in-house programs offered on a monthly basis should include physical activity, music, social groups, spiritual and educational programs, community outings, special events, personal parties, arts and crafts, movies, and current events. Tables 7.2 and 7.3 offer some typical programming standards for independent and assisted living residents.

In the residential component of the community, some shared-cost programs might include spa activities such as massage or fitness trainers. Many retirement communities use travel agents to provide reduced group rates for residents' cruises. One community conducted a series of educational classes on the culture and history of the ancient Maya of the Yucatán peninsula that culminated in a cruise and a tour of the ruins in Mexico. Normally, if a certain number of reservations is achieved by the community, the cruise agent will include discounted or complimentary cabins for management personnel who accompany residents. As this type of program is normally very time-consuming to coordinate and organize, management has tended to allow staff to accompany the residents on their cruise. It should be clear that the community accepts no responsibility for either the residents or the employees while on activities that take them out of their geographic vicinity and that they are taking these trips at their own risk. Also popular are casino and theater trips. The rule for providing programs for independent residents is to *listen, listen, listen*. The residents can be an excellent source of ideas; it is the responsibility of the activity department to act on those ideas and incorporate their leisure interests into successful program offerings.

The in-house recreation services might include such things as a gardening club, bridge afternoons, movies, educational series, arts and crafts classes, and residents' councils. In an effort to capture the interest of residents in continuing education, some

Table 7.2   Sample Activity Programming Standards: Independent or Residential

Program type	Extensive	Moderate	Low
Physical Exercise			
Sitting exercise	3×/week	5×/week	3×/week
Regular	5×/week	3×/week	
Walking group	5×/week	2×/week	
Aquatic exercise	3×/week		
Dance	1×/week		
Social			
Bingo	2×/week	1×/week	1×/week
Birthdays	1×/month	1×/month	1×/month
Lunch out	1×/month	1×/month	
Shopping	3×/week	2×/week	2×/week
Doctor appointments	4×/week	3×/week	2×/week
Cards	2×/week	2×/week	2×/week
Happy hour	1×/week	2×/month	
Movies	1×/week	1×/week	1×/week
Men's activities	1×/week	2×/month	1×/month
Cultural			
Entertainment	4×/month	3×/month	6×/year
Trips—cultural	1×/month	6×/year	4×/year
Art classes	1×/week	2×/month	1×/month
Crafts	1×/week	1×/week	1×/week
Writing	1×/week	1×/month	6×/year
Acting (plays)	4×/year	2×/year	1×/year
Singalong	3×/month	2×/month	1×/month
Mental			
Bridge	1×/week	1×/week	2×/month
Group discussion	1×/week	1×/week	2×/month
Current events	1×/month	2×/month	1×/month
Book review	1×/week	6×/year	4×/year
Spiritual			
Services in-house	2×/week	1×/week	1×/week
Services—external	2×/week	1×/week	
Bible study	1×/week	1×/week	
Planning			
Resident council	1×/month	1×/month	1×/month
Act. steering committee	1×/month	1×/month	1×/month
Special			
Theme events	1×/week	2×/month	1×/month
Intergenerational	2×/month	1×/month	4×/year
Pets	4×/month	2×/month	1×/month
Plants	1×/month	4×/year	3×/year
Speakers—health	1×/month	6×/year	4×/year
Speakers—other	1×/month	6×/year	4×/year
Puzzles	1×/week	1×/week	1×/week

Table 7.3   Sample Activity Programming Standards: Assisted Living

Program type	Typical
Slow exercise	3×/week
Bingo	2×/week
Birthday party	1×/month
Cards	1×/week
Movies	1×/week
Entertainment	2×/month
Crafts	1×/week
Singalong	2×/month
Group discussion	1×/week
Church services	1×/week
Pets	2×/month
Puzzles	3×/month
Kids	2×/month
Plants	6×/year
Walks around building	5×/week
Bulletin boards changed	1×/month
Newsletters (large print)	1×/month
Decorate	1×/month
Transportation	1×/week
One-on-one	7×/week

communities have devised innovative continuing education opportunities.

Today's senior "is a member of the most information-driven segment of U.S. society," according to David Wolfe, one of the foremost experts on the mature market. "They prefer news shows and documentaries to other TV viewing. They are big readers of newspapers and magazines. They travel to expand their horizons, rather than for the escapist reasons that widely motivate young people to travel. They are signing up at colleges and universities by the tens of thousands. They are creative about shaping their lives and are intellectually involved in life."[6]

On average, older adults see themselves as more than 10 years younger then their actual age, according to the *Marriott Seniors' Attitudes Study* conducted by ICR Survey Research Group for Marriott Senior Living Services. "The perceptions of their age correlate to a desire to remain active and vital," the survey found. Asked if they were bored with their lives, most said no (76.3%). Asked what they would do differently with their lives, 68 percent said they would do more to help society and 75 percent said they would get more education.[7]

Many residents consider learning a lifelong activity. Communities that develop courses to address this need for stimulating, enriching programming beyond the "4 Bs" frequently associated with retirement communities will better serve the real interests of their population. For example, in the politically correct climate of the 1990s, ethnicity and cultural origins have provided a rich variety of activity programming. The activity director must look beyond St. Valentine's day to celebrating Kwansaa at the end of December or Hanukkah the first week of the month.[8] These programs can take the shape of week-long events, education, and parties. Often, celebrating the differences and uniqueness of individuals enables a community to become unified and more accepting of others as they may change with age. Other courses might include special studies in religion, native art, and ethnic customs of various geographic and cultural regions of the world. Monthly book or literary reviews are always well received. Classes also provide an environment in which residents can learn from one another; textbook learning comes to life when the residents as students can discuss relevant personal experiences in a relaxed setting.

Classes should emphasize the fun in learning and cover subjects that promote personal growth of particular interest to older Americans. The classes can be taught by volunteer instructors or at a small charge at the residents' expense. As a rule, residents will be willing to pay for special educational courses provided that the cost is generally under $25.

Potential residents can also be invited to attend programs on subjects in which they have indicated an interest, enabling them to interact with residents and experience the companionship associated with community life before moving in. In many cases, the strength of a well-coordinated program can prompt prospects to move in sooner than they initially indicated they would. By making these courses available to the public, the community facilitates a better understanding of the "active retirement living" concept. Once seniors from the community at large meet the residents and experience the high-caliber programs, any preconceived notions they may have had about "institutional activities" are put to rest. Communities should also encourage residents to invite their friends to attend the classes; this helps residents maintain strong relationships outside the community. Healthy inter-

action between residents and nonresidents also helps spread the word about the positive attributes of retirement living.

Each community must develop planning standards of its own that reflect the information gathered from the leisure interest surveys or initial assessments. Actual programming will of course vary widely according to the natural talents and creativity of each activity director. Encourage some form of formalized planning that will aid the individual director in developing her monthly calendar and annual budget. Exhibit 7.2 can be used to assess residents' leisure interests and to match residents with similar interests, rather than planning activities designed to interest everyone.

Operators with Medicare units must be goal oriented to meet the needs of each resident as represented by the MDS and the initial assessment mentioned earlier. The residents' needs are clearly defined on the patient care plan, and activities must incorporate residents' interests into this documentation. For example, Mr. Cameron is admitted to a skilled nursing facility with a diagnosis of congestive heart failure and dementia. In his initial assessment he states to the activity director that he used to enjoy gardening and was an award-winning horticulturist after retiring from his law practice. The activity director writes a specific goal for Mr. Cameron to participate in a horticultural therapy group once a week. Staff interventions might include providing Mr. Cameron with a window garden in his room (per facility policy) or delegating the responsibility to him to water plants in the common areas. Empowerment, choices, dignity, and respect must be represented clearly on the care plan.

Community Programs

Another example of putting the residents first is illustrated by the following program that was coordinated in a care center in Phoenix. This multilevel extended care facility also had an Alzheimer's floor. The problem for the activity director was to mobilize the entire building (all levels) to participate in a holiday bazaar fund-raiser. The activity director was well aware of the ability of her involved Alzheimer's residents. She devised a long banner of paper and taped it to a tabletop; she then added brushes, sponges, paint, and glitter and let the residents literally wander in and out

Exhibit 7.2	**Recreation/Activity Program Initial Assessment**

Resident's name: _____

Admission no.: _____ Room no.: _____

PERSONAL DATA

Diagnosis: _____

Date of birth: _____ Age: _____ Date of admission: _____

Photo release: ☐ Yes ☐ No Special diet considerations: _____

Allergies/medical precautions: _____

SOCIAL HISTORY

Past occupation: _____ Education: _____

Marital status: M S W D Name of spouse: _____

Children: _____ Family, friends, support systems: _____

Resident interested in church services: ☐ Yes ☐ No Describe: _____

INTEREST INVENTORY

(P) *Past interest* (C) *Current interest* (N) *No interest*

_____ Newspaper/current events	_____ Intergenerational programs
_____ Exercise	_____ Trivia/word games
_____ Arts and crafts	_____ Residents' council
_____ Spiritual services	_____ Task time
_____ Cooking club	_____ Gardening
_____ Special events/entertainment	_____ Singalong
_____ Community outing	_____ Talking book/magazine
_____ One-on-one visit	_____ Sensory stimulation
_____ Board games	_____ Music
_____ Bingo	_____ Movies/videos/slides
_____ Black cow special	_____ Reading
_____ Pet therapy	_____ Other

LEISURE ACTIVITIES

Interview residents regarding lifestyle, attitudes, and interests (for example, "Describe a typical day at home."). Interview family, friends, or children for information:

_____

_____

_____

_____

_____

_____

_____

_____

(continued)

Exhibit 7.2 Recreation/Activity Program (*continued*)

COGNITION/COMMUNICATION

Orientation: Self: ☐ Yes ☐ No   Day/date: ☐ Yes ☐ No   Situation: ☐ Yes ☐ No

Attention: 0–5 Minutes ☐   5–15 Minutes ☐   15–30 Minutes ☐   1 Hour or more ☐

Communication system: _____   Dentures: ☐ Yes ☐ No

Comprehension/understanding: _____

Memory: _____

Safety awareness: _____

PHYSICAL

Vision: _____   Hearing: _____

Ambulation: _____   Bowel and bladder: _____

Sitting tolerance: _____   Transfers: _____

Right-handed ☐   Left-handed ☐

SOCIAL/EMOTIONAL

	Yes	No	Comments:
Aware of placement	☐	☐	_____
Responds to 1:1 conversation	☐	☐	_____
Initiates 1:1 conversation	☐	☐	_____
Aware of others in group setting	☐	☐	_____
Seeks social contacts in social situations	☐	☐	_____
Avoids social contacts/situations	☐	☐	_____
Expresses feelings/emotions appropriately	☐	☐	_____
Frustrates easily	☐	☐	_____
Touches others inappropriately	☐	☐	_____

Signature: _____   Date: _____

making their individual contributions to the "mural." After the paint dried, it was cut into smaller sections and given to bed patients to cut into 1 × 3-inch strips, then passed on to another floor to punch holes in one end. Next, the strips went into shoe boxes and to still more residents who tied red and green yarn in one end and bundled them in bunches of 25 gift tags to be sold at the bazaar. It may not sound like much, but this multilevel adaptation involved residents from all functional levels on every floor of the facility to complete the project. Sales of the gift tags earned more than $300 for the residents' council fund! Attached to the back of each bundle was a label stating "made by the Alzheimer's residents of St. Joseph's Care Center." The care center was well represented to the community by this fund-raising activity program and received consider-

able media exposure. Ingenuity and the ability to adapt activities for complex multilevel properties are two desirable traits for an activity director. The challenges in today's retirement communities are endless, and a versatile activity program must be ready for anything.

Everyone benefits from a big project: it has purpose, provides a sense of belonging, and creates a sense of accomplishment. Projects such as this that involve the entire staff can considerably enhance the effectiveness of an enrichment program. Projects that are conceived and well organized with a *purpose* will attract the participation of personal care assistants. If the activity director can devise creative programs designed to be interesting to other staff, it is amazing what can be accomplished. Activities meant to entertain or motivate just the residents or cater to their special interests are usually poorly attended. However, a big project that appeals to everyone has the potential to attract large numbers of participants, residents and staff alike.

■■■■ COMMUNICATION

To evaluate the success of a program, feedback from the residents is just as important as the number of residents who attend. For example, a morning exercise program may have 45 residents outside for a brisk walk, whereas the bridge club may have only four tables twice a week. Each activity is valued and used by the residents with relatively little cost or set-up involved. A theme dinner such as "An Evening in the Tropics" could be open to prospective residents as well as guests of residents and serve both to break the routine of always dining in the same restaurant and to impress marketing guests. Planning a successful special event will require the coordinated efforts of the marketing, maintenance, housekeeping, resident relations, and food and beverage departments. Task sheets, an agenda for the evening, and a menu must all be prepared ideally two to three *months* in advance. This will allow time to develop and print invitations, arrange for any decorations and rental equipment, and research the projected costs. When a special event is successful, each resident and staff member is well versed on the details. The last thing an activity director needs to hear is an aide or concierge answering a telephone inquiry with "I don't know anything about a party here." It reflects poorly on the community and detracts from the image the event was designed to create.

The activity department is responsible for the calendar of events or activity calendars in skilled nursing facilities. These calendars should be posted bedside; given to residents; posted at desktops, in elevators, on bulletin boards, and at nursing stations; and given to all department heads. Additions or corrections should be posted and announced so that everyone has the opportunity to be informed.

The community newsletter is another means of advertising activity programs. Ongoing programs can be highlighted by using residents' interviews or reviews that often spark new interest. Announcements for upcoming classes, trips, and events can all be done in the newsletter. A well-appointed and attractive newsletter can also be used by the marketing department for mailings to potential residents and their families to demonstrate a sense of community and activity. Some communities produce two newsletters, one internally designed for the residents and staff and another for public relations and marketing. Both are effective in communicating the life pulse of the community and sparking interest in programs.[9]

The best and most attractive method to communicate daily activities to the residents is in the elevators. A classic brushed brass or silver 8½ × 11-inch frame, open at the top and mounted on the wall of the elevator car, can "advertise" daily activities with a one-page flyer. The flyer can be decorated with clip art and printed on preprinted or color paper and changed daily (be sure to notify residents who live on the first floor as well).

Most modern word processing programs come equipped with preformatted newsletter wizards or templates. These are very simple to customize and look professionally done. With a little practice almost anyone can become proficient at developing attractive flyers, calendars, and newsletters. Most programs come with clip art images, and for a small additional investment literally thousands of additional images and borders are available on CD-ROM. The new desktop publishing programs are very simple to learn and can add even greater polish to the materials. Much of what it takes to get people involved is internal marketing. If the program looks and sounds attractive, people will come.

■■■■ BUDGET

Activity costs are very difficult to estimate because of many factors. These may include such diverse cultural things as demographics and rural versus urban needs and interests. For example, an activity program in a large city like Chicago would most certainly include fine arts, entertainment, and spa activities, whereas a Utah community might prefer more arts and crafts programs and volunteerism.

In addition to salaries and benefits, the activity budget has several main components. These may include general operating supplies, decoration expenses, general operating services and independent contractors, rental equipment expenses, dues and subscriptions, educational programs, events, and food and beverage charges. When budgeting, break each category down into subcategories such as arts and crafts, seasonal

Table 7.4 **Activity Budget Levels**

Program level	Budget per resident per month
Low	$0–$4
Moderate	$5–$8
High	$9–$11
Extensive	$12+

decorations, exercise videos, and movies; include contracts for music therapists, entertainers, golf pros, aqua aerobics, and equipment, just to name a few. Table 7.4 gives general guidelines for various program levels in a stabilized community. Obviously the scope of the programs offered will depend to a large extent on what the community can afford to provide considering its revenue stream and the interests of its residents. It should be stressed that one does not necessarily need to have a large budget to have a successful activity program. Success depends almost totally on the creativity and energy of the activity director.

NOTES

1. D. B. Wolfe, *Serving the Ageless Market: Strategies for Selling to the Fifty-Plus Market* (New York: McGraw-Hill, 1990), 45–46.
2. W. G. Manning and K. B. Wells, "Use of Outpatient Mental Health Care" (Rand report R-3277-NIMH) (Los Angeles: Rand Corporation, August 1986).
3. *Marriott Seniors' Volunteerism Study* (Washington, D.C.: Marriott Senior Living Services, 1991).
4. Contact Creative Forecasting, Inc., P.O. Box 7789, Colorado Springs, CO 80933-7789, (719) 633-3174, for a comprehensive list of resources and activity ideas.
5. See Chapter 8 for more detail on function sheets and their use in production planning.
6. Wolfe, *Serving the Ageless Market,* 46.
7. *Marriott Seniors' Attitudes Survey* (Washington, D.C.: ICR Survey Research Group, 1990).
8. Kwansaa is an annual national celebration of African American heritage celebrated during the month of December.
9. For a free catalog of copyright-free borders, lettering, corner motifs, and clip art, write to Dover Publications, Inc., 31 East 2nd Street, Mineola, NY 11501. Most Dover books cost under $5.00. Briggs also has a fine catalog of activity supplies, ideas, and games.

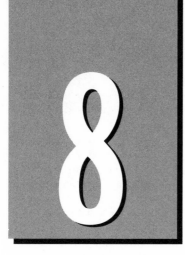

Food and Beverage Service

Over the years, many operators have trekked across the country looking for the esoteric secret to satisfying all residents' tastes and preferences while taking into consideration regional peculiarities and nutrition. After an exhaustive search, I have come to the conclusion that no such secret exists. Seniors' preferences are as different as they are. I am reminded of an incident that occurred while I was visiting a property in Chicago. Residents are not shy about expressing their opinion on everything from how to cook chicken soup to the amount, if any, of ice in the water glasses. While touring the dining room at meal time, I inquired how some residents at a four-top were enjoying their lamb dinner. Three of the residents expressed compliments to the kitchen. A more vocal resident observed that this was the toughest and gristliest piece of lamb that she had ever eaten and that it was totally unsuitable. To that I remarked, "Oh, they *did* give you that piece." She looked curious and asked me what I meant by that, to which I replied, "The kitchen was going to throw it out, but I told them to give it to you because you are the toughest *resident* that we have and if you can't eat it then no one can." She and her companions laughed and said that they thought it suited her; after all, they thought the lamb was excellent. Most of the time, residents are simply interested in being heard about *something* and will criticize the food service to attract attention. People will usually laugh along with you, but experience has taught me that you

had better be well acquainted with the resident before you try to disarm a tense situation with humor.

◼◼ CONCEPT AND DESIGN

The primary decision that will drive the entire food service set-up regards the type of menu plan and service style. This decision will depend on a number of factors. The type of service and cost associated with providing it will be driven by the project's ability to afford it. Conceptually, financial justification of the entire service package is achieved through the development of projections and proformas designed to estimate the potential financial performance of the project. The financial objectives of the owner will dictate the overall assumptions and key criteria for evaluating the project. It is important that any decisions made at the inception and marketing of the project be clearly understood and accepted by all. Once the service package is in place it becomes very difficult to modify when the project becomes occupied, inasmuch as any changes will be viewed by the residents as an attempt to scale back the level of service.

Another factor in determining the level of service of the project will be its relative competitive position in the market it serves. If other projects provide table service, then you may also be forced to incorporate it into your offering. In addition, the potential expenses of hiring food service professionals with a high degree of technical and management skill and the constraints of the local employment market may factor into the service-style decision. As the resident population ages in place, more labor may be required to provide essentially the same level of service than was originally conceived.

This chapter details the various options and methods to provide the most commonly delivered food service in the back of the house or kitchen. There are basically three types of food preparation in congregate retirement projects: tray line or its more upscale derivative, buffet; à la carte; and seatings with dish-up to order table service. Most communities incorporate a combination of two or all three service styles into their food programs depending upon budgetary constraints, level of care, and resident preferences.

■ Buffets

Tray line service and buffets were very popular in the early 1980s, but as the retirement industry entered its growth phase and the residents became more sophisticated, providers were forced to accept the added overhead of a table service operation. Tray lines with their clearly visible steam tables turned into buffet food displays, where providers tried to give a hospitality finish to the project while still saving some staffing hours.

A well-thought-out buffet food service, like any other food product, must be based on a well-written menu consistently prepared and produced from the freshest ingredients available. However, because this food product becomes a movable feast, operators must be prepared to provide a support system with the equipment necessary to keep hot food hot and cold food cold and to meet all local health and sanitation guidelines for mass self-service distribution. These operators must also have a clear plan for resident and staff accessibility, all while enticing the eyes and exciting the palate.

The portion selection of each item on the buffet can be managed using the individual serving size of the selections, location along the line, and even the size of the dish-up utensil. Typically, buffets are organized with inexpensive salads and side dishes first, leaving little plate room for the more expensive entree or carving station at the end of the line. Offering a wide selection of salads and other dishes encourages the diner to try a little taste of each, in effect minimizing the food cost.

The addition of buffet-style dining to an existing dish-up-to-order food-service program can save a community between $10,000 and $15,000 annually in lower labor and food cost while reducing the boredom factor for the residents. Special buffets such as the Sunday brunch, weekday theme dinner, soup and salad bar lunch buffet, and salad appetizer bar at dinner can produce real savings. The addition of these creative meals can also be used effectively by the sales counselors to differentiate your community from the competition. A special meal can also provide an enticement for family members to visit the community, generating additional revenues.

The menu takes on more significance because the distribution of the end product in a buffet is taken over by residents rather than by portion-conscious food service workers. Food cost overruns can quickly absorb any potential savings inherent in buffet service if too many high-cost items are available at the same time. Additionally, significant plate waste is an important factor to consider when selecting items for the center of the plate or entree portion of the buffet. Individuals enjoy trying more items in a buffet situation; therefore, it is important to remember to keep portions small and easily distributed.

Production timetables and work schedules have much more significance when you consider the possibility of several hundred residents lined up for a buffet meal service. Food selected for buffet presentation must be easily mass-produced and have the ability to hold well. Buffet selections that are convenience products (items that can be purchased already prepared) can be dramatic in appearance but inexpensive to produce. They can include such elaborate entrees as chicken cordon bleu with a choice of two serving sizes.

The responsibility of monitoring self-service buffet food is considerable. No matter whether your set-up is portable or permanent, the freshness, healthfulness, and sanitation of the presentation is the first priority, and any operation considering the use of this type of food-distribution system must be committed to training the food service staff diligently in this regard.

As residents' frailty increases with time, the popularity of buffet service declines owing to the physical barriers that it begins to impose. With a more active clientele, buffet-style service aids socialization, giving the residents a chance to chat as they make their way to and from the various food displays. As a community matures, operators may still want to incorporate a certain percentage of their food service as buffet inasmuch as it lends itself well to theme, event dining, and holiday meals. In addition, it can serve as a creative outlet for kitchen staff and break the monotony for the service staff and residents alike.

A la Carte

A la carte dining in an open seating environment, essentially the food service structure available in any fine restaurant, has been widely imitated by congregate operations. This remains the most expensive type of food preparation and service system. The common denominator is that this style of food service is individual. The cooks handle the immediate preparation and cooking of the food from a raw state just prior to the moment when a particular course is ready for distribution. Residents must be committed to dine—that is, to make conversation with their table companions while patiently waiting as each course is prepared to their specifications.

Menus for à la carte dining can be sophisticated, with dramatic presentations. As always, the well-developed menu creates the environment for success. The development of a comprehensive menu whose components are nutrition, variety, color, and texture must also provide for a wide variety of cooking techniques.[1] This allows for smooth implementation for the cooks so that no station on the line becomes overwhelmed. The skill level of the cooks working an à la carte line is considerably higher than that of the typical kitchen prep cook. Decisions regarding degree of doneness, temperature, and the like are made by line cooks hundreds of times each evening. It is conceivable that in a busy congregate dining room using this method of food preparation a diner could spend well over 90 minutes to dine.

Dish-up to Order

This style of food service can be found on most cruise ships. In environments where many diners come to the restaurant within a relatively short period of time, and their numbers can be managed, this service style benefits the diner and management alike. This popular style of food service has become increasingly utilized as former hoteliers have entered the business, offering a way to translate their hospitality expertise to retirement housing. Seatings create a restaurant-style dining experience in a beautiful environment where residents can order off a menu and be served in courses.

A simple time study of the length of time the average ticket takes to be filled or the number of meals dished up per minute will help to clarify the pressure on the kitchen. The plate-up time expectations per cook should not exceed 1.5 meals per minute if the order is to be filled accurately and attractively. Table 8.1 details some average plate-up times by service style. When too many orders hit the line at once, they begin to back up and cause a bottleneck. Establishing two serving times can considerably relieve this pressure.

Clearly, the more customization requested by the resident, the longer the dish-up time. Residents should be advised that cook-to-order (à la minute) selections will involve longer plate-up times than do standard menu selections. Sometimes residents will succumb to peer pressure, knowing that their special order may delay the dinners of their dining companions.

The kitchen is essentially geared toward banquet preparation for all courses; however, some entrees are still cooked à la minute, but now in multiples rather than individually. The food is plated and garnished so that it has the appearance of individual preparation and presentation, but is actually mass produced.

This particular style of service has a number of benefits. First, it provides a rapid dish-up because many of the courses (such as salads, appetizers, and desserts) are plated prior to service. Second, most entrees are prepared ahead of time in components or cooked in multiples, allowing for the accommodation of the diner's personal preference in an abbreviated dish-up. This way, whether served to an early or a late diner, the vegetables and entrees will always be freshly cooked and not taste as if they had been sitting for several hours. Third, because of the economical use of time the dining experience can be compressed, which allows more diners to be served in the same amount of time. A little flexibility on the part of the residents in their meal times can significantly improve their dining experience and utilize kitchen resources more efficiently. Although this style of service appears to serve a number of different masters, it demands a fair amount of planning, preparation, menu design, specialized kitchen layout, and equipment to make it flow.

Kitchens planned for this style of service have considerable areas devoted to the preparation and holding of food, as well as more walk-in refrigeration and more cook-and-hold equipment. Because diners enter together and expect quick service, staging areas in the kitchen and service pantry become essential for loading trays efficiently while maximizing space and minimizing steps for the service staff. Menu design requires special attention to recipe preparation time, a product's holding capacity, and whether recipes can be prepared in component phases to allow for personal preferences.

The single most important issue is a production plan that controls the amount of product prepared and reduces the risk of running out of food, sloppy production methods, and/or inappropriate shortcuts to compensate for poor planning.

Finally, communication between the front of the house (service) and the kitchen is essential to eliminate runs on any of the menu items. Seatings are very fast and can get out of control easily, but when done properly they save considerable labor dollars for the front of the house.

■ MANAGEMENT STRUCTURE

Operating in the competitive retirement housing environment today requires a flexible and fully accountable management team whose members are cross-trained and competent in all aspects of production in the kitchen. The most efficient and cost-effective kitchens are staffed with generalists rather than prima-donna specialists. This trend is evident not only in retirement housing but also throughout the entire hospitality industry. Today's executive chef must not only have experience in preparation and production, nutrition, sanitation, and administration, he must also be adept at managing and motivating his staff in a harsh work environment. Chefs are now being called on to deliver the entire spectrum of food service from concept and design to financial accountability and even working on the line. As food-service operations increase in complexity, dietary managers will become more common. This position bridges the gap between dietitian and food and beverage managers. In certain regulatory environments, the dietitian will need to ensure proper preparation and planning for special diets; however, accommodations for residents with these special needs are not normally made for residents in residential living environments.

Line staffing complements depend not only on the style of the service but also on the physical layout of the kitchen and, of course, the optimum number of

meals to be served daily in the allotted time frame. The amount of staffing in the kitchen should be calculated during peak dish-up hours and is a function of the service style and amount of waiting time acceptable to the diners. In most communities where many diners come to eat at once, it is advisable to have salads and desserts preplated. Another great time-saver is to have the dining room staff make up a sheet pan with preportioned ramekins of the various salad dressings.

Table 8.1 shows the estimated times for plate-up for banquet, dish-up to order, and à la minute service styles. These times will vary depending upon the method of preparation and the number of passes over the plate during dish-up. For example, there will be an initial pass for entree, sauce, starch, vegetable, garnish, rim wipe, cover, and arrangement by table. Plate-up times range from 2 meals/minute for banquet style, where all plates are identical; to 1.5 meals/minute under the dish-up-to-order scheme, in which individual preferences are considered; to 0.13 meals/minute for cook-to-order restaurant-style dining.

The number of cooks will depend on the total covers of output in the desired time frame. In the dish-up-to-order cook staffing example in Table 8.2 of 135 covers, at 1.5 meals/minute (see the previous breakdown), all meals can comfortably be dished up to order in 30 minutes using three cooks at 45 meals per cook. For fewer covers per meal, consider implementing

Table 8.1   Plate-up Times per Serving

Activity	Banquet (seconds)	Dish-up-to-order (seconds)	A la minute (seconds)
Read ticket	0	5	5
Set up plates	5	5	5
Garnish	3	4	4
Meat	5	7	420
Sauce	3	3	3
Veg × 2	5	5	5
Starch	3	3	3
Wipe rim	3	3	3
Check and cover	3	5	5
Total	**30**	**40**	**453**
Meals/minute	2.0	1.5	0.1
Minutes/4-top	2.0	2.7	30.2

Table 8.2   Cook Staffing

	Dish-up-to-order style (peak hours)	
Desired dish-up time (min)	30	45
Total covers	135	135
Total dish-up time (meals/min)	4.50	3.00
Average production (meals/min)	1.5	1.5
Meals/cook during dish-up time	45	68
Number of cooks	3.0	2.0
Plus back-up (if needed)	1.0	1.0
Total cooks	**4.0**	**3.0**

two seatings to reduce staffing costs. For longer meal periods or food service with additional courses, fewer line cooks may be required for the same volume of covers of dish-up times for various types of food service. If management determines that the dish-up time can be extended, then the staffing can be reduced. For example, if all meals are targeted for dish-up in 45 minutes, the number of cooks can be reduced by one to two (three if a backup is required). There will always be a need to accommodate special requests, which may require an additional backup cook for finishing or à la carte orders. Splitting the meal periods into an early seating and a late seating can also help to reduce the number of orders placed in the kitchen at a given time and allow a lower cook staffing complement while maintaining the desired dish-up time.

When we dine, we eat first with our nose as the food is delivered to the table, then with our eyes as it is uncovered, then with our palates. Therefore presentation is a very important component of meal service. The plating guidelines in Exhibit 8.1 can be helpful to ensure a good-quality presentation.

It is incumbent upon the chef or food service manager to train the staff to minimize the amount of movements and utilize their resources efficiently. The key to productivity in the kitchen is economy of time. How the line staff uses its time and organizes its production activities will keep the staff working at a consistent pace with minimal wasted movement. This organization is normally handled through the use of a production plan, which will be detailed later in this chapter. Before implementing the production plan, well-defined job descriptions for each member of the kitchen line staff should be available. In-depth discussion with each member of the team is necessary so that both the manager and the employee are of like

mind regarding the job tasks for each position in the kitchen.

Utility staff in the kitchen are responsible for cleaning and ware washing. However, during the normal course of their day chefs may be training these people in the art of fundamental food preparation. It is critical to first educate the utility staff on proper sanitation practices to avoid any potential cross-contamination. This scenario not only fills the production needs in the kitchen but also provides a logical growth path for junior staff. In fact, many people who have taken that path have proved themselves very valuable and have allowed the chef to avoid staffing an additional position. The end result creates a more cohesive team environment in the kitchen, allowing staff to focus on getting the job done rather than on separation of job duties.

The number of staff required to perform this function will vary according to a number of factors, including kitchen size, dishwasher capacity, number of meals served per meal period, amount of food preparation work required, and even kitchen configuration. As a general rule, a 200-unit community that serves one meal per day will require approximately 8–12 hours per day (1.4–2.1 full-time employees [FTE]); two meals, 12–16 hours/day (2.1–2.4 FTE); and three meals, 16–24 hours/day (2.4–4.2 FTE). Another way to budget this position is one FTE for each 100 meals served. For continuing care communities that operate two kitchens, additional staffing may be necessary to achieve com-

---

Exhibit 8.1   Guidelines for Plating

1. The main portion of the entree is placed at the bottom (6 o'clock) of the plate.
2. The plate should provide a contrast of colors.
3. There should be a contrast of shapes and textures on the plate.
4. Sauces and food must always be wiped from the rim of the plate.
5. Cooking juice must always be drained prior to plating the item (unless the juice is a vital component of the item, such as in a bouillabaisse).
6. Sauce must never be allowed to blend together on the plate (unless an artistic painting of sauces is being done).
7. Remember, simplicity is often better than ornateness.

pliance with nursing-home regulations. Kitchen utility staff should be largely responsible for maintaining the cleanliness of not only all food storage areas and coolers, but also back-of-house areas including hallways and delivery areas. Housekeeping staff should primarily concentrate on front-of-house common areas and resident apartments.

■■■■■ KITCHEN LAYOUT

Kitchen layout depends largely on the style of the product being served. In designing a new kitchen or remodeling an old one, the primary consideration must be traffic flow and the holding of food product. For example, too many people going to the same location at the same time increase the time it takes to complete that particular function. People crossing paths in the kitchen during production or during service may also increase the time necessary to provide meals and expose the staff to potential accidents. Knowing what you are going to serve and the volume of covers will enable the chef to establish work areas and traffic flow to complement rather than interfere with each other.

The kitchen has to be sized to hold food for the maximum number of meals that it is serving so that during either preparation or service employees can be positioned in a station that is self-contained. The kitchen and all its components (purchasing and receiving, dry storage, ware washing and utility, and dining room access) should if possible be set up like the spokes of a wheel whose axis is the production and cooking line. Kitchens laid out in this fashion promote the highest efficiency in serving and production times, which translates to savings in labor costs. Although satellite dining rooms can be very popular among residents in lending diversity to the dining experience, the time needed to set up and service these areas adds costs to the operation.

The equipment selected for the kitchen must be appropriate to the style of food product and to regional preferences. If you are going to employ primarily buffet or tray line service, the kitchen must have steam tables and additional radiant and alto sham ovens—in short, more holding and slow-cooking capacity because there is less immediate cooking. This cooking style will also require more holding space in the coolers or more walk-in capacity; plan on about 18 feet for the cooking line and about 14 feet for the tray line. Overall, a fully appointed kitchen equipment package should not exceed $110,000; add to that approximately $15,000 for kitchen smallwares and tabletop wares.

The food will be mass-produced and held on rolling racks in hotel pans. This type of kitchen requires larger pantry space to accommodate higher quantities of the same type of food coming in regularly. This is in sharp contrast to a typical restaurant set-up. The restaurant may produce 250 covers per night, but it will be served to the clientele from 5:30 P.M. until 10:00 P.M., so that small quantities of food products go through the kitchen and into the dining room a little at a time.

An à la carte set-up will require a standard restaurant line. For our purposes we will use 250 covers of production per night. Such a service style will require two convection ovens, a grill, a six-burner top and oven combination, a steamer, and a fifty-gallon jacketed steam kettle or tilt skillet (a fryalator is also a nice feature in parts of the country where residents like fried food). The front of the line would include two cook's reach-ins, a sandwich station, and a five-compartment steam table. Even for a seating table-service style, it is advisable to set up the kitchen with an à la carte line to provide maximum flexibility. What is then added to complement this arrangement is a banquet-style food-preparation area with additional refrigeration. The best combination is thus available to allow the operator to plate-up banquet style (dish-up to order) and finish-cook to order when necessary. This scenario provides the ability to produce high-volume output while providing the flexibility for handling cooked-to-order foods. This format will lend itself to almost any style of operation in a fraction of the space required for a banquet set-up.

In a banquet or seating operation, the ware-washing area must be much larger than in a traditional restaurant. The meals will all go out within 30 minutes and the dirty dishes will hit the dishwasher all at once. Therefore the area should be large enough for rapid turnaround, including tray breakdown, scrapping, sorting, loading, and unloading, with convenient access to rolling stock-storage areas that do not cross the path of the servers leaving with food to the dining room.

To save time and avoid exposure to theft, the storerooms and loading dock should be as close as possible to each other. The storerooms should be kept locked at all times, and it is a good idea to put the chef's office within sight of this area.

The dining room should have dual access, permitting the creation of a one-way traffic pattern. One door is used to take food out of the kitchen, while the other is used to return the dirty dishes. This system helps the staff avoid accidents and serves to keep the separate functions clear.

Ware Washing and Utility

Table 8.3 details the ware-washing requirements of a typical dish-up-to-order-style kitchen using two seatings. These calculations are for washing times only and do not include scraping (which can be done by the servers) and wash time for pots and pans. It is clear that considerable utility time is available during the non-peak times to assist with kitchen cleaning chores and sanitation practices.

To minimize breakage and maximize the dishwasher's efficiency, servers should break down their own bused trays. Servers usually will have time to do this if they are properly managed. In this way the sorting is done into the racks by the server instead of by the dishwasher. Be sure to remind the servers to wash their hands after breaking down a tray to avoid any cross-contamination.

When setting up the washer for use, the drains should be closed and the water turned on. The heating elements are not normally activated until the machine is full of water. The machine should then be allowed to run for a minute to allow the soap and chemicals to mix with the water. Before running any serviceware through the machine, the operator should check the gauges to ensure that the water in each tank is at the proper temperature. The correct temperature ranges to ensure proper sanitation are as follows:

- Prerinse   110°–120°F
- Wash   130°–150°F
- Power rinse   160°–170°F
- Final rinse   180°–190°F

The final rinse temperature must never be allowed to exceed 190°F or damage to the serviceware may occur. After two hours of continuous washing, the tanks should be drained and the scrape trays cleaned and refilled with fresh water and chemicals. If the machine becomes dirty or clogged, it cannot clean efficiently. Excess levels of grease can react with the detergent to form soap, further reducing the machine's capabilities.

Serviceware can be sanitized with hot water or chemicals. Most communities will have several systems for producing hot water. Domestic hot water will be much too cold for use in the laundry or the kitchen, so booster heaters can be added to the lines running to these areas. Chemical sanitizer baths are just as effective, but hot water does a better job of cleaning soiled dishes and removing lipstick stains.

Dishwashers will normally handle one or two dishracks per load. Two-rack washers are much more efficient in that they have a higher production capacity and can be used to wash virtually all of the kitchen pots and pans. Smaller one-rack washers are not nearly as versatile and will barely accommodate a sheet pan. The dishwasher should not be used as a substitute for the pot sink. A chemically treated, hand-scrubbed pot sink will clean the kitchen equipment more thoroughly and cost less. The average cost to wash a single load in the dishwasher, including chemicals *only*, is approximately 50 cents.

Scale is a gray-white mineral deposit that builds up inside the washing machine when the mineral content of hard water separates from the detergent solution at high temperatures. This scale can build up on the spray arms and rinse jets, reducing the water pressure

Table 8.3   Ware Washing

Wash time:	1.5 Minutes		
Washer capacity:	2.0 Racks		
Covers:	135		

Settings	Units/rack	Number of racks	Rounded
Silver (two runs)	100.0	1.4	1.0
Appetizer/miscellaneous	40.0	3.4	3.0
Glass*	30.0	4.5	5.0
China	30.0	4.5	5.0
Coffee*	30.0	4.5	5.0
Saucer	40.0	3.4	3.0
Soup*	30.0	4.5	5.0
Salad	40.0	3.4	3.0
Bread and butter	40.0	3.4	3.0
Dessert	40.0	3.4	3.0
Total		**36.3**	**36.0**
Turn-around time (wash only)			27.0
Turn-around time (rack only)			13.5
Turn-around time (re-stack only)			13.5
Total			**54.0**

*Handled only once.

and hampering the operation of the machine. A special acid solution can be used with caution to eliminate scale buildup. Operators should never use a bleach solution to clean the warewashing machine because bleach will react with the ammonia found in many cleaning agents to produce a toxic gas.

Washer arm bushings will begin to show signs of wear after the first year of use. As they wear out, the washer arm thumbscrews should be tightened or the dishwasher may rattle.

Flatware, whether silverplate or stainless steel, must receive special attention if corrosion or staining is to be avoided. Soaking soiled flatware as soon as possible loosens food, thus reducing tarnishing and corrosion that result from contact with certain food types. Most chemical manufacturers make available a presoak solution that is specially formulated for flatware. Presoak chemicals should be changed every two hours or they will lose their effectiveness. Additional chemicals should never be added to the solution to freshen it because salts can build up and damage the flatware.

Silverplated flatware can be detarnished at the same time it is being soaked. This is accomplished by soaking the flatware in an aluminum pan or placing a strip of aluminum in the bottom of the presoak pan. The soaking must take place in a slightly alkaline detergent solution where electrolysis can take place, removing the tarnish from the silver and depositing it onto the aluminum. Stainlessware must never come into contact with aluminum or pitting of the stainlessware can result. Therefore care should be taken not to soak stainless flatware with other kitchen utensils.

Flatware should not be allowed to dry between presoaking and washing. It should be washed with the eating surfaces up and stored with the eating surfaces down.

Serviceware is most efficiently stored in the plastic dishwasher racks on castered carts commonly referred to as rolling stock. This storage method minimizes breakage and provides portability both around the kitchen and to functions. In addition, racked serviceware is much easier to count for inventory purposes.

The frequency with which floors are cleaned will depend upon the use they get. Typically only spills and paper or litter are cleaned up immediately, leaving the main cleaning to the end of the day. Hard-surface floors should be stripped of all floormats, which can be steam-cleaned behind the service entry. The floor should be then swept and wet mopped. Some kitchens also use a pressure washer to clean their floors, but management should be certain that the floor has been sealed prior to using this method. The average times necessary to clean 1,000 square feet of floor area are as follows: sweeping, 16 minutes; wet mopping, 55 minutes; and dry mopping, 32 minutes. Pressure washing or steamcleaning can take somewhat longer inasmuch as any water standing on the floor will need to be removed and the floor allowed to dry prior to the replacement of the floormats (floormats can always be replaced by the morning staff).

The hood filters should be cleaned daily, especially if the fryer or broiler is used. Dirty filters can be a fire hazard and are easily cleaned by running them through the ware-washing machine.

Reach-in and walk-in cold storage areas should be thoroughly cleaned at least weekly. The floor and inside doors of the coolers should be wiped down and mopped daily. A critical area that is often overlooked is the fan coil unit. This unit can accumulate mold that is then dispersed by the fan to contaminate the entire contents of the cooler. It is important to remember to monitor the temperatures inside the coolers during cleaning. Occasionally the entire contents of the cooler may need to be removed in order to defrost or clean the shelf units. In this case, never return the food to the cooler until the temperature has returned to at least 40°F.

HEALTH AND NUTRITION

Operators of independent living retirement communities without any continuing care components are not required to provide specifically dedicated diet plans for residents. The process of maintaining a specific diet becomes the responsibility of the resident with the assistance of the food service staff, whose responsibility it is to educate the new resident in the use of the selective menu plan provided by the community. The food service director of a retirement community has the responsibility to provide a menu plan that is healthfully prepared and provides the resident the ability to make selections from a nutritionally balanced menu. Although the nutritional needs of older adults differ little from those of the young, the main difference is a slight reduction in calories, by about 10 percent after the age of 50, according to the Required Daily Allowance concept. Dietitians specializing in senior nutrition generally agree that a typical diet without restrictions for active, healthy seniors should consist of 55–60 percent carbohydrates, 12–15 percent protein, and 25–30 percent fat. It is incumbent upon the meal planner to provide nutrient-rich foods while allowing for smaller portions. An acceptable guideline for the elderly population, according to the *Guide to Normal Nutrition and Diet Modification* of the University of Florida, is as follows:

1. Meat, fish, fowl, cheese, eggs, and milk increase protein, iron, and zinc intake. Legumes and beans can supply remaining protein needs.

2. Carbohydrates, particularly sweets, should be limited to prevent weight gain and possibly decreased glucose tolerance. Whole-grain breads and cereals are helpful in adding fiber to aid elimination. Enriched breads and cereals supply needed complex vitamins and iron to the diet.

3. A variety of vegetables and fruits should be offered in order to replenish stores of vitamins A and C and to add fiber.

4. Six to eight glasses of water are recommended daily for adequate kidney function and to promote regular elimination.

5. Fat intake should be based on the older person's digestive ability and energy needs. Low-fat or skim milk supplies protein of high quality while reducing fat intake.

6. Adequate intake of calcium, iron, and vitamin C should be stressed. For example: vitamin- and mineral-fortified cereals, cheeses, and custards offer these nutrients in a well-accepted, easily chewable form.

Allowances have to be made for individual health, pharmacology, dentition, decreased activity, loneliness or other emotional factors, past eating habits, and decreases in the ability to taste and smell.

The operator and menu writer must make every effort to provide a menu plan that addresses the nutritional needs of this population. Although there are no specific federal guidelines regarding the need for a consulting dietitian, the operators of independent living communities should consider regular menu reviews for any community without a dietary manager on staff.

■ FLAVOR AMPLIFICATION IN FOOD: Catering to Taste and Smell Deprivation

It is not surprising to find that seniors almost unanimously name meals when asked what is the single most important aspect of their daily life in a retirement community. Mealtime brings residents together for socialization and companionship, and for many it represents the only time during their day when they can share their frustrations about the effects of their own aging process with others who can relate to them. This is particularly true for new residents or those with serious medical conditions or ailments. Although many seniors readily accept most of the effects of aging, they can be very challenging for others. Most people understand that as we age, the way in which we experience our world through our senses of sight, hearing, touch, taste, and smell changes as those senses deteriorate over time. As our visual acuity diminishes, we wear corrective lenses; with auditory loss, we wear hearing aids. However, the least accepted and least understood deprivations are those of taste and smell, the two senses that primarily control the body's ability to experience food. Disorders of taste and smell are viewed as affecting the "lower" senses—those involved with sensual and emotional life—rather than the "higher" senses that serve the intellect.[2]

The taste and smell of food have a major effect on levels of food intake and the maintenance of good nutrition. Losses and distortions in these chemosensory mechanisms contribute to a significant degree to anorexia in the elderly. Taste and smell are considered chemical senses because they are stimulated by molecules that contact receptors in the mouth, throat, and nasal cavity. The sense of taste is mediated by taste buds located on the dorsal surface of the tongue and on the epiglottis, the larynx, and the first third of the esophagus. Olfactory receptors are bipolar neurons located in the upper portion of the nasal cavity that project into the limbic system of the brain. The limbic system also processes information associated with emotions, so there is, in fact, a medical explanation for the emotional response we have to food. The olfactory bulb shows considerable degenerative changes during aging, and cross-sections of the bulb often look "moth-eaten" owing to losses in the number of cell bodies of neurons. Those losses are especially profound in patients with Alzheimer's disease.

Because of reduced function in these key chemosensory systems, the natural biochemical responses designed to break down food as it enters the body are consequently also less active. When the body smells, tastes, or simply sees appetizing food, a number of biochemical responses are set in motion to aid subsequent digestion. For example, saliva builds up in the mouth, gastrointestinal juices are released into the stomach, plasma insulin is released into the bloodstream, and the pancreatic system is engaged. All these responses have the combined effect of aiding absorption of food and promoting overall nutrition. As the aging process affects the body's internal response to food, seniors do not enjoy food as much or absorb it as well, and as a result they can become vulnerable to malnutrition, which can contribute further to health problems.

Taste and smell decrements arise not only from the normal aging process, but also from certain disease states, pharmacological and surgical interventions, the effects of radiation, and environmental exposure. Table 8.4 lists some medical conditions reported to affect the sense of taste. Table 8.5 lists some of the drugs commonly taken by the elderly that are reported to affect the sense of taste. Similar medical conditions and drugs affect the sense of smell. For example, most people have experienced the metallic taste of orange juice after brushing their teeth; the chemical in toothpaste responsible for this effect is sodium lauryl sulfate, which is also used to help fat-soluble drugs dissolve. Most elderly persons take their medications with their meals to offset the potentially harmful effects of the drugs on the stomach lining, which in turn affects their ability to taste and smell their food. Their senses are inhibited by these drugs, as is their digestive system, and this effect can at times induce a negative reaction and in severe cases lead to malnutrition.

Table 8.4 Medical Conditions That Affect Taste and Smell

Medical condition	Taste	Smell
Alzheimer's disease	✓	✓
Multiple sclerosis	✓	✓
Parkinson's disease	✓	
Tumors and lesions	✓	✓
Cancer	✓	
Liver disease (cirrhosis)	✓	✓
Cystic fibrosis	✓	✓
Hypertension	✓	
Psychiatric disorders	✓	✓
Radiation therapy	✓	✓
Diabetes mellitus	✓	✓
Influenza-like infections	✓	✓

Table 8.5 Effects of Drugs on Taste and Smell

Classification	Drug
Dental hygiene	Sodium lauryl sulfate
Diuretics, anti-hypertensive agents, and drugs for angina	Acetazolamiode
	Captopril
	Diazoxide
	Enalapril
	Ethacrynic acid
	Nifedipine
	Nitroglycerine patch
Hypoglycemic drugs	Glipizide
	Phenformin

Many medications commonly taken by the elderly are prescribed to be taken with food. Typically, residents in a retirement community will take their medications in the privacy of their rooms before coming down to the dining room for a meal. By the time their meals actually arrive at the table 30 minutes or more could have passed, giving the medication taken on an empty stomach ample time to be absorbed into the bloodstream and the opportunity to adversely affect the residents' ability to taste and smell their food. Simply advising residents to take their medications *after* they eat rather than before can have a profound effect on their overall dining satisfaction. In fact, at one community, after the residents were educated about this concept, resident satisfaction in food and beverage service increased by 10 percent over the previous survey, while perceptions of all other conditions remained constant.

Measurements of taste and smell dysfunction in older adults reveal a progressive decline with age. Those losses tend to begin around 60 years of age and become more severe in persons over 70 years of age. In most retirement communities, the chef and cooking staff have an ability to taste and smell that is more than twice as acute as that of the people for whom they are cooking. In one study, persons between the ages of 20 and 70 had approximately 206 taste buds each. This number was reduced to 88 taste buds for persons between the ages of 74 and 88 years.[3] The average age of residents in retirement communities today is about 82 years. Therefore even the best-qualified chefs working with the freshest natural ingredients are working at a considerable disadvantage, and they will express their frustration in trying to address this problem using conventional methods. Residents may inadvertently harm themselves by trying to amplify the flavors of their food by using too much salt at the table, or by eating too much dessert because they can still enjoy the sweet taste of many of these offerings. Compensating in these ways, however, only leads to nutritional imbalances and could be in direct conflict with doctor-prescribed dietary guidelines.

Recent studies suggest that the amplification of foods and beverages with naturally produced flavors can increase preference ratings as well as subsequent intake and absorption in elderly persons with known chemosensory losses. These commercially produced flavor enhancers, which are inexpensive (adding less than a penny to the per-meal cost), are made by reducing food such as chicken and capturing and concentrating natural flavor and odor molecules. The concentrate can then be attached to a "carrier" (such as water, oil, or flour) and added to the food. This added flavor contains no fat, salt, or other harmful products traditionally associated with flavor enhancement. Table 8.6 gives the percentage of elderly persons who preferred flavor-enhanced foods in one study at Duke University Medical Center.

Flavor-amplified foods not only are preferred from a sensory standpoint, but also can influence the body's natural biochemical response to food, actually pro-

moting better absorption and, as a result, improving the immune status of elderly persons. In a study by Schiffman and Warwick in 1993, elderly persons were offered regular food for three weeks, then flavor-enhanced versions of the same food. Blood samples were taken before and after the use of the flavor enhancement. They showed an increase in levels of T and B cells (white blood cells), the body's natural defense agents against disease and injury.[4] Schiffman's research confirms that as the body's biochemical absorption of food improves, so do nutrition and immune status. This research suggests that the addition to recipes of natural flavors that increase the perceived flavor intensity would improve satisfaction with the food and compensate for chemosensory losses due to normal aging, diseases, and prescription drugs. It can be argued that the use of flavor enhancements can actually promote better health as well as improve resident satisfaction.[5]

Learning that deprivation of taste and smell is a normal part of their aging process and that changes can be made to compensate for it becomes as natural to residents as wearing glasses to augment failing eyesight. Additionally, residents become aware that their enjoyment of food is enhanced by this flavor-amplification technique. It is also gratifying for them to see that management is willing to combine this knowledge with its culinary expertise to create a more tailored and flavorful dining experience.

The increased preference for flavor-enhanced food is extraordinary. In fact, many manufacturers of convenience products, such as Stouffers and Tyson, now list natural flavors among their ingredients. When a convenience product and its scratch-made counterpart are served, the convenience product is often better received than the homemade one. This is simply because the commercial product is higher in flavor than the homemade product as a result of added natural flavor. Certainly natural products are important and should represent the primary ingredient source. The addition of fresh herbs and spices and pretreating with marinades should not be abandoned. We walk a fine line, however: for if too many herbs and spices are added, the seasoning then overpowers the main ingredients. Often residents' delicate digestive systems become agitated when aromatic herbs and spices are not used in moderation.

Flavor enhancement improved food intake in 20 out of 30 foods tested. Research has confirmed an improved

Table 8.6 Preference for Flavor-Enhanced Foods by Elderly Persons

Food type	Unenhanced	Enhanced	Flavor used
Vegetables			
Carrots	25%	75%	Carrot
Green beans	17%	83%	Bacon
Green peas	6%	94%	Pea, bacon
Potatoes	39%	81%	Potato, bacon
Meats			
Beef (ground)	6%	94%	Bacon, beef
Beef (casserole)	37%	83%	Bacon, tomato
Chicken	40%	80%	Bacon, chicken
Soups			
Chicken	22%	78%	Chicken, bacon
Tomato	16%	84%	Bacon, tomato
Vegetable	17%	83%	Bacon, tomato, pea

immune status as measured by the total level of blood lymphocytes, which help to fight diseases inherent in the elderly population. In addition, residents feel better about their dining experience, and opioid (endorphin) levels increase as residents' ability to sense their food improves. It has actually been proven that residents become physically stronger as well. With flavor enhancement, residents are less interested in fatty foods and in adding salt to their entrees, and thus they are better able to adhere to their doctor-prescribed dietary guidelines.

PLANNING

The meal plans and budgeted expenses for each of the components of the menu plan should be determined at the time the proforma is written. The menu plan should address the number of meals a resident will receive per day as part of the service package included in their rent, any à la carte meals not included in the rent, the question of whether these meals are full-course or abbreviated meals, and the issue of full-course hot breakfasts versus continental breakfasts. It is important to note that at the planning stage it becomes very attractive to build many different meals and mini-events into the plan as a means of showing off the community and impressing guests. However, it should be noted that although there is an initial cost directly associated with the food, a more pervasive expense will be the labor and benefit costs associated with serving it. Once the basic number of meals per day has been determined and the budgeted food cost for each of those meals established, creativity and technical skill take over.

Breakfast

Breakfast is a great time in any retirement community. There is always plenty of activity and much conversation among residents discussing their plans for the day. When breakfast is offered and is included in the monthly service fee, residents will come. Additionally, in colder climates where there is less access to the outside at certain times of the year, the dining room becomes a congregating point for residents and breakfast an event. Many retirement communities use a combination of different breakfast offerings; for example, a basic continental breakfast of fruit juice, breakfast pastry, and a hot beverage will be available with an abbreviated à la carte hot breakfast menu. This allows the property the chance to produce a little revenue from the meal period to offset some of the additional cost, while offering some variety to residents.

A la carte breakfasts alone normally do not attract enough residents to justify their cost and will add little marketing advantage. The costs associated with the purchase of breakfast pastries will far exceed those associated with some hot breakfast items. Although use of a self-service breakfast will save on wait staff, the opportunity for residents to take a little something extra for a midmorning snack can escalate costs if the breakfast is not properly supervised. Whether the property offers a simple continental breakfast, an enlarged continental breakfast, or a hot breakfast, the most important issue governing breakfast is not its impact on food cost but the impact on labor and dining room maintenance.

Continental breakfasts are a very popular alternative to the à la carte breakfast. A continental breakfast can be offered "light" (coffee, juice, and muffins) or "heavy" (including hot cereals and a selection of fruit or breakfast meats). Many congregate retirement communities offer a light to medium continental breakfast to their residents and include the cost in their monthly service fee. A very nice buffet-style continental breakfast with an assortment of juices, pastries, fruits, hot cereal, and chef special of the day can normally be produced for under $1.00 per person. Although costs may vary in different regions of the country, efforts should be made to limit the definition of *continental*. A true continental breakfast should not require the presence of a cook behind the line during this meal period. The fruit can be sliced the day before and left covered in the walk-in cooler, and the opening server can easily be instructed in the fine art of making hot cereals.

It is a good idea to label different types of coffee, milk, and juices for easy identification by residents. Cold cereals can be purchased in bulk and stored in self-serve glass containers. Self-service juices and milk can be pre-poured into one-liter plastic carafes and kept cold in an iced cambro bin designed for this purpose. Avoid the use of single-serving cereal boxes because they can be conveniently removed from the dining room. Toasted items do not hold well but can be prepared in small quantities for serving in a heated hotel pan. Servers should avoid taking specialized toasting orders, inasmuch as they can create delays in the kitchen.

A continental breakfast buffet can be set up conveniently close to the kitchen entrance doors on skirted banquet tables or preferably on a built-in breakfast bar. It is a good idea to provide some type of floor protection or install special slip-resistant tile adjacent to the breakfast bar area.

Lunch

Lunch is also an excellent time to add revenue with the addition of an abbreviated à la carte menu. Always a favorite of the community's marketers, lunch provides some of the residents who like to entertain in the afternoon a chance to show off their home to friends, family, and associates. This program should be strongly considered during the fill-up stage of a new community. If dining-room space is limited as the community becomes fully occupied, residents can be encouraged to take their main meal at noon. Menus should be on the small side, feature chef's specials, change frequently, and be priced consistent with the going street rate for restaurant lunch meals. Depending on the climate, the community's proximity to other restaurants, and the independence of residents, lunch can be a money-making endeavor enjoyed by all.

Another lunch option is the shared menu concept, which allows residents the opportunity to have their main meal either earlier in the day or in the evening. Older, less active populations find this an attractive option, and the kitchen has an easier production plan for the day. This can also be a very economical option.

Some communities offer lunch as the main meal of the day, with a soup and salad bar set-up at the dinner meal. Many residents actually prefer this arrangement, choosing not to go to bed after a big meal. Many have found that this arrangement facilitates better digestion of their food during the day and better sleep at night. Operators may also find it easier to staff full-time positions with employees from breakfast through to lunch, rather than the typical short shifts in the evenings. In tight labor markets, operators have found that many people who are looking for part-time work prefer this arrangement over working the dinner hours, when they would rather be home with their families. With the main meal at dinner, many operators are forced to hire high-school students who are marginally reliable and who may go off to college about the time they become fully trained and proficient in their jobs. Long-term employees who are willing to work the evening shift and come to work in the dining room from another full-time job are usually more stable.

Dinner

The dinner menu is normally the critical menu plan of the day. There are a number of alternative methods in designing a menu for this meal period, beginning with the menu rotation. Writing a menu for retirement dining is different from the process in other venues in that your clientele is a captive audience. Overcoming boredom is the greatest challenge; therefore, the daily food and beverage program must offer variety, and this requires considerable planning on the part of the person writing the menu.

Menu rotations must consider the following factors: number of total menu days, number of courses per day, and number of selections per course; product availability, color, texture, and variety; staff schedules and skill level; style of service; and scratch cooking versus the use of convenience products. When evaluating a menu plan, no two entrees should come off the same position on the cooking line; if they do (e.g., two grilled items or two sautéed items), timing complications can ensue. Good results can be achieved with a two-, three-, or four-item entree selection. Fewer selections make achieving the necessary variety somewhat more difficult and may require implementing a number of standing menu items. A four-item entree selection that includes braised, roasted, sautéed, and grilled items creates diverse selections for residents, who can choose from a number of cooking techniques with optional accompaniments and sauces. This pattern of organization also maximizes the distribution of the workload throughout all the cooking positions in the kitchen.

Once the entrees have been selected, the other courses can be determined; they should complement the entree course. Most retirement communities offer the resident the opportunity to select among menu items, and it thus becomes the responsibility of the menu writer to develop a menu with side dishes that complement one another.

THE MENU

A well-written menu is the key to a cohesive food service operation. Not only does it provide a satisfying dining experience to residents, it also affects overall food costs, kitchen and dining room labor costs, and reputation. Menu writing is a learned skill dictated by residents' preferences, their ability to digest the type of food prepared, the budget available to produce the food, and its availability—all driven by the technical skill of the staff actually responsible for the daily production. It is important for the chef to have an understanding of the nutritional needs of the elderly combined with a sensitivity to their diminished senses of taste and smell. In the absence of such experience, management may choose to employ the services of a qualified consultant to develop menu plans until such expertise can be acquired by on-site staff. However, generally speaking, it is much better to survey the residents to determine their likes and dislikes, and then to design the menu around their preferences, than for an outside consultant to second-guess.

The availability and projected cost of the menu items selected become particularly important, especially if the property is working with a menu rotation. Selections should match the seasonal availability in the wholesale food market to minimize food cost. Each individual entree item in the cyclic menu should also be put out to bid and negotiated. In this way, the chef can ensure that the lowest price available in the market can be incorporated into the menu. Companies with several communities can take advantage of group purchasing strength by developing corporate menus, with each entree specified by price and vendor code number for ordering. For example, the corporate food and beverage director can negotiate the use of broken shrimp for seafood casserole at $5.40 per pound rather than buy whole shrimp at $7.10 per pound. Savings such as these really add up over the course of a four-week cycle. If the vendor order code and price are specified when the food orders are placed, the menus will have a very good chance of coming in within a few cents of the budgeted food cost.

As the menu begins to take form, careful consideration must be given to the color and texture of each of the components to eliminate the possibility of combining food products that are too similar in nature; for example, the all-white menu would include too many light-colored soups, sauces, poultry, vegetables, and starches. Another pitfall in cohesive menu planning is a menu that uses dishes with the same preparation method or accompaniment. For example, the stuffing menu—stuffed tomato salad, baked stuffed pork chops, stuffing for the starch, and baked apples stuffed with a dried fruit mélange—can become very repetitive. Although these selections may sound slightly far-fetched, writing a five-week menu cycle with two soups, two salads, one appetizer, four entrees, two vegetables, two starches, and two desserts offered per day can translate to 70 soups, 70 salads, 35 appetizers, 140 entrees, 70 vegetables, 70 starches, and 70 desserts. Although some repetition is acceptable, the sheer number of items in each of the categories can be somewhat difficult to manage. The menu plan is further complicated by the addition of garnishes and sauces.

As the menu plan continues to unfold, staffing issues must be addressed, including the depth of skill of the staff and the necessity of producing each menu item consistently each time it is offered. One sure recipe for disaster in menu writing is developing a menu that is too labor intensive or that requires culinary expertise far beyond the basic skill of the kitchen staff. Simple, well-prepared, "home-cooked" food consistently presented is what most people are used to eating, and it will normally be far better received than a half-hearted attempt at competing with the culinary trend of the moment. Certainly we never want to limit the creativity of our kitchen staff; however, consistency is infinitely more important in any food service, especially where the clientele returns to the same location to dine daily. Standardizing core recipes and in some instances entire menu plans is another essential tool, but it is important to remember that this tool is only as good as the accuracy of the standardized recipes and the amount of training available in the kitchen, to ensure that all the cooks are comfortable with the preparation methods employed.

Equally important—because it is directly associated with the amount of labor required in the kitchen—is the subject of scratch cooking versus the use of convenience products. We have discussed the need to use the best products available. It is also important to recognize that kitchen staff will do more than just cook during their shift. Daily food deliveries to be put away, sanitation, deep cleaning, in-service training, and administrative tasks all must be addressed during the average day. In addition, the menu planner should be aware of the many different products available on the market and where they fit into the budget, nutritional needs, and culinary orientation of the property.

PURCHASING

Once the menu has been designed, the next step is to develop a cohesive purchasing plan. There are different ways to purchase: contract buying, triple-bid purchasing, use of specified product directives, or a combination of all three. No matter which method of purchasing is used, it is critical at the project planning stage to allocate sufficient funds to purchase the appropriate goods for the style of food service contemplated.

Prior to any actual purchasing, specifications for each of the primary product categories and their planned use should be prepared. For example, what grade of meat will your property use—commercial/select, choice, or prime? Will you use fresh, frozen, or canned vegetables? Any of these are acceptable as long as they fit the market that has been selected and meet budgetary criteria.

Instead of using the highest grades of meat, consider using other cuts that still give high quality. For example, no-roll 109 prime rib at $2.45/pound versus choice at $2.74/pound, flat iron steak at $3.47/pound versus flank at $4.00/pound, and ground turkey at $1.36/pound versus ground beef at $1.72/pound. Though these differences seem small, the savings are $17.40 for 60 pounds of prime rib, $13.25 for 25 pounds of flat iron steak, and $14.40 for 40 pounds of ground turkey. Different cooking methods can also enable the chef to substitute a cheaper cut of meat. Alto sham ovens that use moist heat to cook can produce a very tender product with minimal shrinkage. Shams are also useful for holding food from one meal period or seating to the next without drying the product out.

Using a bid process with several different purveyors can also help to stretch your food budget. The chef should at a minimum use four meat, fish, and poultry and two produce purveyors. Case prices on produce can result in differences of from $0.25 to $6.00 for the same items. Purveyors will also feature weekly specials that can allow the chef to adjust menus to lower costs.

Consider the introduction of convenience products into your menu. These are labor-saving products, such as ready-cut produce and portion-controlled meat, fish, and poultry. These are not necessarily precooked products, but raw products that have been partially prepared. In no way do these products compromise the quality of your offerings. Rather, their use serves to enhance the production power of the kitchen by freeing chefs and cooks to do what they were trained to do—cook, not break down vegetables and butcher meat, fish, or poultry. Their use can also save money. Concentrated fruit juice can be up to 35 percent cheaper than canned juices. Vitality will even install a dispenser at no additional cost. Freshly squeezed orange juice costs about $0.16 per four-ounce serving compared with $0.08 per four-ounce serving for concentrate, a 50 percent savings.

Convenience products such as precut vegetables, frozen medley vegetables, and top-quality center-of-the-plate items are meant to augment the menu plans. These products have been available in the marketplace for at least ten years, and in that time much has been done to eliminate the negatives previously associated with them, such as flushing the vegetables with chemicals or gas to retard spoilage. Savings for precut carrots can add up to 40 percent. These items help to reduce waste from raw product preparation work, help to control labor costs, and give your food service a consistency that is sometimes lacking owing to absenteeism, administrative duties, sick days, vacations, and other labor shortages. The convenience-product industry has made tremendous strides to make products that meet the high standards demanded in fine restaurants. Although convenience products are not always the answer to runaway food costs, they can help to bring immediate consistency to the food-service product and require a minimum skill level to prepare. Resident response to these products, as to everything else, is mixed, and this is why it is always important to limit the appearance of such products to no more than 20 percent of the menu. The following example compares community-prepared items with Sysco's Classic Brand:

Chicken Cordon Bleu, 4 oz., 36 pk, no. 1624329	$31.78	
4 oz, $0.95 raw ingredients + $0.20 labor	$ 1.15	
Sysco Cordon Bleu	$ 0.88	
Savings	$ 0.27	23%
Stouffer's Vegetable Lasagna, 4 pk/case, no. 1013978	$39.17	
One portion $0.80 raw food + $0.20 labor	$ 1.00	
Stouffer's	$ 0.78	
Savings	$ 0.22	22%
Sysco New England Scrod Cod, 40 pk, no. 1782549	$16.00	
One portion $0.83 raw food + $0.15 labor	$ 0.98	
Sysco New England Scrod Cod	$ 0.75	
Savings	$ 0.23	23%

Convenience items should be introduced only when the pricing is comparable with or less expensive than the total cost of the raw product plus preparation-labor costs. Communities that can save 8 to 12 cook-hours per week through the use of these products will ultimately realize an annual savings of $4,000–$6,000 in kitchen labor.

Other cost-saving strategies include better utilization of leftovers. For example, one can freeze leftover fish to use in newburg dishes, stir-fries, and stews. In a 300-unit community the average cost for the fish entree for one evening can run to $250.00. Using leftover fish one night per week can save $1,000 in food costs per month or $12,000 per year.

When and how often you purchase is contingent on the available storage space and the depth of the menu offered. It is important to remember that there must be sufficient lead time between the actual purchasing and the proposed date of use to allow for receiving, storage, and preparation of the products. One rather simple rule of thumb is that the entire inventory should be turned over every five to seven days. Along the same line, budget dollars used for purchasing food that is not readily used and will remain in inventory for more than seven days are money not well spent. Excessive inventory resulting from poor production planning is normally the main contributor to cost overruns. Inventory in dry storage and coolers should not exceed 10–12 percent of the monthly food budget: a well-devised purchasing plan will help to keep this level in check. All deliveries should be made to the community during nonproduction times, allowing the order to be verified against the purchase order and properly checked in. It is also a good idea to check on the cost and availability of products as the menu plan is being created. Locally created menus can take advantage of regional price breaks and vendor specials—savings that a corporate menu plan can often fail to realize.

Communication is the next important issue in purchasing. As food-service staffs are downsized it is important to emphasize the need for written communication. Weekly vendor bid sheets and purchasing logs that include a complete listing of items purchased—specifying vendor, accepted price, amount of product, day ordered, and delivery date—should be routinely prepared by the chef to maximize the value achieved from budgeted dollars. At no time should there be a question regarding the status or location of

the food products to be used. Exhibit 8.2 itemizes additional cost-saving strategies.

PRODUCTION PLANNING

Remembering the importance of clear communication, and that operating a good food service operation requires the management of a multitude of details, brings us to the necessity of having a cohesive production plan. While much of what we do every day is the taking in and processing of verbal information,

---

Exhibit 8.2   Cost-Saving Tips for the Kitchen

1. Establish low-labor emergency menus in case you lose an employee for a day or more.
2. Always prepare food one day in advance.
3. Plan vacations. Prepare some foods ahead and freeze items such as breaded items, quiche, and pesto.
4. Plan menus with labor balance. If you have high-labor entrees, use low-labor vegetables and salads.
5. Buy foods competitively. Use at least two purveyors for each fish, produce, meat, and grocery product.
6. Use leftovers in attractive lunch specials, employee meals, or soups.
7. Take advantage of purveyors' insights into fluctuating markets.
8. Forecast menu items so that you do not overprepare.
9. Adjust preplanned 30-day menus to eliminate overpriced items. When raspberries are $42 and strawberries are $10, switch to strawberries.
10. Slow-roast expensive meats to increase yield and tenderness.
11. Install soap dispensers in dishwasher and pot sinks to minimize waste.
12. Train all personnel to care properly for all equipment and utensils to maximize life.
13. Keep the kitchen and food storage areas locked at night.
14. Minimize the number of entrees. More entrees mean more inventory and more expense.
15. Minimize food inventory in the walk-ins and dry food storage areas. Inventory should not exceed 10–12 percent of the monthly food budget and should be turned every five to seven days.

none of us has the ability to remember everything we are told. Again, the written message takes on a new significance. As a matter of course any food service manager must plan the day's production, and she should also take the time to communicate to the entire staff the needs of the day and the parties responsible for the work. Kitchens and dining rooms are exceptionally busy places, and in the rush of activity much can happen to distract individuals from their primary tasks.

A well-written production plan (Exhibit 8.3) creates the database for many of the daily functions of the food service department. Initially it should list the menu items being prepared during the initial time frame, the amounts of raw product, the number of portions, the size of cooked portions, directions and standard recipe, the time of completion, the name of staff member assigned to the task, the quantity of any remaining items or a notation when the item ran out, and the planned use of any items remaining at the end of the service. The production plan not only specifies the quantity of each item to prepare, it also serves to document consumption. One of the key challenges facing the chef

---

Exhibit 8.3   Meal Production Planning

STANDARD PRODUCTION SHEET

Site: _____   Day: _____

Date: _____

Menu item	Quantity to prepare	Total # of raw portions (oz.)	Cooked portion size (oz.)	Directions	Time ready for service	Leftover amount	Run-out time	Leftover disposition	Supervisor	Prep person
Entree 1 Sauce: Garnish:										
Entree 2 Sauce: Garnish:										
Entree 3 Sauce: Garnish:										
Alternate										
Soup										
Salad 1										
Salad 2										
Starch										
Vegetable 1										
Vegetable 2										
Dessert 1										
Dessert 2										

is to predict accurately the amount of each entree that will be ordered. The balance between the amount of food to order and the risk of running out of a particular entree is critical to resident satisfaction and managing food cost. Historical data on resident preferences and volumes ordered is extremely beneficial when used by the managers as they create new menus and purchase, schedule, and review the staffing and supervision needs of the operation. In this way the chef can keep track of resident tastes and patterns of consumption when ordering and planning for future menu rotations.

Chefs can become very skilled at managing their budgets through menu planning based upon historical production plans. For example, they can put a high-cost entree on the menu with a very popular lower-cost item to minimize the number of high-cost orders. They can also include a popular item on the menu on the same night that they try out a new creation or a new convenience product. Careful menu and production planning is the hallmark of a seasoned chef.

If there was ever a phrase to describe the production of food for any type of hospitality operation—be it a restaurant, a hotel, or a retirement community—it would be "timing is everything." If the production plan in the back of the house has not gone well, all the dining room ambiance and clever, diplomatic conversation on the part of wait staff and managers will not cover for the fact that the kitchen is "in the weeds" and the food is not ready or the orders are backed up. There is no turning back, especially in a dining setting where the clients are *living* with you. A bad or inefficient production timetable wreaks havoc with budgeted staffing schedules in both the front and the back of the house while jeopardizing resident satisfaction, which can ultimately affect your marketing effort. Most residents are understanding of an occasional bad meal, because even in their own homes when cooking for themselves they have known disaster. They will certainly tolerate this when it happens, provided it is the exception rather than the rule. Yet they will also always react when they begin to see trends headed in the wrong direction, because they have a vested interest in the quality of food service: they are simply unable to dine elsewhere. In addition, because most residents will have paid for these meals in advance at the beginning of the month, they pay for a meal whether they like it or not. No one can guarantee perfection; however, good production planning can help to minimize mis-takes. The planning and responsibility for its preparation fall to the executive chef; the cooks, prep staff, and utility staff follow and rely on the lead of this individual. They expect that all of the appropriate steps will have been taken to provide them with the tools they need to produce the food within the necessary time frame.

Although we can all agree that the preparation plan and timing are critical to the success of the operation, there is another, equally important facet of the implementation process: the actual dish-up. Once the style of food service that the property will provide has been determined, the organizational skills of the chef and cooks at those times when the dining room is full become critical. Economy of time requires that every movement of the line staff, whether cooking à la minute or dishing up to order, be analyzed to maximize their efforts. A well-designed steam table with like foods grouped together promotes a logical dish-up progression, facilitates the quick and smooth filling of orders, and is the key to good service in the dining room. Every item necessary to fill any of the menu orders must be prepared and available before the opening of each meal period.

INVENTORY SYSTEMS AND COST CONTROLS

Several methods are commonly used in the industry to calculate food costs. Some companies calculate their costs very simply at the end of each month using the direct method, while others track their daily food cost by splitting their inventory into direct and indirect items and using a storeroom requisition system. There are advantages to each system.

Under the monthly system, all expenditures during the course of the month are totaled on a receiving report or collected from a weekly food vendor invoice. As these items are delivered and stored, the cases and individual items are marked with their corresponding cost. This can be found on the extended vendor invoice and should include shipping charges.

It is also essential to keep a daily meal count summary for each and every meal that leaves the kitchen. These meals include breakfast, lunches, dinners, guest meals, marketing meals, and employee meals. At the end of each day, week, and month, the meal counts are totaled. The true cost calculated per meal is only as good as the accuracy of the meal counts: too low a meal count (which is normally the case), results in an artificially inflated cost per meal.

An inventory is taken on the last day of each month, priced, and extended. The increase or decrease is calculated based on the inventory of the preceding month. Decreases are added to the total food costs from the receiving invoices, and increases are subtracted. Normally the chef will reduce the food cost based on the raw food costs incurred for banquets and parties, which are events with associated nonmeal costs. The adjusted total is then divided by the total number of meals served to reach a cost per meal (see Table 8.7 for an example).

The monthly system has the advantage of minimizing paperwork and the associated error that inevitably enters into the system. All food purchased each month and used is considered a direct charge to the food cost. The daily system is considerably more complicated, but it can produce a daily food cost that enables chefs to manage food cost and budget over the course of the month rather than wait until the month's end to discover that they have missed the target.

Under the daily system, all food items received are classified as either direct or indirect. Direct foods are generally perishables that will be used during the course of the month in which they are delivered. Direct foods can include fresh meat; deli meat; frozen convenience entrees; frozen meat; fish and poultry; all fresh produce; all dairy products; dispenser juice and coffee; ice cream, sherbets, and yogurts; fresh herbs; and fresh breads and rolls. Direct purchases are not requisitioned as they are used; rather, they are accounted directly to the food cost for the month in which they are received from the vendor. Indirect products are those that generally have some significant shelf life and are requisitioned from the storerooms. Indirect foods can include any product in the dry storeroom and all frozen desserts, frozen vegetables, and frozen breads and muffins.

Under the daily food cost system, a running or perpetual inventory is kept on the indirect food items using a requisition form. When indirect items are removed from their secure storage area by the chef, they are itemized on a requisition form. The daily inventory is calculated by using the closing inventory from the previous month, *plus* inventory purchases that are put into storage each day, *less* requisitions to equal the closing inventory. The difference gives the daily total food cost. In other words, the gross daily food costs are equal to the daily direct purchases plus inventory requisitions. This figure will fluctuate on days when deliveries

Table 8.7 Calculating Food Costs per Meal

Monthly purchases	
Meat and fish	$ 17,867.60
Dairy products	$ 4,702.00
Fruits and vegetables	$ 4,231.80
Other food costs	$ 20,218.60
Total all food costs	**$ 47,020.00**
Inventory	
Beginning	$ 4,274.68
Ending	$ 3,792.68
(Increase) decrease	$ 482.00
Adjustment	$ 47,502.00
Less banquet and party raw food cost	$ 195.00
Total adjusted monthly food cost	$ 47,370.00
Total meals served	18,808
Monthly cost per meal	**$ 2.52**

occur, but it has a tendency to balance out as the month progresses. Total daily costs are divided by the daily meal counts in the same manner as the monthly system to yield the daily cost per meal. A full inventory of all indirect foods is performed on the last day of each month to calculate an ending inventory and make any adjustments to the monthly food cost. Goods in production (items already requisitioned out that day) and direct issues (perishables) are not included in the inventory.

The main advantage to the daily system is control, but with control comes complication. The system can easily break down if food is improperly classified, or if the chef fails to requisition the issues from indirect storage, or if storage areas are accessible to other staff members. The daily system is useful for communities that are in the fill-up stage, in which costs to feed the growing population are constantly changing. Once the community has stabilized, however, the daily food-cost system becomes more trouble than it is worth. It is a difficult system to teach new employees, and it can be a real source of frustration to the accounting department, which normally performs the daily calculations.

Another method of calculating food cost is by recipe cost. This is done by multiplying the potential recipe cost per portion by the number of portions served. This method is useful to cost out an individual entree or menu, and it is often used to estimate banquet, special function, or catered meal costs. Under this system, portion control is vital. If there is too much variation in the size of the individual portions, then the total estimate will be inaccurate.

Potential recipe costs can be provided with computer-generated recipe cards, taking care to ensure that the ingredient costs are current. Portions served are determined by noting the number of attendees at the meal and by keeping accurate meal abstracts. The cost per portion multiplied by the portions served and then divided by the total number of portions served will yield the average cost per meal.

Cost per meal is often confused with daily food cost. Depending on utilization, a continental breakfast costing approximately $1.00 per person to produce, combined with a dinner that may run as high as $3.69, can yield a combined daily food cost of $4.69, but when averaged on a per-meal basis, the cost is only $2.35 per meal. When comparing food costs from different communities, it is important to be sure that the data compare apples to apples: many variations in food service package and meal count methods may occur, and some may not always translate well to your program. For example, many communities also include kitchen labor costs in their per-meal calculations, which can add from $1.00 to $1.50 per meal to the cost. The industry average food cost per meal for congregate care for a low-end program will be $1.60–$1.80 per meal; a moderate program will range from $1.80 to $2.25; and a high-end program can run from $2.50 all the way up to $3.00 per meal. These ranges will of course depend on the number of meals offered per day, and they can be a blended rate of dinner and breakfast or lunch and dinner. Finally, some chefs will back out guest and employee meal revenues from their food cost to reduce further their per-meal cost.

To break down food cost per meal to each meal period, multiply the food cost per meal by three (for a three-meal-per-day program), then divide by two because half of the total daily food cost will be dinner or the main meal. The other half should be split one-third for breakfast and two-thirds for lunch. For example, a food cost per meal of $2.28 translates to $6.84 per day; dividing by two sets the main meal cost at $3.42. Dividing the other $3.42 by three sets the cost of breakfast at $1.14, and the remaining $2.28 will be the approximate cost of lunch. The actual costs may vary slightly in proportion, depending on the menu selections at each meal.

■■■■ SANITATION AND SAFETY

The importance of a well-designed, well-managed, and well-implemented sanitation and food safety program supersedes all other facets of a food service operation. It is incumbent upon the operators to set well-defined policies (with appropriate training) that meet and even exceed federal and local standards. A food handling and safety training program is intended to safeguard the health of residents and employees alike. Food must be undamaged, clean, free from adulteration and contamination, and completely suitable for human consumption. Residents expect to be served safe, appetizing food that has been prepared and handled in a sanitary manner in a clean environment. The food service supervisors and managers are responsible for knowing, understanding, and enforcing the standards and practices called for by the program. Additionally, most states have certification programs for food handlers, and some of these are mandatory. A certified food-service supervisor should be available during all operating shifts in both the front and the back of the house. Therefore the chef, sous chef, food service director, dietary manager, or dining room managers, or all of these personnel, should have local certification.

Although it is extremely difficult to run a perfect operation, supervisors must be aware of their employees' practices, the condition of the equipment, and the ability of the food service staff to adhere to the required policies at all times and to take immediate action, when and if a problem arises, to correct it. The good food-service team looks for ways to raise standards, and careless attitudes should not be tolerated. All food-service staff should be encouraged to clean up as they go, as well as to maintain themselves and their work areas in a clean and efficient manner. All employees should receive training within their first week of employment to eliminate the possibility of acquiring any inappropriate food-handling and safety habits. Thereafter employees should be scheduled to review the program as part of an ongoing training and review process. The cost of these efforts is minimal compared with that of transmitting a food-borne illness, which could devastate the community's hard-earned reputation and significantly hamper marketing efforts. The tasks required to handle and prepare food safely are a learned behavior. Employees performing those tasks should feel that they are a natural part of their work routine. Their supervisors are ultimately responsible for the success or failure of any food safety standards program.

Table 8.8   Shelf-Life for Common Fruits and Vegetables

Apples, fresh	Store in fruit or vegetable box three weeks to a month. Inspect daily to remove rotten fruit so that the balance will not be contaminated. Watch for blue mold or black rot.
Apricots	Easily stored for one to two weeks.
Asparagus	May be kept in refrigerator one week after ripening.
Bananas	May be kept at 50 to 60 degrees and used within two to three days after ripening. Do not store in the cooler at any time.
Berries	All fresh berries can be kept for a week to 10 days. However, it is recommended that these be used as quickly as possible for best flavor.
Broccoli	Can be stored for eight to ten days.
Cabbage	Early variety will keep about two weeks. Late variety is much sturdier—will last two months.
Cantaloupe	Inspect daily for ripeness. When ripe, may be held in the cooler for one week.
Carrots	If in good condition, they may be kept in the storeroom for a few days. Under refrigeration, they will last three months.
Cauliflower	May be kept for two weeks if the leaves are not cut away. After the leaves are removed, it deteriorates rapidly.
Celery	Should not be kept longer than a few days. If it is wilted, placing in water will freshen it.
Corn	Corn is one of the most sensitive of vegetables and should be used within 24 hours of arrival.
Cranberries	May be stored in a vegetable box for as long as two months.
Cucumbers	These are not sturdy and should be used within one week.
Eggplant	Should not remain in storage for more than a week.
Garlic	Can be kept for about two months at temperatures from 55 to 66 degrees. In vegetable cooler at temperature from 32 to 36 degrees, garlic will last four months.
Grapefruit	Will last six weeks at 32 to 36 degrees.
Grapes	White seedless or red Tokay grapes will keep for four weeks. Red Emperor, obtainable in fall, will keep for two months.
Kale	At temperatures from 32 to 36 degrees, kale will remain in good condition for three weeks.
Lemons	May be kept from one to two months at 50 to 60 degrees.
Lettuce, Iceberg	If in good condition and inspected regularly, iceberg lettuce may be kept for four weeks. The leaves should not be removed until the lettuce is to be used, unless they have begun to rot. However, to obtain maximum quality, lettuce should be used as soon as possible after arrival.
Limes	Will not last in storage more than two weeks.
Melons	May be stored for a maximum of three weeks. However, it is recommended that they be used as soon as the proper degree of softness is achieved.
Mushrooms	Fresh, should not be kept more than one or two days.
Onions, Green	If kept under refrigeration, will last a week or 10 days.
Onions, Yellow	If stored in a cool, dry place, unrefrigerated, will last three months.
Oranges	Should be used within a week if possible. If necessary they may be held in a reasonably good condition for a month or six weeks.
Parsley	Will last for a week. Keep well iced.
Parsnips	Can be stored two to three months at 32 to 36 degrees.
Peaches	Most varieties will last about a week; the yellow cling variety will last about two weeks. Must be inspected and sorted each day.
Pears	Summer or Bartlett variety—before ripening, may be kept three weeks at 65 to 75 degrees; after ripening, must be refrigerated and used within a few days. These require gentle handling to prevent bruising and must be sorted every five days. Bosc or Comice variety may be kept six weeks before ripening if sorted weekly.
Tomatoes	Should not be kept more than a week after ripening. They require daily sorting for ripeness.
Turnips	Will keep 10 days to two weeks without refrigeration. Under light refrigeration, will last three months.
Watermelon	May be held a week to 10 days.

Food Safety Standards and Practices

- Employees should not be allowed to work with food when they are sick.
- All cuts and abrasions should be cleaned with soap and disinfectant and covered with a bandage or waterproof protector.
- Employees may not work with a wound that may be infected.
- Employees should bathe daily and use deodorant.
- Employees should wear freshly cleaned outer clothing or uniforms daily.
- Employees must restrain or cover their hair at all times.
- Employees may not smoke, chew gum, or eat around food work areas.
- Employees must wash their hands regularly in warm water (110°–115°F) and soap

  When entering the kitchen

  After using the restrooms

  Before and after any food, coffee, or cigarette breaks

  After handling garbage

  After handling any soiled equipment

  After handling raw food products, such as meats, poultry, and cooked foods

  After coughing or sneezing

  After handling hair, facial hair, soiled uniforms, or any skin

- Hand sinks are used for washing hands, not for working with food.
- Sanitize all equipment after each use.
- Frequently sanitize all food contact surfaces.
- Do not wipe food contact surfaces with kitchen rags.
- Always have sanitizing solution available at each work station.
- Always use the proper color-coded cutting boards for each food product.

Government-approved concentrations for sanitizer solutions are as follows:

Surface: 100 ppm min.   200 ppm max.
Dip: 50 ppm   100 ppm

A concentration of 200 ppm is 1 tablespoon of bleach, 5.25%, in 1 gallon of water.

All food products coming into the facility should be checked immediately to ensure that they meet the community's standards and returned to the appropriate vendor if they are in any way questionable in quality or freshness. Dry foods should be stored out of their original packaging. Raw foods should never be stored above cooked products. Spoiled, returned, damaged, or otherwise unwholesome food should be held in separate storage areas. Ice for human consumption cannot be used for any other purpose. Food requiring refrigeration must be cooled to an internal temperature of 40°F or below. Cooling time for cooked food should never exceed four hours. Frozen food should be stored and maintained at 0°F or below. Table 8.8 outlines shelf-life for common fruits and vegetables.

Chemicals must always be stored separate from food. All stock must be rotated to allow the use of the oldest products first. A pest control program must be implemented immediately upon operation of the food service.

It is generally the responsibility of any food service supervisor to contact the local authorities and take immediate action if necessary to protect the health of the community.

Training can be performed in a number of ways: in-service meetings, videotaping of correct procedures, display of work-area posters depicting proper sanitation and food-handling techniques, or individualized attention such as daily sanitation-side worksheets.

NOTES

1. The National Association of Nutrition and Aging Services Programs (NANASP) publishes national standards for congregate and home-delivered food services and programs as well as a newsletter entitled *Many Hats,* which includes tips for site managers and has activity updates. They also sponser regional and state training seminars on senior nutrition and programming. The organization was formerly known as the National Association of Title Seven Directors. They can be contacted at 2675 44th Street SW, Suite 305, Grand Rapids, MI 49509. Phone (616) 530-3250, fax (616) 531-3103.
2. C. Lucas, B. W. Pearce, and S. S. Schiffman, "Reactivating Appetite," *Contemporary Long Term Care* 17(12) (Dec. 1994): 55.
3. S. S. Schiffman, "Taste and Smell in Disease," *New England Journal of Medicine* 308 (1983): 1275–79, 1337, 1343.
4. S. S. Schiffman and Z. S. Warwick, "Effect of Flavor Enhancement of Foods for the Elderly on Nutritional Status: Food Intake, Biochemical Indices, and Anthropometric Measures," *Physiology and Behavior* 53 (1992): 395–402.
5. For more information on research on and availability of flavor enhancements, contact the Flavor and Extract Manufacturers Association of the United States (FEMA), 1620 Eye Street NW, Suite 925, Washington, DC 20006. Phone (202) 293-5800, fax (202) 463-8998.

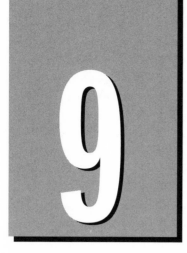

9 Dining Services

The most important event in the daily lives of the residents in a retirement community is their dining experience. No single aspect of the operations in any community receives more attention than the food service. Most people consider the *entire* dining experience when they evaluate the quality of their meal and their overall satisfaction with the services the community has to offer. An occasional bad meal can be overcome by good service, and a quality dish can counteract the effects of some bad service. But when poor service is combined with an inferior food product, residents will react. The degree to which the dining room operation meets or exceeds the resident's expectations can affect the community's reputation more than almost any other aspect of the operation.

The style, interior design, and even architecture of the building will establish a certain expectation about the operations housed within it. If the building is lavish and upscale in appearance, the residents and guests will expect top-quality food service. If the food service is unable to live up to the expectations established by the building, the residents and guests will not speak of the property positively within the community. On the other hand, if the food quality and service meet or exceed the residents' expectations of what the building communicates, then they will say so.

When the residents enter the dining room, they seek something more than merely to satisfy basic hunger or thirst. "They are seeking an 'experience'—a sensory envelope of sight, sound, taste, smell, touch, that matches a mood or reinforces an image of self."[1] In addition, this may be one of the only times during the day that they socialize with other residents. During their dinner they will look for things they have in common to discuss, and their current dining experience will be a popular topic.

FOOD AND BEVERAGE SERVICES

Each community organizes its service package according to the local market, the needs of its current and target resident population, and its budget. Some communities provide food services à la carte, whereas others bundle food within the monthly service fee. Assisted living communities generally offer three meals a day, whereas congregate or continuing care retirement communities generally offer an allotment of meals, usually 30 a month. For most communities, a light breakfast and a two- to three-entree dinner is sufficient. A cost-benefit analysis should be done before any consideration is given to adding a midday dining option. Most assisted living communities have little choice about this midday meal, but other retirement communities with a less frail population should consider this option very carefully. The lunch meal will have the biggest impact on labor cost by converting short four-hour morning shifts into eight-hour shifts. Unless this additional cost can be recovered from the residents through à la carte billings or a general rent increase, the implementation of a midday meal will have the effect of decreasing the operating margin of the community.

Most communities offer breakfast daily, either full service or continental. The breakfast can be served buffet style or in a combination of table service and buffet. The typical continental breakfast will feature hot beverages; assorted juices; fresh fruit; dry cereals with skim, whole, or lactaid milk; a pastry and bread selection; and a hot cereal.

Some communities prefer to serve the main meal at lunchtime, with a soup-and-sandwich dinner. Residents of these communities would rather have their larger meal at noon than go to bed after dinner with a full stomach. Others prefer a light meal at noon and reserve the evening meal as their main dining and socializing time. For the lunch meal, offering the soup du jour, the chef's daily hot or cold entree, standard alternatives, salad selections, the daily dessert special, and beverages should be adequate to meet the residents' expectations.

The dinner meal will, of course, attract the most attention. The standard dinner menu should feature a choice of soup or salad, a choice of two entree items (to include meat, fish, poultry, or the chef's addition), and the chef's selected dessert or ice cream. All primary meals should be served with fresh rolls and butter, as well as a hot or cold beverage selection. Residents are permitted to have seconds, or they may order a smaller portion. A chicken or fish alternate should also be available, cooked à la minute. Some communities offer premium alternates—such as shrimp, filet mignon, or prime rib—and add an up-charge to the resident's bill through a check or chit system. Some communities have managed to generate as much as $13,000 per year in additional revenue from their premium foods.

In addition to the normal daily food service, most communities sponsor special events, such as a Wednesday afternoon tea or a weekly cocktail hour. These events encourage residents to mingle and socialize or welcome new residents. They are generally staged in one of the common rooms and feature finger sandwiches, cookies, and pastries presented on silver trays. Residents are served tea, coffee, or punch and a snack item determined by the local food service director. During weekly cocktail hours, residents provide their own liquor, while the community provides mixers, limited garnishes, ice, glassware, and dry snacks.

A resident volunteer or activity director generally provides bartender services.

The ability to offer the residents alcoholic beverages will depend on state and local licensure requirements. Most states and municipalities require that a community possess a liquor license in order to sell alcoholic beverages to residents. If the community is located near a local school or library, this activity may be prohibited altogether. Residents can, of course, consume their own spirits in their own apartments or in common areas. Many residents enjoy a before-dinner cocktail or wine with their meal. Residents can decant their own wine or have an employee who is of age do so. Liquor sales in larger communities can be a significant source of income to the property. One 340-unit congregate community in Chicago had a bar service that yielded $900 per month in additional revenue to the project without any additional labor costs. They were able to attract 20 percent of their residents to the lounge daily, with each visitor consuming an average of 2.5 drinks. Residents generally pay for their drinks by signing a chit that is posted to their monthly accounts. Of course good security and portion control of the liquor are essential to running a successful bar.

SERVICE STYLES

There are three basic service styles in the dining room. The dining room can be opened continuously, opened for a specified dining period within which all residents can be served, or opened and closed for short periods using prearranged seating times. Generally speaking, the longer the dining room is open to the residents the higher the cost in labor for both the front and the back of the house. Longer time periods within which the dining room is open provide maximum flexibility for the residents and lessen the institutional feel of a community. Residents who were used to eating whenever they wanted before moving into the community typically have some difficulty adjusting to predetermined dining times.

The problem with open seating times in the dining room is that most people come down to eat at the same time, so that the dining room must be operated like a restaurant. Restaurants are very inefficient in feeding large amounts of people in short amounts of time. They are typically open for dinner from 6:00 to 10:00 P.M. and count on the fact that their customers will arrive to eat at times more or less evenly distributed over the evening. If all of their customers were to arrive in a two-hour period, seating, service, and production capacity would quickly be exhausted. When the restaurant reaches capacity, it simply turns people away or asks them to wait. This can never happen in a retirement community where residents have *already paid* for their meals through their monthly service fees.

The two-seating dining concept has proven a more comprehensive way to give top-quality service within a limited time frame and with limited staff. This concept can be applied to one or all meals. The dining room is closed for 30 minutes between seatings to allow the food service staff to reset the room and the cooking staff to fire the next set of entrees and vegetables. The advantages of the two-seating arrangement include the following:

Operating costs are lower. Staffing levels are necessary only to serve one-half to two-thirds of the population. Normally 60 percent of the population will choose the first seating when offered a choice.

Food is plated and served more quickly. Far fewer orders are placed at one time, eliminating the bottleneck that normally occurs behind the line when the majority of residents come to the dining room and place their orders within a one-hour period. Typically, food service programs that experience numerous complaints about slow service suffer from too many orders being placed in too short a time. The kitchen responds by rushing each order through the line, which increases the potential for error. Restaurant-style service in the dining room is not well suited to the senior clientele, which generally comes to eat at the dining room en masse. It is more efficient to serve a group of residents who are seated at one time.

Food is fresher. The kitchen can prepare the food in two batches, which reduces the tendency for certain dishes, especially vegetables, to become overcooked as they are held for long periods in the steam table. Resident selections of alternates that may need to be cooked to order can also be more easily accommodated. In addition, if the kitchen experiences a run on one entree, then additional alternates can be prepared between seatings to avoid running out of food.

Residents do not have to wait to be seated. The dining room is totally set and ready for the residents to seat themselves at the beginning of the seating time. They do not have to wait until a dirty table is bused and reset to take their seats. The dining room can be completely cleaned, bused,

and reset between seatings using all service staff, the utility staff, and any available nurses' aides. Diners at the second seating receive the same quality of food and service as at the first seating.

Two seatings separate resident profiles. In most communities, there will exist active and frailer residents. Often the two profiles do not mix well, particularly at meal times. The typical senior-living dining room has two types of diner: those who are lined up outside the dining room 15 minutes before opening, and the leisurely diners who may start the evening off with a cocktail. The early diners are generally interested in *eating;* the late diners are generally interested in *dining.* Whereas the early diners will normally eat and leave the dining room within 45 to 60 minutes, the late diners will generally relax with coffee and dessert, taking up to 90 minutes to complete their meal. This phenomenon allows management to split the seatings into two distinct dining times, one starting at 4:45 P.M. and ending at 6:00 P.M. and the other starting at 6:30 P.M. and ending at 8:00 P.M. The dining room is closed from 6:00 to 6:30 P.M. to bus and reset the tables.

In this way half of the resident population can be served at each dining time. Under this arrangement, instead of having, for example, 100 orders hit the kitchen line within a 60-minute period, 50 orders are placed at each of two separate times. Residents will normally receive their orders hotter, more quickly, and more accurately when the line is not as rushed. Management will require far fewer employees to dish up and serve the food for 50 covers at a time rather than 100 covers.

Increased resident satisfaction. Resident perceptions regarding staffing and food quality are improved once their needs are addressed within two smaller groups, instead of one large one. The system maximizes the efficiency of the kitchen, while providing the residents with the service and promptness that they expect and deserve.

LAYOUT

The design and layout of a dining room should allow for as much flexibility and service efficiency as possible. Architects should remember that most residents will eat two to three meals per day in the dining room seven days per week. Variety in design and culinary presentation can significantly contribute to the diner's satisfaction. Dining rooms that are segregated into smaller dining areas, or communities with country kitchens or cafes in addition to their main dining areas, give their residents some choices. These areas can also be used for theme dinners and special occasions. The layout of all dining areas should take into account traffic flow and be designed to afford a clear and unobstructed path to and from the kitchen. The kitchen should ideally be the central hub of a wheel whose spokes feed into and out of the various dining and activity areas. Designers should examine the kitchen layout and service path to determine the best location for the servers' station, keeping in mind that the longer the distance service staff walk, the more time it will take them to fill each course order.

The dining areas should also be easily accessible. Designers should avoid the use of booths and bench seating because residents have difficulty seating themselves. They should also minimize the use of room dividers and planters, which can obstruct efficient service and may collect trash.

Seating capacity should be designed to accommodate at least 75 percent of the number of stabilized units *plus* double occupants *plus* 10 percent capacity for resident and marketing guests.

Larger or remote dining rooms should be equipped with side stations. These are areas within the perimeter of the dining room that can accommodate a coffee warmer, soup kettle, chafer, desert tray, condiment storage, and a small busing area. Remote storage areas for linens, paper goods, silver, and glassware are also very helpful to improve staff efficiency, reduce costs, and improve service to the resident diners and their guests.

▃▃▃ EQUIPMENT

When determining the type of equipment to use in the setup of the dining room, the owner or operator should consider (1) the initial cost, (2) whether the items are "stock" routinely carried in inventory by the supplier and thus can be easily replaced in a matter of days, (3) the durability of the item for its intended use, and (4) ease of cleaning and storage. Some operations use customized china, silverware, and glassware, which may lend a touch of class to the dining room and discourage theft. Yet these customized items are almost always more expensive and must be inventoried by the community instead of the supplier. Some suppliers will offer to customize china with the community's logo for a small additional charge, which enables them to do special runs for larger orders that they do not have to stock themselves.

A quarterly inventory of china, glass, silverware, and linen should be performed to evaluate shrinkage and loss. The house stock (items in inventory at the community but not in service) should be counted and kept in a secure location. As the working stock of items in service becomes depleted, the dining room manager can then remove inventory from the house stock by checking it out piece by piece and deducting the amounts from inventory. In this way the entire inventory will not need to be counted at once. Count only the working stock and add to it the house stock less any removals. Operational losses for all equipment should not exceed 25 percent annually. Individual loss expectations are noted below.

▃▃ China

As in restaurants, the food and beverage operation of a retirement community may be considered part of the sales department. The resident purchases meals (and service) in advance as a part of a monthly service fee. For many businesses, packaging is everything, and packaging in food service involves the presentation of the meal on the plate. How residents perceive this package preconditions their acceptance or rejection of the product itself. Therefore, the quality of the tabletop setting must be consistent with or better than that of the food product that will be plated onto it.

Good restaurant china is very resistant to breakage, chipping, and scratching. In fact, some manufacturers like Villeroy and Boch will guarantee certain china against chipping and replace at no cost products that become chipped. China is usually broken by hitting other china. Seventy-five to eighty percent of all breakage occurs in the soiled dish area and may be traced to careless servers or utility staff. In many cases, china is broken accidentally by staff because the warewashing area was not designed with a spot to land a tray full of dirty dishes, forcing the buser (server) to empty trays on top of other soiled dishes or in a sink. In some cases in which it would appear at first to be cheaper to switch from existing china to another more durable, less expensive, and manufacturer-stocked item, it is a good idea to use some of the china on a trial basis for a number of months prior to the initial purchase to try it out. Heavy or thick plates are not necessarily more durable or resistant to breakage, but they do tend to hold heat longer than thin plates. Plates with borders are much better for sight-impaired residents, have a tendency to frame the food on the plate, and make small portions appear plentiful. Avoid plates with colored borders or gold rims (they are painted on after glazing), as they deteriorate over time in the 180°F final rinse cycle of the commercial dishwasher. Also, plate designs are at times confusing to residents with dementia or other cognitive impairments.

Functional considerations include durability; chemical composition; thickness and weight; engineering and construction; resiliency to shock; resistance to warping, scratching, and fading; porosity; cleanability; thermal characteristics; microwave and salamander/broiler usage; and breakage patterns.

The initial purchase of china is a most important step for a facility. The cost per plate setting for china can run anywhere from $20 for cafe china to $60 for Lenox. All decisions must consider what the primary market prospects can afford, for every dollar of capital expenditure (or savings) will have an impact on the residents' monthly service fee. Operators must focus pragmatically on where to save capital and where to invest prudently to provide the best value for the residents.

China is normally the single most expensive investment of the dining operation, both at the initial purchase and for ongoing replacement. China will have a shorter life than silverware but a longer life than glassware. Annual china losses should run under 10 percent for operations with a good grade of china and well-designed warewashing and storage areas in the kitchen. A well-trained dish crew following proper guidelines for loading, unloading, sorting, and stacking, as well as incentives for reducing breakage and loss, is essential.

Glassware

The considerations for china also apply to glassware. Glassware is generally less durable than china, especially if it has a stem. For retirement communities, a place setting consisting of a 10.5-ounce goblet for water, multipurpose wine glass, and 5-ounce juice glass works well for most applications. (Residents prefer goblets for water and wine. They are lighter than a highball glass and more versatile for residents with arthritic contractions.) In addition, a sherbet cup for desserts, octagonal salad plate, and matching cereal bowl will provide the most versatility and require the least storage space and expense. These items should all be

microwave safe and should not "pond" water when inverted in the dishwasher. Glassware that is safely stackable is much easier to store and handle.

Most restaurant operators purchase glassware that is mass produced (or pressed) and consequently lower priced than either hand- or machine-blown or custom-made crystal. Mass-produced glassware is usually thicker than blown glass and much more durable. It is best to select glasses with sturdy stems, weighted bottoms, and rolled rims—the points where most breakage occurs. Blown glass is generally less durable, especially if it has a beadless edge, and will often contain trapped air bubbles that can expand and shatter the glass in high-temperature dishwashers. Costs for good-quality, durable glassware will run from $0.50 to $3.00 per stem. Some operators will use the same glassware for all purposes. Although this may save on storage and inventory costs, the food cost will tend to increase because the water goblets will be used for juice or wine, with higher associated costs.

Some manufacturers will guarantee their stemware against chipping and loss of serviceability for over 50 washings. Like china, most glassware is broken in the soiled dish area. Designing the warewashing area to include an upper rack shelf allows servers to rack their own dirty glasses rather than push them into a heap on the dirty dish counter.

Tabletop items—which include salt and pepper shakers, creamers, sugar caddies, bud vases, and cruet sets—should experience losses in the 5 percent range. Salt and pepper shakers should be of the tower variety with smooth surfaces that do not collect food particles. Sugar caddies will need to be large enough to hold regular sugar, Equal, and Sweet and Low. Bud vases should be short and weighted on the bottom so that smaller (and inexpensive) flowers and greens can be used to decorate the table without blocking the residents' view of one another. Cut glass with a simple design works best for the tabletop items because they are easier for the elderly to grip. They are, however, harder to keep clean.

Silverware or Flatware

The selection of flatware is also an integral part of the packaging of the food product. The feel of a utensil and its appearance on the table can either enhance or detract from the message of quality. The selection of silverware or flatware is much easier than that of glassware.

Silverware is five to ten times more expensive than stainless steel flatware. Most restaurants use silver-plated flatware, which is considerably less expensive than sterling but more expensive than stainless. Good-quality stainless is preferred over plated flatware, which tends to chip and peel over time. The quality of stainless is measured by its relative chrome and nickel content. "Lower quality stainless steel flatware contains roughly 13% chrome, while high quality . . . contains 18% chrome and 8% nickel."[2] Recently manufacturers have introduced an 18/10 flatware with an even higher nickel content, which makes the flatware more resistant to corrosion, harder, and more scratch resistant.

When selecting a pattern, the operator should consider the weight of the utensil, its pattern, and its functionality for seniors with limited grip strength. Larger knives with rounded handles work well, for example, when they are hollow and not too heavy. Salad and dessert forks are often too small to handle and can be replaced with a larger dinner fork to serve the same purpose. Complex patterns with too many ridges are harder to clean and have a tendency to pit. In general, the larger and the lighter the better. As the size of the flatware increases, it becomes easier to grip but heavier to hold. This is especially true for the new 18/10; the 2 percent increase in nickel content makes it only slightly heavier than the 18/8, but it *feels* more substantial.

Losses in flatware tend to be greatest and can be as high as 30 percent annually. For a small 90-unit community, replacement can run as much as $1,500 per year. Flatware is easy for employees to steal, is often left in residents' apartments from tray service, and most frequently gets thrown out by servers who scrape food waste into the garbage barrels. Some operators have controlled losses by asking residents to use their own flatware for room service, providing incentives to staff to control losses, affixing magnets to their trash bins, or periodically dumping the trash barrel and sorting through the food waste from the night's meal service.

Table 9.1 itemizes typical tabletop requirements for a 90-unit community.

Tablecloths and Napkins

Many high-end retirement communities use tablecloths and cloth napkins at some or all meal periods. Historically, white tablecloths were a symbol of elegance in fine dining. White is still considered the color of choice for formal service, but with the advent of colorfast dyes, many restaurants have begun to use colored tablecloths and napkins to match their decor. Whites were so often used in the past because the dyed fabrics could not withstand the excessive use and commercial cleanings that were required.

The two primary natural fibers for use in tablecloths and napkins are cotton and linen. Mercerized cotton is relatively inexpensive, has a good sheen, starches well, and has a long life since it holds up well to soaps, bleaches, and detergents. Yet 100 percent cotton fabrics wrinkle or crease easily unless the cotton fabric is treated to be wrinkle free. Linen is relatively expensive and does not have as long a life as cotton. It has a moderate sheen and crisp texture (it wrinkles and creases more easily than cotton), but linen absorbs moisture well, sheds dirt easily, and is lint free. Polyester fibers (Dacron) are usually combined with cotton (50:50 or 60:40) for even greater serviceability. This fabric resists wrinkling, but it may produce an excessive amount of lint. Because of Dacron's no-press, no-iron characteristics, some communities purchase "wash-and-wear" tablecloths and launder them in house. The higher the percentage of cotton, the better the item holds starch for fewer wrinkles and creative napkin folding. Napkins made of Dacron and cotton are not as absorbent as those of 100 percent cotton or linen, and they tend to spread water or spills around rather than absorb them. Service cloths or side towels should be very absorbent, lint free, and capable of withstanding excessive bleaching. They are normally made of cotton, linen, and rayon or combinations thereof.

Most tablecloths will need to be replaced after each seating or after a kosher meal. Some, however, can simply be reversed and used for the next seating. Another option is to use a Lexan or Plexiglas tabletop over a tablecloth to extend its useful life. Residents will also accept the use of cloth placemats and paper napkins for breakfast and lunch provided the tabletop itself is attractive. Paper placemats are used as well in some communities and can now be purchased in a variety of attractive and classic colors and even seasonal designs. The use of paper will, of course, communicate a message of its own and should therefore be carefully considered in the overall "packaging" of the meal.

All linen should be counted and sorted nightly. If linen is given to an outside laundry service, it should be inventoried before it is sent out. All deliveries should then be counted to verify the delivery receipt. This step

Table 9.1   **Typical Tabletop Requirements for 90 Units**

China   Villeroy & Boch: Geo

Item	Model	Price/dozen	Price/unit	PAR	Units	Total
Dinner plates	51.4271	$105.36	$8.78	2.5	225	$1,975.50
Bread and butter plate	51.4161	$50.50	$4.20	2.5	225	$945.00
Bouillon cup	51.4724	$60.36	$5.03	2.5	225	$1,131.75
Coffee cup	51.6524	$64.80	$5.40	2.5	225	$1,215.00
Saucer	51.6525	$45.96	$3.83	2.5	225	$861.75
Total china			**$27.24**			**$6,129.00**

Silver   Villeroy and Boch: 18/10 La Coupole

Item	List price	Price/dozen	Price/unit	PAR	Units	Total
Dinner knife	$147.00	$62.84	$5.24	3	270	$1,413.96
B&B knife	$120.00	$51.30	$4.28	3	270	$1,154.25
Bouillon spoon	$40.00	$17.10	$1.43	3	270	$384.75
Coffee spoon	$61.00	$26.08	$2.17	3	270	$586.74
Salad fork	$61.00	$26.08	$2.17	6	540	$1,173.49
Total silver			**$15.28**	**405**	**4860**	**$4,713.19**

Glassware   Libbey Duratuff

Item	Model	Price/dozen	Price/unit	PAR	Units	Total
Goblet—10.5 oz	17132	$23.66	$1.97	3	270	$532.35
All-purpose wine	3957	$15.50	$1.29	2	180	$232.50
Sherbet cup	5162	$7.65	$0.68	3	270	$183.60
Cardinal salad	8068107	$22.75	$1.90	3	270	$511.88
Cardinal 5.5 juice	8003048	$9.00	$0.75	3	270	$202.50
Cardinal cereal	8063173	$16.30	$1.36	3	270	$366.75
Total glassware						**$2,029.58**

| **Total china, silver, glassware** | | | | | | **$12,871.77** |

alone can save the operation several hundred dollars per year—rarely are linen delivery counts accurate.

Function and Banquet Equipment

Folding tables for continental breakfast, theme meals, parties, and special events are an essential element of any food service operation. These tables can be purchased in a variety of sizes, eight feet being the most popular. Wishbone-style folding legs allow maximum seating compared to pedestal or straight legs. Knock-down cabaret tables with pedestal tops (center-column) and bases offer considerable flexibility, but they are not as sturdy when set end to end for heavy items like ice sculptures. These tables can be covered with standard square tablecloths from the dining room and skirted with matching cloth. These skirts are best attached to the tables using plastic Velcro clips. The corners of the banquet table can be accented with an accordion-folded colored napkin for added flair.

Stackable chairs are a must for large events and parties. The chairs should be one piece, without mechanical or folding devices that will eventually wear out and fail. Chairs to be used by seniors should have arms and be lightweight and durable. It is very helpful if the chairs can be moved using a furniture dolly or chair cart. Ease of storage is another important consideration: these chairs, if left out when not in use, will make the common areas look cluttered. Quality stacking chairs are designed to be stacked without becoming marred.

Buffet and display equipment can enhance the marketability of the food service even more than the china, silver, and glassware discussed earlier. This equipment must be highly functional and durable. Its awkward shape does not lend itself well to storage, and it tends to receive rough treatment. Chafing dishes and soup tureens can be purchased in silverplate, chrome, stainless steel, or crockery and are priced according to the design and the material. A large silver chafing dish with stand, insert, and lid may cost more than $1,000. Stainless steel is much less expensive, and silverplated equipment can be replated for a fraction of the cost of new equipment. Chafing dishes can be heated with canned gels, liquid fuel, denatured alcohol, bottled gas, or electricity; most use canned gels. The heat source is only needed to maintain the heat of the food product. As the temperature increases, or after the cover is removed for service, the food will not hold well.

Other equipment—such as mirrored or glass gourmet display trays, beverage housings and ice trays, ice carving pedestals, drip collectors, cake tiers, cubes and columns, various baskets, large shell bowls, serving stones, and rainbow glows—can add a significant touch of elegance and professionalism to any buffet. When garnished with fresh greens and edible flowers, the entire display becomes enticing. Molds for ice sculptures can be rented or purchased and the sculptures created on site. Many ice companies have a catalog of designs to offer, or can custom-create a specialty sculpture. A large vase with exotic flowers at the top makes a dramatic statement at the dessert station for only about $125 delivered and set up. I have also done clamshells filled with 12-count shrimp and an ice crab with a bowl carved out of its back filled with cocktail crab claws. There is nothing like ice and carved fruit to add distinction to the food display.

Not only are buffets a great way to save money on food and labor, they also generate family and guest participation for additional revenue. Family members are often thrilled with the food and the displays, and this response helps to ease their sense of guilt about their parents living in the community as well as mitigate any complaints they may receive about the food. For employees, buffet displays can be a great learning experience and, when completed, generate a sense of accomplishment and pride in the organization and the executive chef and dining room manager.

For regional operations, ice-carving or gingerbread-house competitions or other "cook-offs" can be a fun and creative way to generate publicity for your community and help offset the old-folks'-home image of the retirement housing industry within the local community. One such competition was hosted by our community in Dallas, Texas, to create a gingerbread village in our lobby. All of the other local retirement communities were invited to participate, and the contest was judged by a board of prominent restaurant chefs,

hoteliers, and instructors at the local culinary school. The gingerbread houses were then auctioned off to local businesses (one was purchased by the Dallas–Fort Worth airport and displayed with our name during the Christmas holidays), and the proceeds were donated to seniors in need.

Chairs

Chairs with sturdy frames, arms, and high backs with casters on the *front legs only* are best for residents with handicaps. Chairs with casters on all four legs can be hazadarous on some floor surfaces, as residents use them to steady themselves. Be sure to incorporate a walker and wheelchair storage area adjacent to dining areas, to improve staff efficiency and reduce the risk of accidents. Purchase chairs that are designed with casters, inasmuch as the addition of casters to existing chairs can effect the structural integrity of the chair and void any manufacturer warranty. Chairs should be selected that are without piping, cushions, or other pockets in which food scraps can accumulate. The upholstery should be washable or protected fabric with a *firm* cushion. Wooden chairs seem to work best because they are easily repaired, recovered, and refinished. Chairs must be light enough for residents to draw themselves to the table, yet sturdy enough to last for many years of hard use. Composite chairs have recently been introduced into the marketplace that are extremely durable and maintain their finish indefinitely.

Tables

Many residents will prefer tables for two (deuces 30" × 36"), especially when they first move in and have not yet found regular dining companions. The other tables should be either four-tops (42" × 42", 36" × 36", or 30" × 42") or tables that can be converted from square to round to accommodate additional diners. Round tables should be large enough for six diners (54" diameter). In addition, it is useful to have several 29-inch-high tables that can be raised to 31 inches to accommodate wheelchairs. Order several banquet tables and half- or quarter-rounds to be used for theme parties and events.

Tabletops should be selected that are attractive when left uncovered. In this way the tables can be used with or without a cloth and can also be available for other purposes, such as games, crafts, and cards.

When setting up a dining room there should be a minimum of 2 feet of aisle space between the backs of two adjacent chairs plus 18 inches for each chair. Therefore, the total distance from the edge of one table to the next should be 5 feet (18 inches + 18 inches + 2 feet).

MANAGEMENT AND STAFFING

The management of the dining room operation can range from a lead server in small operations to a dining room manager and hosts in large communities. Any operation serving more than 70 covers at a time will need to have a dining room manager to help seat residents and manage staff: this means communities with open seating that are 70 units or larger or with two seatings that are 140 units or larger. Once the residents have been seated, the dining room manager can assist with beverages, ensure proper communication with the kitchen, and monitor resident satisfaction. During shortages, the dining room manager should be prepared to take on a station and serve the residents directly.

Between meals, the dining room manager is responsible for scheduling; employee selection and training; ordering supplies; linen management; inventorying china, silver, and glassware; planning functions; setting up events; sanitation in the dining room; and side work. As with the executive chef, the dining room manager should consider him- or herself a *working manager*.

See Exhibit 9.1 for cost-saving ideas for the dining room.

Sidework

Sidework task sheets should be distributed to each person during scheduled shifts. Tasks are identified with predetermined completion times, and each employee is checked out by the manager or shift supervisor before the end of the shift. The manager and the employee sign off for the work completed each day. Sidework includes vacuuming; wiping down and sanitizing furniture; cleaning side stands, counters, and cabinets; removing any and all dishes and serving equipment to the utility area; resetting all tables; restocking all tabletop equipment; and restocking any side stations with nonperishable food or equipment necessary to operate the food service at the next shift. In this way the nonserving time during an employee's shift is fully utilized to prepare the dining room for service. Properly completed sidework will significantly improve the efficiency of the servers during the meal period. Resident requests are more easily accommo-

---

Exhibit 9.1   Cost-Saving Ideas for the Dining Room

1. Schedule utility staff and personal care assistants to help with the set-up work whenever possible.
2. Call in replacement personnel who do not require overtime.
3. Send morning servers home early on slow days.
4. Schedule buffet lunches to cut two servers 3 hrs/week—a total of 24 hr/month.
5. Charge $40 per server for private parties of eight or more to cover additional costs.
6. Have BBQ buffets once per month to reduce 12 server hours per month.
7. Schedule meetings and training at nonserving times during the shift so staff is not called in just for training.
8. Hire personnel carefully to minimize turnover and training costs.
9. Schedule dining hours to accommodate staff who may have two jobs.
10. All sidework should be complete before each meal so that part-time servers' shifts can be spent serving.
11. Keep buffet equipment cleaned, stored, locked, and inventoried.
12. Monitor the consumption of supplies such as paper cups, doilies, etc., to discourage theft.
13. Train all personnel to properly rack and stack china and glassware.
14. Create a contest to minimize losses in china, silver, and glassware with quarterly prizes. Periodically check garbage cans for lost silverware.
15. Require residents to use their own silverware for room-service orders.
16. Use disposable products for tray deliveries.
17. Use doilies as underliners to reduce breakage.
18. Launder and press your own linen.
19. Use part-time help and split shifts.

---

dated and fewer trips are required to the kitchen, allowing servers to spend more time in the dining room at their stations rather than in the kitchen, out of sight and inaccessible to the residents. The dining room functions more effectively in the front and the back of the house when it is designed to maximize staff-resident interaction and minimize service intervention in the kitchen. Additionally, minimizing the servers' steps during the meal service and grouping equipment are essential to successful operation. To that end, sufficient equipment and an adequate number of well-placed and fully stocked service stations are necessary. The dining room manager should walk through the dining room before opening and after closing at each meal period to correct any deficiencies.

The cold station in the kitchen should include all food and equipment necessary for an entire meal service without having to restock. This includes all pre-plated salads, cold appetizers, and condiments such as salad dressings, cottage cheese, apple sauce, cranberry sauce, mustard, and ketchup. Dessert items for that evening's service should be trayed and ready on rolling racks in the walk-ins. The server's station should be located in an area of the kitchen as close as possible to the walk-in cooler. The area should have enough available space to locate a stainless-steel work table for trays of plated cold food as well as several rolling racks of plated cold food. Any underliners such as bread and butter plates, utensils such as salad forks or spoons, doilies, creamers, teapots and teabags, and the like should also be stored here. During service a line cook or utility person (but not a server) should continue to refresh and restock the area as needed. This station should be totally set approximately 15–30 minutes before the opening of each meal service (Exhibit 9.2).

Service stations in the dining room should adhere to the following guidelines:

1. Each station should allow two but no more than three servers to work out of that station.

2. Each station should be equipped to handle 30 covers for a second seating:

50 salad forks	15 coffee cups
30 water glasses	15 coffee saucers
30 bread and butter plates	10 bread and butter plates with doilies
30 soup spoons	1 turn of correctly sized table linen
30 teaspoons	
30 butter spreaders	30 napkins in the appropriate fold

3. All stations are to be supplied with a complete line of condiments: ketchup, Worcestershire sauce, mustard, oil and vinegar, cracker baskets (5), lemon slices.

4. In addition, at least two soup stations inside the kitchen must be maintained and equipped for easy server access as follows:

100 soup cups	2 soup wells
100 soup saucers	2 soup ladles
50 extra soup spoons	2 ladle rests (bread and butter plates)

Exhibit 9.2   Sidework Checklist

- ❏ Replenish all the silver on assigned stations.
- ❏ Check on glassware.
- ❏ Refill all cracker baskets and sugar caddies.
- ❏ Restock coffee cups/saucers/bread plates.
- ❏ Clean the coffee and juice machines, service station refrigerator and milk machine.
- ❏ Collect/inventory all teapots and stainless creamers and wash them manually.
- ❏ Wipe down chairs and tables on assigned stations.
- ❏ Clean all the kitchen countertops.
- ❏ Clean the microwave and the salad station.
- ❏ Collect all the flower vases from each table and keep them in the reach-in refrigerator.
- ❏ Organize all trays and breadbaskets.
- ❏ Empty the garbage receptacle in the dining room.
- ❏ Polish all the flatware used for the shift.
- ❏ Replenish all the flatware on every station to be used for breakfast set-up.
- ❏ Replenish all the linens and napkins in the dining room including every station.
- ❏ Replenish condiments in the kitchen including soup station.
- ❏ Maintain the bread warmer. See that there are enough rolls/bread for the shift.
- ❏ Refill and wipe down all salt & pepper shakers individually. See to it that salt & pepper shakers are emptied and washed at least once a week.
- ❏ Set up flatware, glasses, china, and tabletop on every table.
- ❏ Wipe down and refill oil & vinegar sets every night.
- ❏ Organize all specialty beverages, juices, sodas, and milk inside the service refrigerator.
- ❏ Wipe down all the menu holders, or update menu board.

In this way a little preparation can ensure that during the evening's service all equipment is immediately available to the server at the station, without forcing the server to leave the dining room to replenish supplies. Closing sidework must include completely restocking these service stations. The key to this type

Table 9.2   Staffing Model for a Three-Meal Dining Room, 112 Residents

Covers/month	$112 \times 3 \times 30.5 =$	10,248		Breakfast	7:30–8:15	or 8:30–9:15
Guest meals	2×30	60		Lunch	11:00–12:00	or 12:30–1:30
Total		10,308		Dinner	4:15–5:15	or 5:30–6:30
Daily		344				

		Covers	Two seating	Servers	Persons	Rounded
Breakfast	33.3%	114.42	57.21	1:12	4.77	5.00
Lunch	33.3%	114.42	57.21	1:12	4.77	5.00
Dinner	33.3%	114.42	57.21	1:12	4.77	5.00
	100%	**343.25**			**14.30**	

Shift	Serving hours	Nonserving hours	Total hours		Hrs/day	Hrs/wk	FTE
5 Servers (7:00–2:30)	2.00	5.00	7.00 hrs	=	35.00	245.00	6.13
5 Servers (3:45–7:00)	3.00	0.50	3.50 hrs	=	17.50	122.50	3.06
	25.00	**27.50**			**52.50**	**367.50**	**9.19**

of service is the server's ability to service multiple tables at one time.

Staffing

Staffing congregate or continuing care retirement community dining rooms will require approximately a 1:30 ratio of servers to residents for a continental breakfast and 1:16 for all other table service. These ratios provide each server with four tables, which, with the proper premeal sidework and a dish-up-to-order service style, should permit efficient service. Assisted living communities will require a higher ratio of servers to residents (1:12) because some residents will require assistance with their meals. Communities with Alzheimer's residents will require 1:5 or 1:7 ratios of servers or care managers to residents (Table 9.2).

These staffing ratios will produce quality service to most resident populations provided the right training, sidework, and premeal setup have been done in advance. Salads and desserts can be preplated and stored on sheet pans covered on a rolling rack in the walk-in cooler. Salad dressings can be prepoured into plastic ramekins and kept on a shelf in the server's reach-in cooler. Soups can be dished up in the kitchen at the server's station or in the dining room from an electric soup tureen at a side or busing station. The entire operation must be organized so that server trips to the kitchen are minimized and time with residents at their stations is maximized. Servers should not float around the dining room catering to all residents' needs. They should be assigned primary residents or a specific work station, in much the same way as the personal care aides are assigned residents. Thus servers can learn the individual preferences of their assigned residents and optimize the chances that the food that reaches their residents is what they ordered and expect. This approach builds resident satisfaction in the food service operation and confidence in management.

Some large congregate or continuing care retirement communities use busing staff or assistant servers. These people can perform beverage service, plate removal, table cleaning, and resetting and sanitation. For operations with open seating serving 300 or more covers per night, the staffing required is staggering. Assistant servers can be hired at a lower rate, learn the fine art of service, and expedite the delivery of the food product. The disadvantage to having assistant servers is that the senior servers may become lazy and not bus their own tables, sometimes even making an empty-handed trip to the kitchen to direct a buser to their station.

Labor cost and overtime in a food service operation can significantly affect the total delivered food cost and ultimately the bottom line. Nonserving hours should be utilized efficiently for sidework, tray deliveries, sanitation, dishwashing, inventory, and functions. In addition, servers who also have the flexibility to work short or split shifts can save the operation thousands of dollars annually.

ORIENTATION

Orienting servers to the special needs of an elderly population can provide staff with the insight they need to avoid a potentially embarrassing or offensive situation. It is impossible to comment about all possible special situations, yet a few general comments in several categories might be helpful. Seniors tend to know exactly what they want and how they want it. They are value conscious (many were reared during the Depression); they may have money but be more frugal; and they are less easily influenced by others. Their behavior may be perceived by the staff as demanding. When servers are assigned specific residents and become accustomed to their individual needs and preferences, communication becomes much easier; the chances that resident requests are misunderstood or neglected are minimized; and when servers get to know residents by serving them every day, they are more likely to recognize when the residents may not be eating or feeling well and alert management.

To cater better to seniors, menus should have large, easily read typefaces, should have significant contrast between the type and the background paper, and should not have a surface that produces glare.

Ill residents should be offered any assistance necessary to comfort them. Do not move an ill resident. The lead server should summon professional assistance quietly, and servers should try not to embarrass the ill person or arouse commotion in his or her immediate area. Any accidents should be quickly wiped clean to avoid ruining the appetite of other residents.

Blind or sight-impaired residents should be treated with as little extra fanfare as possible. If unescorted, they should be led to their seats by the hostess or their server. Most blind guests will follow by grasping the lead's elbow. A blind guest may ask to have the menu read and should be verbally notified when being served. The server should assist as necessary, and it may be necessary to cut or portion larger items for the blind guest.

Should a deaf or hearing-impaired resident ask for a menu explanation, the server should explain the menu while directly facing the resident. Many deaf persons can read lips, but they need to see the other person's mouth. A gentle nudge or a visible approach to the table should be used so that the deaf resident realizes that he or she is going to be served. Some deaf residents may be able to speak (sometimes in monotone), and others may need to point to specific menu items in order to place an order.

Late-arriving residents who arrive near closing time deserve the same, high-level service as residents arriving at the opening, and management should plan for late customers. If possible, the residents may be served in a separate dining area or in their rooms so as not to be disturbed by staff cleaning or resetting the dining room. If a resident arrives near closing time, the hostess or server may do several things: (1) Politely inform the resident that you have closed, but you will make every effort to serve him or her. (2) Politely inform the resident that you must check with the manager or the chef to see if he or she can be seated. The hostess or server may delay briefly in the kitchen and then inform the resident that he or she can be served. This sets the stage for politely asking the resident to leave as soon as he or she has finished eating. (3) Inform the resident that you are closing and that you will have something prepared quickly; serve promptly.

Inebriated residents should not be seated if this can be accomplished without giving offense. Remember that the other residents in the dining room deserve a quiet meal, and a drunken resident can ruin their evening as well as yours.

Residents with short-term memory deficits will often forget what they ordered, or see an alternate entree ordered by their tablemate and request the same. Any refused food should be promptly returned to the kitchen. The server should never try to sell or raffle off food that the resident does not want. Residents may also be confused about which meal they are eating. Some will even order breakfast items at dinner. Many of these requests can be easily accommodated by the kitchen. The objective is to get the resident to eat. Well-fed residents are generally healthier and happier than those who may leave the table hungry and cranky, and who will then return directly to their apartment and place a call to a daughter or son to complain about it. Do not argue with residents. Accommodate them. It is much easier in the long run.

Even in the finest restaurants or your mother's kitchen, occasionally an entree will turn out bad. Every effort should be made by the kitchen staff to recognize and intercept it *before* it hits the dining room. Residents do not expect perfection, but they do expect a generally consistent food product and service. They will only become upset if they perceive that the food or the service is becoming consistently bad and that their opinions are not respected.

Always check with the diner, soon after the entree is served, to ensure that everything is satisfactory. This courtesy must be extended by the server, and the food service manager should also address all residents at least once during their meal. When food is rejected by a resident, substitution for the refused item should be done immediately. Under no circumstances should kitchen personnel seek to justify or explain away the resident's complaint or argue with food service personnel about the incident. The food should not be thrown away before inspection by management or supervisory personnel. The dining room manager should be notified immediately.

All incidents and noteworthy occurrences during the course of the day should be documented in the food service log book. The log book should be hardbound with sequentially numbered pages so that a continuous, unalterable record can be kept. A log of all resident reactions to the food and service can be very useful in reconstructing events and tracking residents' complaint patterns and staff reactions, returned meals, resident preferences, comments made by residents or changes in their behavior, training needs, and daily meal counts or resident guests. This enables the supervisor to track resident patterns and workload and follow up on resident questions and incidents. The log is also helpful in documenting and prioritizing requests while ensuring that all residents are heard.

Children require additional or special service. Their ages will dictate how much special attention they require, but children generally enjoy being treated as adults, and the server should try as much as possible to do this. Do not ignore a child, and do not resort to baby talk. Offer a high chair or booster chair if required. Suggest a child's portion of a popular dish—spaghetti, hamburger, hot dog, or peanut butter and jelly sandwich—and bring it to the table as quickly as possible. If the child is irritable, food may sometimes quiet him or her. The server should never reprimand the child for misbehavior.

International guests or residents may not speak or understand the language. The guidelines for blind or deaf residents can be used for international residents as well.

VIPs deserve special service considerations, but this should not be observed by other residents in the dining room lest they come to feel like second-class citizens. VIPs should be served in private dining rooms to the extent that this is possible, or in areas of the dining room that are not readily visible to other residents. VIP guests should be given the best available server,

never someone who has not been exposed to advanced server training.

The efficient performance of a dining room operation cannot be left to chance. We have all had the experience of bad service. We know what it looks and feels like. Everything that an employee brings to the job is inherently his or her own—attitude, friendliness, smile, willingness to serve—but the techniques of proper service can be taught. The dining room manager thus must hire for attitude and train employees to work *smart,* not hard. Use Exhibit 9.3 to test your servers' skill level.

A service plan should be developed by the dining room manager that details the overall operations. The service plan should include a description of each meal service, whether it is buffet or table service, how the dining room will be split among the servers, and the numbered stations and assignments. A complete description of the setups for each side station in the dining room and in the kitchen (including approximate numbers of each of the items in the side station) should be given. The plan should also include policies and procedures, such as nonserving time, guest meal policy, reservation policy, telephone etiquette, kitchen rules, sanitation practices, minimum training standards, standards of professionalism, a quality audit, resident preferences and dietary restrictions (by station if known), and dress code and uniform guidelines. In this way, when the dining room manager is absent or there are policy questions, the service plan can be opened as a resource. This is also a good place to establish premeal and sanitation sidework schedules and assignments that can be agreed upon with the staff. The servers should play a key role in developing the plan so that their opinions and ideas are reflected in the operations. The likelihood that they will support and follow this plan is greatly increased if they play a part in its development.

Premeal meetings should be held by the chef or lead cook and the dining room staff *before* each meal service. This gives the kitchen the opportunity to explain to the servers important information about the meal before they offer it to the residents. The premeal meeting should detail each food item on the menu, from the soup and salad to the entrees, alternates, and dessert options. The main ingredients, anything special about the way the dishes are cooked or taste, sauces available and how they were made, portions available, special requests, and how long alternate items will take to prepare if they are requested should all be described.

Exhibit 9.3   Skill Training for Dining Room Servers

Site: _____

Dining room manager: _____

Server: _____

Date: _____

1. What type of service is available at retirement communities? (choose one)
   ___ a) American Plate Service
   ___ b) French Service
   ___ c) Carte Service

2. When approaching a table, what do we ask the guests first?
   ___ a) Their names
   ___ b) What they would like for a beverage
   ___ c) How they are today

3. When do we begin to take the residents' orders?
   ___ a) After they ask what the soup is
   ___ b) When they stop talking to one another
   ___ c) After we return with their beverages

4. How do you get information about the day's menu?
   ___ a) By asking other servers
   ___ b) By reading the menu before the service
   ___ c) By attending the premeal meeting and asking questions

5. When taking an order, whose order is taken first?
   ___ a) The person closest to you
   ___ b) The person facing the kitchen door
   ___ c) Ladies' orders are always taken first

6. Beverages are always served from which side?
   ___ a) The side closest to you
   ___ b) Either side of the guest
   ___ c) The right hand side of the guest

7. Food is always served from which side?
   ___ a) Either side of the guest
   ___ b) Always reach across the guest
   ___ c) From the left side of the guest

8. When extra silver is required at the table:
   ___ a) We take it from another table
   ___ b) We hand it to the guest
   ___ c) We bring it on a linen napkin

9. When a meal is not up to the guests' liking we:
   ___ a) Tell them everyone else liked it
   ___ b) Say it's too bad and walk away
   ___ c) Apologize and offer to replace it immediately

10. When assembling a tray, we always try to:
    ___ a) Make it pretty
    ___ b) Have everything appropriate to the order on it at one time
    ___ c) Keep the order small

11. When carrying a tray, we always try to:
    ___ a) Show how good we are at balancing
    ___ b) Keep the tray at shoulder height
    ___ c) Carry it with the other hand

12. When you are busing a table, always remember to:
    ___ a) Scrape the dishes in the dining room to help the dishwasher
    ___ b) Leave the dishes until everyone in the room is finished
    ___ c) Bus dishes to a tray and remove them to the kitchen immediately

13. When serving coffee, what condiments are always served?
    ___ a) None
    ___ b) Cream and sugar
    ___ c) Let the guest ask for condiments

14. When should the correct condiments be served with menu items?
    ___ a) Only after people ask
    ___ b) When the items are served
    ___ c) We don't serve condiments

15. Should a server know the daily desserts?
    ___ a) No, that's why we have a printed menu
    ___ b) The dining room manager should tell the guests
    ___ c) Servers should know all the daily desserts

16. When or by whom is the sidework in the dining room done?
    ___ a) By the last person serving
    ___ b) By the dining room manager
    ___ c) Preceding the opening and after the closing of the dining room

17. Table settings are considered complete when:
    ___ a) Every place setting is complete as well as the table center
    ___ b) You set them with whatever is available
    ___ c) When they all have about the same thing

18. How often is a tablecloth changed in the dining room?
    ___ a) Each time the table is used
    ___ b) When the spots are noticeable
    ___ c) Once a week

19. Is your name tag considered part of your uniform?
    ___ a) Only when you are waiting on someone you don't know
    ___ b) Yes, always
    ___ c) Only when there are big parties

20. When writing the ticket for food, how important is it to write clearly?
    ___ a) It's not important; you can always tell the chef
    ___ b) It is important to write legibly
    ___ c) It's not important; only the server has to read the ticket

TOTAL SCORE: _____ /20 = _____ %

The servers should also be made aware of any "heart-smart" items with low fat, sodium, or cholesterol, along with the diabetic choice for dessert. Some chefs will even plate up a sample of each entree and allow the servers to taste each, with sauces, so that they are prepared to represent the meal correctly to the residents on first-hand experience. By spending a few minutes with the servers before each meal, the chef will be creating a partnership with the servers who will be representing (selling) his creation to his clients (residents) in the best possible way. Consequently, the residents will be more likely to receive what they expected and be satisfied with their dining experience.

When serving begins, it is up to each server to make sure that the food plated by the cook is exactly what was ordered by the resident. Every cover must be lifted and checked against the order to ensure accuracy. If it is incorrect, the server should refuse the meal. The servers do not work for the chef or cook; during serving times, the cook works for them.

Any breakdown in communication between the front (dining room) and back (kitchen) of the house can negatively affect resident perceptions about the quality of the food. Servers have the power to sell the meal to the resident. The smart food service director or chef will recognize that the servers are as important to please as the residents. Once the food leaves the kitchen, there is little the chef can do to influence its reception by the residents. When residents complain about the food, the servers must accept responsibility for correcting it, not blame the kitchen.

Only through a spirit of partnership and communication between the servers and the kitchen will the image of food quality be positively managed by the employees. How the food is served and represented is as much a part of the overall perceived quality as are its ingredients and preparation.

STANDARDS OF PROFESSIONALISM

To help ensure that each resident experiences pleasant community living and is the recipient of first-class, resident-oriented service, all employees are expected to follow certain general guidelines. Adherence to these guidelines will provide the kind of service that enhances residents' community-living experience and makes for long-term success (Exhibit 9.4). The keys to this service are alertness, attention to detail, and follow-through. (Exhibit 9.5 details the keys to *poor* service.)

Exhibit 9.6 lists tips for safety and accident prevention.

General Service Guidelines

1. When encountering a resident, be sure to initiate the greeting. Be courteous and cheerful, and maintain proper posture during the greeting.
2. When dealing with a resident, maintain frequent eye contact. Do not look down or away.
3. Smile at the resident.
4. If another resident is waiting, smile and say that you will be right with him or her.
5. Always maintain a pleasant tone of voice when talking with a resident.
6. Answer any questions a resident may have. If you do not know the answer, apologize and inform the resident how to obtain the answer. Any resident who appears to be in need of assistance should receive it immediately from any nearby employee.
7. Do not eat, drink, smoke, or chew gum or tobacco in an area where you may encounter residents. This includes the concierge area and lobby, other public spaces, and the restaurant. These activities should only occur during lunch or breaks in designated employee areas.
8. When a resident has a complaint, acknowledge it and apologize. Then determine what you can do to solve the problem. If you can help, do so enthusiastically. If not, inform the resident as to who can solve it, or inform that individual yourself. (See Chapter 5 for more on handling complaints.)
9. Be sure to inform management of any problem that may disturb resident satisfaction, or any resident problems you may have dealt with. Try to anticipate problems whenever possible.
10. Never argue with residents. If a problem arises, a manager should be summoned immediately.
11. Always refer to the resident by name if it is known. Take the time to learn residents' names. Nothing sounds better than our own name when someone remembers it.
12. If a resident appears to be confused or in need of assistance, cheerfully inquire as to how you may be of service.
13. Never make negative remarks about the property, fellow employees, management, or residents in the presence of a resident.

Exhibit 9.4 **Some Tips for Good Service**

1. Never stand around. Always look for something to do for the residents and be available to them. Waiting for your order in the kitchen does not make it come up sooner.
2. Always greet your residents. Introduce yourself, make eye contact with guests, and smile.
3. Avoid talking to other employees, especially in the presence of residents.
4. Do not shout or give loud orders in the dining room or kitchen.
5. Never argue with anyone, especially a resident.
6. Do not mop your face with the side-towel. Never carry a side-towel under your arm or on your shoulder.
7. Replace your towel now and again.
8. Use a clean, sanitary towel to polish silver or glassware only before opening the restaurant or when out of residents' view.
9. Do not lean on chairs or put your foot on a chair rung. Stand erect or bend from the waist to hear. Do not crouch down or bend at the knees.
10. If the resident spills something or you spill something on a resident, apologize, clean it up, and advise the dining room manager or supervisor.
11. If a resident drops a napkin or piece of silverware, replace it with a clean one. Do not rob from adjacent tables!
12. Never use profanity.
13. Take resident complaints to your supervisor, or better yet solve them yourself.
14. Never hurry your residents.
15. Never eat during service or in the kitchen.
16. Do not carry pencils, books, etc., where visible, i.e., in pockets, in your hair, behind your ear, etc.
17. Carry menus in your hands—not under your arms or in a shirt, blouse, apron, jacket or inside your pants or skirt.
18. Do not lean on walls or sidestands. Do not rest anything on the resident's table. Do not perform any functions on the resident's table, such as stacking dishes, placing soiled silverware on plates, writing the residents' orders, and so forth.
19. Do not put your hands in pockets or on your hips.
20. Do not cross your arms in front of your chest. Grasp your hands in front or behind you.
21. Do not complain about food to kitchen personnel—tell your supervisor.
22. Do not blame the kitchen for slow service. Accept responsibility for the entire food service operation.
23. Do not point in the dining room or gesture at a table.
24. Always be courteous.
25. Walk briskly, but never run. Do not walk briskly when leading residents to their seats.

Service Protocol

Dining in retirement housing will differ slightly from dining in a typical restaurant. The following guidelines should help clarify some important points regarding service protocol for the elderly.

Many elderly persons experience uncontrollable shaking or palsy. Therefore, beverage glasses and cups should only be filled to within two or three inches of the rim. Coffee cups should always rest on a saucer unless mugs are being used. Warm tea should be served with hot water in a cup on an underliner. A lemon wedge should be on the underliner. A selection of three teas, including regular tea, should be offered by the server when the tea water is delivered. Milk should be verbally offered since milk (not cream) is a traditional

accompaniment of English tea. Soft drinks typically are unpopular among seniors. A limited selection should be available upon request. Sugar-free soft drinks are often popular with diabetics. At least three flavors of fruit juices should be available for all meals. Orange and grapefruit juice should at least be a frozen concentrated

---

Exhibit 9.5 **Seven Sins of Poor Service**

1. Apathy
2. Brushoff
3. Coldness
4. Condescension
5. Robotism
6. Rulebook
7. Runaround

Exhibit 9.6   Safety and Accident Prevention

1. Be alert for tripping hazards, such as chairs pulled away from tables, briefcases or purses near tables, unexpected motions of diners, and so forth. Be especially aware of residents pushing chairs from the table as you walk.
2. Always make sure residents know of your presence before you begin serving a table.
3. Clean up spilled food, drink, and ice immediately. The rule is "Clean as you go." Use a service towel to wipe up spillage from tables and chairs. Use a rag to clean the floor.
4. Do not hold water glasses between fingers so that rims touch. This method does not offer enough support, and glasses may slip from your hands. Always hold glasses by the base.
5. Always close drawers that you have opened. Someone may hit an open drawer while passing by, resulting in injury.
6. Hold hot plates with a clean, dry side towel to avoid burns. Remember to warn the residents when plates are hot.
7. Clean up any broken items immediately. If items are broken near food, make it known to others.

If this occurs in or near the ice, the ice bin should be covered with a tray immediately. New ice should then be brought in an ice pail to use until the bin is clean and refilled. Never pick up broken items with your hands. Always use a towel or dustpan and broom.

8. Always use a metal ice scoop to fill glasses with ice. *Never* scooop up ice with the glass. (Glasses may break in the ice. Because glass looks like ice, the whole bin must then be emptied.)
9. If you discover broken or chipped glassware, or ragged or bent silverware, take it out of circulation. Give it to your supervisor.
10. Avoid overfilling containers with food and liquids, especially those that are hot and may cause burns.
11. Bend at the knees when picking up heavy items. This will give you more support and guard against back injury.
12. Always return all items to their proper place.
13. Be familiar with fire protection and evacuation procedure.
14. Know the location and contents of the first aid kit.

---

brand. Clear juices such as cranberry and apple juice are good for the urinary tract; these are very popular with seniors and can be ordered for diabetic diets. Tomato juice and V-8 juice should always be served with a lemon wedge (all lemon wedges should be at least 1/6 count, and they should be fresh).

Most retirement communities offer American-style plate service. Thus food is dished onto plates in the kitchen, and not at the table from a silver tray (Russian service) or a guerdon (serving cart) (French service). Oval trays should be used to carry food to the tables. This is done for many reasons: many items can be carried at one time, thus saving trips to and from the kitchen; entree plates can be carried and stacked with plate covers, thus keeping food warmer; carrying a tray requires less skill than professionally carrying three or more entree plates with side dishes; and an oval tray is then available to bring dirty dishes back to the dish room.

All trays brought from the kitchen should be covered with an open napkin so that if the tray is damaged or stained, it remains sanitary and fresh looking. When extra flatware is brought to the table, it should be on a cloth napkin on a side plate. Flatware should never be taken from one table and given to another.

If food or beverages are spilled on a diner's clothing, then the dining room manager or server should approach the table, apologize, and offer the diner a signed, dated cleaning ticket (if appropriate). If the diner cannot get the stain out with normal cleaning then he or she must bring the article of clothing to the dining room manager with the cleaning ticket so that the clothing can be professionally cleaned at the facility's expense. All spillage incidences should be recorded in the dining room daily log book, noting the server's name, so that any patterns can be traced. Often excessive spillage is a result of poor training.

Most residents will want to take food from the dining room back to their rooms. This is especially true if they are on a two-meal program or have a pet or a guest. The retirement community should develop a firm policy that "doggie bags" are not permitted: residents may eat as much as they wish at the table, but no food may be taken to their apartments. This is a condition of most insurance coverage. When food leaves a restaurant's premises, the restaurant is no longer responsible for its safety. Yet because residents rarely leave the premises, we are still responsible for the quality of the food product while it is in the building. Tray deliveries are our responsibility as well, and all uneaten food should be disposed of. The removal of food from the dining room can cost an operation thousands of dollars over the course of a year. I have even seen some residents line their purses with plastic wrap and slip entire slices of prime rib inside! Although we want to encourage residents to eat as much as they can to stay healthy, especially if they are on medications that may cause stomach upset, the risk of food-borne illnesses increases with food leaving the supervision of the food service department. Unpeeled fruit can be the exception to this rule and is a good source of fiber, but even in a small community, this translates to another couple of cases of bananas or apples each week. Often residents will take food from the dining room for a snack if they are unable to purchase food outside the property. A trip to the local grocery store or arrangements for groceries to be delivered can provide residents the opportunity to stock their own kitchens.

Servers should make their approach to a table sincere but not "canned." Try to make the resident feel at ease and comfortable. Never sound as if the resident is a bother. Use the resident's name if it is known. Take orders in a systematic manner, and try to get ladies' orders first. Repeat each order to the resident to make sure it has been understood correctly and to minimize mistakes. Never auction off food at the table: the server should be sure he or she knows who gets which items before delivering them. Do not wait until a resident's glass is totally dry before offering a refill: approach the table for rebeveraging when one glass is two-thirds empty. Make sure foods look appetizing. Always use clean and correct plates and glassware. Always use fresh and appropriate garnishes. Always use the proper accessories. Try to take orders and serve from one point at a table unless it is necessary to move to another point to reach all of the parties. Exhibit 9.7 outlines questions to ask yourself to test your service quality.

Never leave a table empty-handed. Always remove all empty glasses, plates, condiments, sipstix, and the like, and all crumpled paper and dirty napkins. Change the ashtrays. A server should always ask if a resident is finished with a drink before removing the glass. Nothing infuriates a resident more than having her drink or plate taken away before she is finished.

Write guest checks legibly. Abbreviate only where there can be no confusion. Always write as if someone else will be reading the check. The chef should designate abbreviations for each entree during the premeal meeting.

Servers should spend as much time in the dining room at their stations as possible to be available to their residents. Waiting in the kitchen for an order to be plated does not make it appear any faster. Always be alert to guests' signals: they can sometimes be as slight as a nod or a wink. Respond quickly. Servers should never walk with their eyes on the floor, but should always look at their residents to see if someone needs them. Residents should never have to get up, snap their fingers, shout, or throw things to get a server's attention.

When taking an order, the server should approach the table with a smile and be prepared to answer any questions about the items on the menu. A friendly and pleasant personality will help create a warm atmosphere, enable the server to be a better salesperson, and help meet the goal of total resident satisfaction. When filling out a check, the server should be sure to complete the top of the check with the date, his or her server number, the table number, and the number of guests. The person sitting with his or her back to the front entrance should be designated guest #1 (use his or her name if the kitchen knows the guest's preferences). The rest of the people in the party will follow in sequence clockwise. (Remember, ladies' orders are always taken first, regardless of position at the table; continue with the men clockwise.) Hot items are normally written on the top portion of the check, which then goes to the hot food section of the kitchen. Cold items are written on the bottom portion of the check, which likewise goes to the cold food section of the kitchen. Desserts, beverages, and soups are also written on the bottom portion of the check. When picking up an order, the server must pick up *cold items first,* then hot food. Whenever possible, a tray should be stacked so that the food that will be served first is on top. Female diners should always be served first.

■■■■ ORDER OF SERVICE

1. The dining room manager or host greets residents at the door, seating them at the appropriate table. Assist residents with their chairs, placing the first guest in the seat facing the door.

Exhibit 9.7 Sixty Questions for Great Service

1. Are salads chilled and not room temperature?
2. Are water glasses automatically refilled?
3. Are hot food and beverages served on hot plates or in hot cups?
4. Is hot food served hot and cold food served cold?
5. Is apartment delivery service timely, as quoted?
6. Are residents put on hold for less than 30 seconds?
7. Are apartment delivery trays picked up in less than three hours?
8. Is all equipment retrieved?
9. Are dishes or glasses free of chips?
10. Is the flatware on tables polished and free of spots?
11. Are the glasses free of spots or streaks (hold them up to the light)?
12. Are the menus or placemats free of rips, stains, or smudges?
13. Are the bread and rolls fresh?
14. Are there enough menus for the residents?
15. Do the continental breakfast or special events have any "razzle dazzle"?
16. Are the residents acknowledged within one minute?
17. Is the food picked up without sitting in the window too long?
18. Is there enough china, flatware, or glassware?
19. Is the flatware set straight on tables?
20. Are sugar bowls clean inside? (Take the sugar packets out and look.)
21. Are the salt & pepper shakers free of grease (touch them) or half empty? Are the ketchup bottles clean and full?
22. Is there enough prep to assure that you will not run out of any items?
23. Do the service personnel have pleasant attitudes?
24. Do the service personnel follow the prescribed order of service?
25. Is proper service etiquette, as trained, observed?
26. Do meal periods start on time?
27. Are debris, bits of paper, and food *immediately* picked up from the carpets or floors in the dining room?
28. Does a resident get top-quality food and beverage for his or her money? It may be included in the monthly fee, but residents will always be evaluating.
29. Does the resident get exactly what the description on the menu reads?
30. Does the food service director or host speak with each table during a meal period?
31. Are chairs and booths free of dirt, stains, or crumbs?
32. Do residents get coffee immediately on being seated?
33. Does the coffee steam?
34. Is each entree garnished?
35. Is the garnish fresh and appealing to the eye?
36. Are the continental breakfasts or specialty buffets replenished quickly?
37. When orders arrive, are they complete? Do the service people know who gets what without asking?
38. Are the coffee cups free of stains?
39. Are the tables and chairs solid? Do they wobble?
40. Are clean fresh towels used to wipe down tables, not paper napkins?
41. Are the residents recognized by a smile, a hello, or eye contact when they arrive at the door of the dining room?
42. Do service personnel clean as they go?
43. Does a resident get a menu that is clean, dry, and presentable?
44. Are uniforms clean and attractive?
45. Do all employees wear name tags?
46. Do all employees abide by grooming standards?
47. Are special requests for food items honored when ingredients are available without a hassle from the server or kitchen?
48. Are servers familiar with the product they serve (i.e., soups, daily appetizers and desserts, entree items)?
49. Is there consistency in glassware and china?
50. Do servers assist residents when necessary?
51. Are tables crumbed after the entree?
52. Are all sauces and dressings presented in a ramekin on the side?
53. Is extra flatware presented on a cloth napkin and underliner?
54. Are napkins refolded when residents leave the table during a meal?
55. Does everyone know the table numbers in the restaurant?
56. Does the food service director personally inspect the continental breakfast at least once a week?
57. Is glassware always touched by the stem or at the base?
58. When not picking up a food order, is the server tending the station?
59. Does the food service director or host detail all stations and tabletops before opening?
60. Are the servers responsive to resident requests? Are residents' expectations managed?

2. A clean, fresh-looking menu will be set at each place setting.

3. The server acknowledges the table within one minute.

4. The server approaches the table with a friendly greeting within three minutes, pours cold water, and presents a signature breadbasket and butter. The server explains the daily menu and offers to get beverages and margarine.

5. The server returns with beverages and asks if there are any menu questions.

6. The server returns to the table after two minutes to take orders, starting with the women and moving clockwise around the table. The order is taken on a captain's order pad, with person #1 (chair with back toward the front door) at the top of the list. Each order includes appetizer or soup, salad, and entree. All questions must be addressed in a patient, friendly manner; substitutions are possible when ingredients are available.

7. The first course (salad) is served, serving women first, from the right with the right hand.

8. Clear the first course when everyone at the table finishes, not as the diners are individually finished.

9. Check the water and beverages.

10. Serve the salad or appetizer course, remembering to bring the requested salad dressing on the side in a separate ramekin. Extra sauce for an appetizer should be placed at the left of the setting.

11. Offer freshly ground pepper.

12. When everyone is finished, clear the salad course, from the right with the right hand, always clearing the women's places first.

13. Check the silverware for the entree. Is any fresh flatware needed?

14. Serve the entree, remembering that any sauces are to be served at the left of the entree plate, in a ramekin on an underliner. Present the entree with the main (meat) item closest to the diner. Again, serve women first, from the left with the left hand.

15. Since a captain's order pad was used to take the order, using the seat number method of order taking, there should be no question regarding who gets what.

16. Offer to replenish the breadbasket as well as the beverages.

17. Do not rush the diners, regardless of how busy the dining room is. This meal is the primary social event of the day, and the diners' experience must never be compromised.

18. Residents should never leave a primary meal hungry. Thus if a resident wants another little taste of something, it should be provided, served on a salad plate.

19. Clear the entree once all diners have stopped eating. It is important to clear anything that will not be needed for dessert: entree plate, bread and butter plate, bread basket, side dishes, and salt and pepper shakers. Never stack dishes or scrape plates in front of a diner.

20. Crumb each place setting.

21. Offer the dessert presentation, and remember to mention that ice cream is available in addition to the chef's special dessert (some properties may present a dessert tray). Serve dessert to the women first. Offer coffee and decaffeinated coffee. Decaffeinated coffee must always be freshly brewed. Because many residents are required to drink decaffeinated coffee for medical reasons, it is absolutely essential that regular coffee never be mixed with decaffeinated.

22. If a guest is present, then a guest meal ticket must be given to the resident for signature. Once the dessert course has been served, the server should bring the check to the resident in a check presenter or face down on a salad plate. All guest checks must be filled out correctly with the resident's name, apartment number, number of guests, price, and totals.

HOW TO BUS AND RESET A TABLE

1. All tables are to be bused onto trays, which are placed on tray jacks, and never into bus tubs. No trays should be placed on tables or chairs.

2. Remove all soiled items from table and load the tray properly: glassware in the middle for stability, flatware around the edges, the soiled tablecloth on top.

3. Thoroughly wipe the tabletop, salt and pepper shakers, sugar caddies, and candleholder or vase.

4. Wipe chairs and pick up litter and debris from around the table.

5. Squat and lift the tray with the leg muscles and return the tray to the stewarding area. Place the tray in a predefined location.

6. Remove condiment bottles and linen napkins from the tray and store them properly.

7. Gather all necessary items for proper table setup from the service station.

8. Promptly return to the table and set it properly. Pay attention to detail.

▬▬▬ TABLE SETTING

All tables should be covered with a clean tablecloth, falling evenly, with the seam side down. All tables will have the following items in their "centerpieces":

  1 Clean sugar bowl with bleached sugar, raw sugar, Equal, Sweet and Low

  1 Clean, full set of salt and pepper shakers

All tabletops should be set according to a sketch provided by the food service manager (Figure 9.1). Such a setup is based on the dining room layout.

All place settings will include

  Polished, spotless flatware:
    1 Salad fork
    1 Dinner fork
    1 Dinner knife
    1 Teaspoon
    1 Soup spoon
    1 Bread and butter knife

  Clean, spotless glassware:
    1 Water goblet
    1 Wine glass (optional)
  Clean china:
    1 Bread and butter plate
    1 Coffee cup and saucer
  Linen:
    1 Linen napkin

▬▬▬ Place Setting

1. Imagine a dinner plate, 10½ inches in diameter, placed in front of the diner (a show plate or set plate may or may not be used).

2. Flatware is to be set half an inch from the edge of the table with the tips of all handles level (do not stagger the utensils). Be careful not to touch the eating surfaces of the flatware with your fingers. Setting from the imaginary plate toward the left, place the dinner fork, then the salad fork. Setting from the imaginary plate toward the right, set the dinner knife, blade facing to the left, then the teaspoon and soup spoon. All flatware should be set straight and close together.

3. The bread and butter plate is to be placed above the salad and entree forks so that the right plate edge is in line with the left edge of the entree fork. A but-

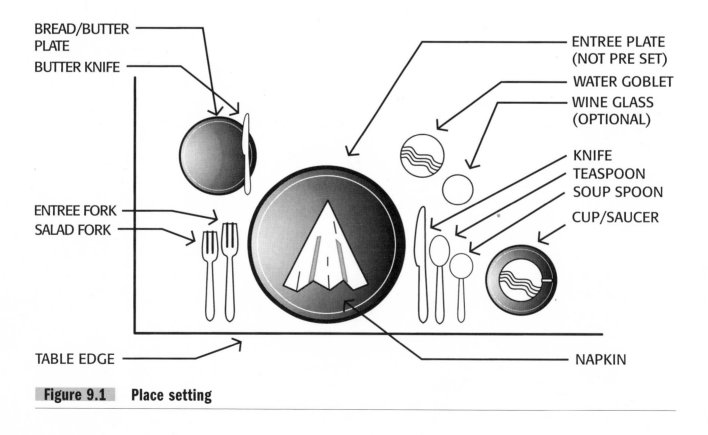

BREAD/BUTTER PLATE
BUTTER KNIFE
ENTREE PLATE (NOT PRE SET)
WATER GOBLET
WINE GLASS (OPTIONAL)
KNIFE
TEASPOON
SOUP SPOON
CUP/SAUCER
ENTREE FORK
SALAD FORK
TABLE EDGE
NAPKIN

Figure 9.1   Place setting

ter knife is set vertically on the right edge of the bread and butter plate, with blade facing to the left. The coffee cup, sitting on a saucer, is placed to the right of the soup spoon, so that the saucer almost touches the soup spoon. The coffee cup should be placed so that the handle is at three o'clock. The coffee cup should never be inverted.

4. The water goblet is set upright, at the top of the knife tip. If one is present, a wine glass is set upright, to the right of the water goblet, above the spoons.

5. A clean, starched napkin is folded at each place setting. The type of fold should be changed periodically to add variety to the place setting.

NOTES

1. S. Colgan, *Restaurant Design* (New York: Restaurant and Hotel Design International Magazine, 1987).
2. J. Durocher, "Flatware," *Restaurant Business Magazine,* May 1, 1991, 200.

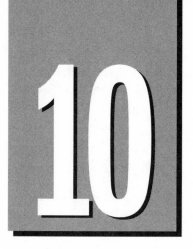

10 Housekeeping

An organization is only as good as its frontline staff. Often housekeepers are treated as "invisible" staff, when in fact they *are* the frontline staff to your residents. No one understands this better than the Disney Corporation. At Disneyland theme parks, management knows that the cleanliness of the park is of paramount importance to a quality experience. They also know that the cleaning staff, which is constantly cleaning, sweeping, and polishing the park, will handle more guest inquiries than any other employees. Management has recognized the importance of extensive guest relations training to equip these employees to *add* to the guests' experience. They are among the most thoroughly trained employees at the parks, second only to those portraying the Disney characters in costume.

The housekeeping department plays a vital role in meeting the cleaning needs of the resident and providing weekly companionship. Many times the housekeeper is one of the resident's only regular visitors, and the resident will often look forward to cleaning day for the company it provides. In many cases, strong friendships can develop between the resident and housekeeper. It is important to recognize that the housekeeper often may be the main information conduit between community management and the residents. After all, the housekeeper is spending more one-on-one time with the resident than any other single staff member. It is therefore critical that the housekeeping staff be trained to represent the community well. Residents will typically test out rumors on their housekeeper and pass on the response to many other residents. Weekly sessions with staff at the beginning or end of the shift can be a valuable tool to manage resident satisfaction and expectations. The housekeeping staff should be rehearsed to give appropriate answers to the questions most frequently asked by residents and families. Often, residents or their families will ask the same questions of different individuals to test how the responses may vary. In addition, frequent surveys of all employees can help to identify dissatisfaction in the ranks and allow management to address issues before they may be communicated to the residents.

COMMUNICATION

Resident referrals are a vital (and inexpensive) source of leads for the marketing staff. Care should be taken to ensure that all community personnel understand the importance of these referrals and what they each can do to promote them. Managers will want to be certain that the message being delivered by the sales staff reflects reality in the operations and is consistent with the views of the housekeeping staff in particular. Consistency equals credibility. The more consistent staff are in communicating the features and benefits of the community, the more credibility the entire operation will demonstrate to the residents.

Another major function of communication among the housekeeping staff is to alert management to the changing health conditions of the residents they visit each week. Often this can test the employees' loyalties inasmuch as residents will normally attempt to hide such problems from community management for fear of being asked to transfer out of their apartments to a higher level of care. This phenomenon is common in communities with independent apartments, assisted-living facilities, and even life-care communities, where a resident's greatest fear is nursing home placement. The importance of early detection and reporting of a resident's change in health status must be stressed to the housekeeping staff. It is ultimately in the resident's best interest to receive the treatment that he or she may need as health deteriorates. This proactive approach can and does normally lead to more comfort and independence for the resident, not less.

Any change in a resident's health status should be reported to the housekeeping supervisor so that it can be shared with the appropriate management staff at department-head meetings, or sooner if it is significant. The housekeeping supervisor should ask the housekeepers weekly about their residents and should conduct inspections of their work in all the resident apartments at least quarterly as a part of normal supervision. In extreme cases, residents have been known to tip their housekeeper to protect their anonymity. Periodic inspections by the supervisor can help to minimize this practice. Most companies strictly prohibit the acceptance of tips by employees; violations can lead to disciplinary measures up to and including termination. When approached with a tip, employees should thank the resident for the gesture and remind the resident of company tipping policy. The employee might suggest that any contributions be made to the employee appreciation fund, where they can be shared by all of the employees whose combined efforts bring the service package to life.

▰▰▰ RESIDENT ROOMS

Early on in the planning of a community, decisions should be made on housekeeping and laundry services. There are many options to consider, including frequency of housekeeping visits to the apartments, tasks performed at each visit, annual deep cleaning, linen and laundry service, pest control, air conditioning filter maintenance, and scheduling. These services are not eas-

ily reduced after the community becomes occupied without creating the perception that the entire service package is being eroded.

It is much easier to keep a clean facility that way than it is to to be continually cleaning a dirty facility. If management allows the community to become dirty over time, then dirty becomes the standard. Once established, it is very difficult to raise the bar or improve cleanliness standards with existing staff, because they will always feel as though they are being forced to work harder for the same pay. However, once the community is clean, it becomes much easier to keep it that way. It is the dirty facility that gets noticed; no one ever notices the clean one, unless the standard of clean is greater than expected.

The frequency of visits to any given apartment will largely depend on the level of care of its occupant. Independent-living residents may require a housekeeping visit every week or two. Assisted-living residents may require a visit once or even twice per week, and skilled-nursing residents daily. Owing to the smaller size of the assisted-living apartment, the length of time to clean should be less, allowing housekeepers to complete up to nine apartments per day. From a scheduling standpoint it becomes important to segment the population as much as possible to promote the most efficient use of staffing. Be sure to step up the housekeeping staffing as the level of care increases. Also, it is a good idea to schedule one housekeeper Tuesday through Saturday, and one Sunday through Thursday to allow for weekend coverage to accommodate housekeeping emergencies if they arise. This is particularly important in communities that offer assisted living or higher levels of care.

Most independent residents do not require a weekly visit unless the competition for residents in the area demands this frequency. Bimonthly visits are much more efficient and cost effective. For example, in most communities, a housekeeper should be able to clean seven or eight apartments (nine or ten assisted living rooms) plus hallway carpets, empty trash rooms, and coordinate linen replacement each working day. Therefore, a 200-unit community should require 28.5 employee-days per week or 114 employee-days per month to clean all apartments weekly (including nonresident apartments, for example, guest and model rooms). The same 200-unit community cleaned bimonthly at five apartments per day (1.5 hours per

Table 10.1   **Housekeeping Staffing Analysis**

Cleaning apartments	Total apartments	Per day	Per person	Total FTE	Hours daily	Hours weekly	Hourly wage	Cost per apartment	Monthly cost
Weekly	200	40	7	5.71	45.71	228.57	$6.00	$6.86	$5,485
Bimonthly		20	5	4.00	32.00	160.00	$6.00	$9.60	$3,840

apartment) plus the extras will only require 20 employee-days per week, or 80 per month. At $6.00 per hour, the monthly savings amount to $1,632 or 30 percent. Add payroll taxes and benefits of 23 percent and the annual savings amount to $25,000. Communities with smaller apartments should be able to stretch their housekeeper productivity to six apartments per day. This scenario will require only 67 employee-days per month, which will yield $27,264 annually or 41.5 percent in savings over the weekly visit arrangement. During difficult economic times, many residents on fixed incomes are ill equipped to accept continual monthly fee increases. Options such as this have received widespread support among residents, allowing them to trade housekeeping frequency for lower monthly fee increases, which can ease their financial burden. Some communities that have converted to bimonthly housekeeping offer it as an option at lease renewal. Obviously, communities that can offer the bimonthly arrangement from the start are at a distinct advantage operationally. Table 10.1 illustrates the same principle in full-time equivalents.

Most communities normally run their housekeepers on eight-hour shifts. In most circumstances, the same productivity of seven apartments per day can be achieved in 7.5 hours. Using the 200-unit community weekly service example above, the shift difference amounts to an additional $342 per month or 6.25 percent savings, which translates to $4,100 annually. This is a relatively painless option when spread among all housekeepers, but it may not be reasonable in tight labor markets. In any event, all work schedules should be planned at least one week in advance by the housekeeping supervisor and posted. These should also include all nonresident apartments, including vacancies, guest apartments, models, and marketing units, which should be scheduled for and consistently cleaned on a routine basis. The last thing you need is for a sales representative to show a vacant apartment to a prospect only to find a big bug on the carpet. Many communities assign pest control in the resident apartments to the housekeepers.

Residents should never be promised that any specific length of time will be allocated to their apartments for cleaning. It is normal for many to expect at least an hour each week, more if their apartments have more than one bedroom. Most apartments can be thoroughly cleaned in about 30–45 minutes, depending on the square footage, if the department is well organized. The residents should be told that the housekeepers are on no specific time schedule, but rather that they are expected to clean a number of apartments per day following a task list for each apartment. This policy should be spelled out by the sales representative during the initial tour and then again in writing in the resident handbook. Residents should be advised to expect *light* housekeeping each week. The daily production expectations of each housekeeper should, however, be planned in advance and appropriately assigned. If the community also provides an annual or spring cleaning (Exhibit 10.1), then the resident should be informed as to what specifically to expect from this visit as well. Each community should design cleaning specifications for resident apartments, guest rooms, and common areas (Exhibit 10.2) along with the frequency of cleaning, estimated time for completion, and cost. At the end of each shift, the housekeepers should quickly walk the entire building with a damp rag and trash bag to ensure that the property looks fresh.

All staff should be instructed to be especially considerate of residents. They should always knock before entering the apartment and greet residents as they are invited inside. This is particularly appropriate in a health-care setting or in a skilled-nursing facility. Both in the apartment and in the common areas staff should watch their equipment and electric cords and courteously ask residents to move if they are in the way or at risk. Staff should be instructed on how to assist residents to move, including the body mechanics of transferring a resident in the event that it becomes necessary. Staff should always be friendly and *patient* with residents and be reminded that ultimately they are employed by them.

Exhibit 10.1   Annual Cleaning Checklist

1. Clean windows, inside and out if possible, and shutters, if any.
2. Remove and clean drip pan under refrigerator, then slide refrigerator out, unplug it, and clean behind and underneath. Also clean front coils, plug refrigerator back in, and slide it back into place.
3. Vacuum draperies and/or vertical louvers with appropriate attachment (make sure vacuum attachments are clean before using).
4. Vacuum corners of all rooms vertically and horizontally, removing all cobwebs.
5. Move all pieces of furniture as possible and vacuum/clean baseboards and carpet behind furniture. Use a wet towel with a small amount of cream cleanser to remove scuff marks from baseboards. *Never* use bleach water; it will discolor the carpet.
6. Clean sliding door tracks or the patio door frame using a dark-colored rag.
7. Clean/vacuum screens on porch and balconies. Vacuum/sweep corners vertically and horizontally to clean walls or stucco.
8. Vacuum mattress and flip mattress after cleaning bedsprings, frame, and slats under mattresses of all beds.
9. Clean baseboards in all closets using the above procedure, exercising care not to touch resident clothing and shoes.
10. Clean all shelves in all closets. If shelves are very sticky, use mineral spirits.
11. Vacuum upholstered furniture. Do not spot clean—advise resident to hire a professional.
12. Thoroughly clean all fans, vents, light fixtures, and chandeliers with resident permission.
13. Clean slats on louvered doors. Use a wet towel with a small amount of cream cleanser to remove dirt from around door handles and all switch plates.
14. Vacuum, spot, and shampoo all carpets, including porches, if any.
15. Clean range and oven. Wipe down all appliances, including kitchen cabinets and countertops.
16. Check kitchen cabinets for supplies from the community dining room and return them to dining room manager.

Apartment: _____

Date: _____

After the resident has moved in, the housekeeping supervisor should meet with him in order to schedule a time and day for housekeeping service. The housekeepers should be instructed to follow a weekly checklist for each apartment with at least the following duties: vacuum all carpets; clean kitchen sinks; wash countertops; damp-wipe cabinets in the kitchen; dust closet and entry doors; mop kitchen and bathroom floors; clean and disinfect tubs, showers, and bathroom fixtures; dust windowsills, light fixtures, and furniture; remove trash; sweep patios; clean balcony/patio doors and entry door windows; change bed linens (where clean linen is provided); and spot-clean carpets. It is important to have a list of what is included in the weekly visit and what constitutes additional services that can be billed. Housekeepers should not be permitted to touch or move breakable personal items. Decisions should be made by residents during their initial interview by the housekeeping supervisor as to what items will not be cleaned. Residents with personal articles that may have a high monetary or sentimental value should be informed that management is not responsible for their cleaning, damage, or loss and should be advised to have them appropriately insured. In addition, housekeepers should not move heavy pieces of furniture or turn mattresses. The housekeepers will supply all cleaning materials unless the resident has a special request and wishes to supply cleaning materials.

For special tasks, the resident should fill out a work order request at the concierge desk. The housekeeping department can then contact the resident regarding the request and arrange a time to perform the service. Residents are notorious for requesting spur-of-the-moment maintenance and housekeeping "favors" of staff, who may find it easier to accommodate them than argue over a chargeable service. The only real way to manage this is to offer the residents service in 15-minute increments, provide incentives to housekeepers and maintenance employees to share in ancillary revenue generated, and tightly schedule the employees so that

---

Exhibit 10.2 **Housekeeping Checklist**

Weekly or Bimonthly

Kitchen

___ Clean refrigerator: handle, door, top
___ Clean backsplash, countertops, cabinets
___ Clean window and windowsill
___ Clean dishwasher door
___ Clean stovetop, range, and hood
___ Clean sink (do not wash dirty dishes)
___ Sweep, damp-mop floor
___ Remove trash
___ Clean garbage disposal guard

Living Room

___ Dust furniture and pictures
___ Clean windows, tracks, sills, and screens
___ Vacuum and spot-clean carpet

Public Areas

___ Clean elevator floors, walls, and ashtray
___ Clean fire extinguisher, inside box, and door
___ Clean hallway light fixtures and exit signs
___ Clean doorbell, door frame, and entry shelf
___ Vacuum hallway carpet
___ Clean handrails
___ Clean stairwells
___ Clean trash rooms
___ Clean housekeeper storage rooms and carts
___ Clean resident storage rooms

Porch

___ Clean porch furniture
___ Clean mildew
___ Vacuum cobwebs
___ Vacuum carpet
___ Wipe down porch rails

Laundry Rooms

___ Damp-wipe washer
___ Damp-wipe dryer and clean lint trap
___ Clean floor
___ Clean louvered doors

Bedrooms

___ Dust furniture and pictures
___ Vacuum and spot-clean carpet
___ Clean windows
___ Remove trash
___ Clean louvered doors
___ Change bed and ticket laundry

Bathrooms

___ Clean sink and counter
___ Scrub toilet
___ Clean tub or shower including door tracks
___ Polish mirror
___ Polish all chrome fixtures
___ Remove trash
___ Clean louvered door

Housekeeper: _____

Apartment: _____

Date: _____

Checked by: _____

---

there is little time in their day available for such favors. Charges can then be assessed to the residents if they request extra housekeeping or services, based on current rates, with the appropriate work order to support the billing.

It is the responsibility of the housekeeping supervisor to organize the staff for the most efficient operation. All housekeeping carts should have an inventory list of supplies and be properly stocked at the beginning of each shift. Because most housekeepers have individual preferences and can become somewhat territorial, carts should be assigned to each person. Be sure to order lightweight Rubbermaid or other nonmetallic carts for easy cleaning, mobility, and durability; these fit into your housekeeping closet or storage areas.[1] Metal carts are heavy, tend to leave marks on hallway walls, can rust through, and are not easy to restore after they become worn. All mops, brooms, and ladders should be fitted with rubber caps on the handles to keep them from leaving marks on the walls.

SCHEDULING

Normally the most efficient method of scheduling room cleaning is by floor. In this way the housekeeper can vacuum the hallway carpet and clean fixtures and hand rails as she moves from room to room. Resist the urge to attempt to accommodate resident requests as to when they would like to have their apartment cleaned. This can have the housekeepers spending nonproductive time running all over the community from one floor to the next at the residents' beck and call. Rather, tell the residents that the most efficient way to clean the apartments is as it is done in hotels: starting from one end of the hallway and systematically working to the other end. When residents move into their apartments, they should be advised that apartments in their wing will be cleaned at set times, for example, on Thursdays in the morning between the hours of 8:00 A.M. and 12:00 P.M. or in the afternoon from 12:30 to 3:30, depending on the apartment's location down the hallway, and that it is management's preference that the resident be there when the apartment is cleaned (or sign a waiver to permit access to the apartment if the resident is absent). Each housekeeper will arrive about the same time each week, and a routine will quickly develop so that the resident will know when to expect the housekeeper. Housekeeping schedules normally become disorganized in multilevel communities during fill-up when occupancy is scattered all over the building. It is critical to set the rules early on to achieve the maximum flexibility, or residents will totally control the timing and delivery of this service. The more flexibility for the housekeepers, the more productive they will be. If they are moving randomly throughout the building, they may only be able to clean five or six apartments during their shift.

The housekeeping supervisor should assign each staff member a number of apartments and common areas to clean daily in a posted master housekeeping schedule. This way all staff are aware of how the workload is distributed and arrangements can be made to cover for employees who may call in sick or are no-shows. The supervisor should hire a few "on call" part-time employees to ensure vacation and sick coverage and handle other unexpected staff shortages. These are people who are available on a temporary, per diem basis. They can already be signed up and on the payroll so that when they are called they can come right to work. This practice can save the department costly overtime and the use of expensive temporary agencies. Many communities will also cross-train concierge, dining room, personal care, or driving staff to cover when shortages occur. Be sure to back out their time so that it is properly reflected on the budget of the department in

which they worked. The cross-trained worker should be paid the same rate of pay in each department.

SECURITY

Residents should be encouraged to secure their valuables during visits by community employees or outside vendors and guests. Residents can be very security-conscious, and operators need to evaluate the potential for theft. For a small fee, each housekeeper can be checked through state police records at hiring to determine if he is appropriate for this level of security. It is important to note that the personnel department may not be required to perform these checks on all staff hired, only those who have similar access to the residents' apartments. Many times, however, it can be the longstanding employee who learns the ways of the resident and how to take advantage of them.

Any loss reported by a resident or her family should be investigated immediately by two or more community management staff and documented. Depending upon the severity of the loss, it is also a good idea to recommend that the resident or family contact the local law enforcement authority with as much discretion as possible. It is human nature to lose or misplace things frequently as we grow older. Operators must be aware of and guard against the potential wave of complaints that can surface when a community theft problem has been identified. Things that have been misplaced for months can be reported stolen, and then word gets out that there may be a problem. Management should never set a precedent by reimbursing a resident for lost or stolen articles, for this can set in motion a chain of events that is not easily reversed. Residents should, however, be reasonably reimbursed for any damages they may sustain as a result of the community's negligence. All such matters should be fully investigated according to community policy and turned over to local police and the resident's insurance agency. Resident handbooks and agreements should not accept any responsibility for residents' valuables (unless required to do so by law), and residents should be encouraged to obtain the appropriate renter's insurance and such other coverage as they may deem desirable. The community should also establish key control policies and issue keys to housekeepers for the apartments they routinely clean.[2]

Consent should be granted in the residency agreement to allow management reasonable entry to the apartment to make necessary repairs, alterations, or improvements; to supply the agreed-upon services; and to show the apartment to prospective or actual purchasers, mortgagees, or tenants. In addition, emergency access for cause without the resident's prior consent should be arranged in advance when concern for the resident's health exists, or if management believes that the resident has damaged the apartment.

Many operators rotate their housekeepers to prevent abuse of the housekeepers' time as bonds develop and to alleviate boredom among the staff. Although this has been successful for some, as residents age they experience a heightened sense of vulnerability and are very suspect of a new housekeeper. At times, misplaced valuables will be reported stolen and it becomes difficult for management to reassure the resident or isolate the theft if there is a problem. Rotation does, however, have a number of advantages. It allows for variety and breaks the monotony of cleaning the same apartments month after month. A housekeeper who cleans too long in one place can overlook things that a new set of eyes may catch. In addition, if residents become attached to a housekeeper and that employee leaves the community, separation anxiety may result. The employee turnover rate also does not become known to the residents as readily with monthly rotation. Rotation discourages favoritism on the part of the resident and the housekeeper. Working relationships are more likely to stay on a business level while tipping, moonlighting, gossip, and cliques are minimized.

As mentioned earlier, residents can be among the best vehicles for advertising a community, and although rotation has some advantages, residents generally will become more satisfied with the same housekeeper each week, whom they can get to know and trust. In addition, regardless of what may be on the task list, many residents are very particular about *how* they like things to be cleaned. It will take any new housekeeper weeks to learn these nuances.

COMMON AREAS

A master housekeeping plan that incorporates the cleaning frequency and intensity for all areas in both the front and the back of the house should be developed. The plan should specifically cover how each room, furnishing, and fixture should be cleaned and specify the appropriate cleaning agent. It is up to the housekeeping supervisor to take the guesswork out of the job and define specific expectations. Each cleaning activity should be identified and a time study conducted to evaluate the appropriate time allotment for each job. Obviously, there will be a need for such a plan to be flexible, but its very composition can be quite informative. To put such a plan together will serve to clarify the expectations of management and employees alike. Management will generally have a greater realization and appreciation of what it takes to clean a community and be better equipped to allocate their budgeted funds. Employees will be able to reach an understanding of what is expected of them by management and can negotiate expectations that are perceived to be unrealistic.

The housekeeping needs of a community change as the building fills. As the first residents move into the building, a variety of tradespeople attend to last-minute details as the punch list is completed. These workers are notorious for leaving large, conspicuous messes that the housekeeping staff are expected to clean up. Many operators underestimate the amount of staff time needed to keep the project looking sharp during this critical time. They wrongly assume that without residents, only a skeleton housekeeping crew will be required to keep up the common areas. In addition, all resident apartments will need to be cleaned before they can be showed or occupied. Typically, the carpet installers are the last contractors to visit the apartment, and they rarely leave it in move-in condition. During periods of heavy move-in activity, hallway carpets and corridors will need more than weekly attention, as will elevator cars and back-of-the-house areas. Finally, as the project reaches full occupancy, the entire community will need to be policed daily to keep it looking fresh. It is important to remind *all staff* of their responsibility to help the community look its best. It is everyone's job to take pride in the community and treat it as if it were his or her own home.

Some areas—such as the dining room, kitchen, maintenance areas, and other back-of-the-house locations—may be cleaned by employees other than housekeepers. For example, the lobby may be the responsibility of the lobby attendant; the kitchen and back-of-house areas are normally cleaned by utility staff from the kitchen; and the dining room may be cleaned by the servers.[3]

CLEANING PROCEDURES AND INFECTION CONTROL

The housekeeping staff is responsible for completing daily, weekly, monthly, quarterly, and annual cleaning procedures in accordance with proper sanitary practices. Proper sanitary practices are defined differently in every community according to the housekeeping supervisor's background and biases. In any case, due to the somewhat frail nature of the tenants, extreme caution should be exercised in defining what a clean facility looks like. The apartments and food service areas in particular must be kept clean and as free as possible of germs and other contaminating agents at all times, not just during the weekly visit. Proper and safe methods for cleaning, disinfecting, and sterilizing all areas, surfaces, and equipment should be taught to all related department staff. In addition, there may be mandatory procedures and rules for the cleaning of apartments whose residents may be suffering from contagious diseases, to prevent their spread to other residents.

Knowing the definitions of and procedures for cleaning, sanitizing, disinfecting, and sterilizing is the first step toward good communication and compliance. The following definitions are normally applied in a health-care setting, but they will also suffice for our purposes:

Clean—To remove dirt, impurities, or extraneous matter from a surface. *Examples:* sweeping, mopping floors, damp-wiping, vacuuming, laundry, and so forth. *Amount of bacteria removed:* Moderate.

Sanitize—To clean thoroughly enough to promote healthful surroundings. *Examples:* All of the above cleaning examples. Germicide may or may not be used. *Amount of bacteria removed:* Moderate amount depending on the cleaning agent and the thoroughness of cleaning.

Disinfect—To kill or inhibit the growth of disease-causing bacteria by cleaning thoroughly and then using a disinfectant spray, a disinfecting cleaning solution, or boiling water. *Examples:* All cleaning tasks using water and detergent germicide, disinfectant spray, or boiling water. *Amount of bacteria removed:* A significant amount, depending on the strength of germicide (disinfectant) used and thoroughness of cleaning.

Sterilize—To kill all living organisms on an item or surface by using intense heat or steam under pressure. *Examples:* Autoclave, bedpan sterilization, dry heat sterilizer. *Amount of bacteria removed:* All.

Cleaning in health-care facilities always will mean to clean and disinfect, because a detergent or detergent-germicide combination cleaning product should be used in every cleaning-water solution. Although this is not normally required for residents' apartments, it is a good habit to establish with staff. Disinfectant sprays should be used on all surfaces that cannot be cleaned with water and detergent germicide, such as cloth, upholstered furnishings, or mattresses.

The cleaning of tile floors should include vacuuming or sweeping thoroughly, paying close attention to corners and areas near or under furniture, then wet-mopping with water and added detergent germicide, and posting warning "Wet Floor" signs at both ends of the wet area. The same methods are employed when using a floor-cleaning machine; staff should follow all directions posted on the machine. Following cleaning, a thin coat of floor wax can be applied with the floor wax applicator. It is important to use only *non-skid* waxes. Again "Wet Floor" warning signs should be posted until the floor dries. Wax should be stripped from the floors approximately every six months. Follow the directions on the wax stripper container or manufacturer's recommendation.

Before cleaning carpets, all furniture should be removed and the carpet vacuumed thoroughly. Carpet shampooers vary in the amount of water they use, so be sure to follow the instructions on the machine carefully. Operators should be sure to fill the machine with the correct amount of water and a carpet-cleaning product that contains some sort of detergent germicide. Be careful not to oversoak the area; spot-clean dirty areas first. Shampooing of common areas should be done during evening hours, when most residents will be in their apartments, to avoid slipping and tripping hazards and to allow the carpet to dry normally without tracking wetness to other areas. Do not allow staff to vacuum wet carpets with a standard vacuum, or they may be electrocuted. Water leaks and overflow problems can be handled safely with a wet/dry or shop vacuum. Dry-cleaning systems can also be effective to spot-clean heavy-traffic areas during normal business hours. It is important to remind staff never to use a bleach solution when cleaning baseboards above carpeted areas, as it may permanently remove carpet color pigments.

When cleaning windows and glass, a solution of water and nondetergent cleaning ammonia can be used. Caution should be exercised because some ammoniated products have been found to be toxic to those with upper respiratory conditions. When such conditions exist, an alcohol-based window cleaner can be substituted. The windows should be washed, rinsed, and dried thoroughly. Detergents or soap solutions not intended for windows or glass will leave a residue. Never use a squeegee or an ammonia product on windows with tinted film.

Damp-wiping should use a solution of detergent germicide in water following the instructions on the container. Staff should be instructed to dip their cleaning cloths in the solution and *squeeze them out thoroughly* to avoid damaging adjacent woodwork or upholstery. In addition, they should pay particular attention to corners, ridges, and hard-to-get-to areas by cleaning them *first*. The solution should be changed regularly. A small amount of concentrate and a measuring cup should be kept on each housekeeping cart to allow the housekeepers to refresh their solutions without making return trips to the supply areas.

Public and private restrooms are normally most at risk for the potential spread of bacteria. Therefore, extra attention will be necessary to ensure proper disinfection of these areas. All surfaces should be cleaned thoroughly, especially the toilets and urinals, paying close attention to the sides and back and under the rim. All rust and stains should be removed, and all surfaces should be dried and the chrome polished. All other areas should be damp-mopped and all dispensers refilled. Residents should be provided with soap for their handwashing sink on move-in only. In public washrooms, sealed dispensers are the most sanitary and economical to maintain. A cup dispenser is a good idea for residents who may need a drink with their medications, and a box of tissues can be helpful if residents are not inclined to walk off with them. Most common-area washrooms have floor drains to protect the outside areas from flooding in the event of a plumbing clog or malfunction. As with all drains, they have a P-trap beneath the drain cover, which when filled with water creates a barrier to prevent sewer gases and insects from entering the bathroom from the drain system below. Over time, especially in warm climates, the water barrier in the P-trap can evaporate; bugs in the bathroom or a sewer smell is a sure sign that this has happened. The problem is easily resolved by pouring a glass of bleach water down each floor drain. In fact, as a pre-

ventive measure it may be a good idea to have the housekeeper responsible for cleaning this area water these drains routinely.

Normally the wait staff are responsible for cleaning the dining room, with the exception of polishing glass and mirrors and shampooing the carpets. The dining room should be vacuumed after every meal period. It is a good idea to first remove all debris from chairs, tables, and table bases before vacuuming. All tables should be washed and dried and all chairs damp-wiped, including the removal of scuff marks on the legs. Scuff marks are more frequently the result of vacuum bumps and casters than of resident abuse. When vacuuming the dining room, all chairs should be moved each time and tables shifted at least weekly. Failure to remove all food debris properly will result in insects in the dining room. If a problem already exists, a treatment of boric acid will work exceptionally well. Boric acid is a nontoxic, odorless powder that has no harmful effect on humans. It is normally applied, using a bulb applicator, in the evening and vacuumed up in the morning.

The kitchen area is primarily cleaned by the kitchen utility staff; however, a deep cleaning of all equipment, walls, food storage areas, and floors should be performed at least quarterly. The housekeeping staff should be enlisted to assist in this major undertaking. Kitchen cleaning parties (KP parties) can usually be coordinated after the evening meal and should be organized with cleaning-task lists by individual in advance. Many staff will enjoy the extra hours, and it will not seem too bad when 10–12 people pitch in to get things done. A pizza break sometime during the night can provide a morale boost as things wind down. During the takeover transition of new properties, we have conducted such parties to bring the new project up to our standards. This serves two purposes: first, it communicates the expectations of sanitary standards to the employees and sets the stage for the new manager, and second, it serves to weed out those employees who may not be as committed to their community or their job. At the end of two or three nights of cleaning until the wee hours you are left with an immaculate kitchen and a proud staff with a sense of accomplishment and the commitment necessary to keep it that way.

The housekeeping supervisor should attend all meetings of the infection control committee, if there is one, or learn proper infection-control techniques.

Through in-service training, all housekeepers should be informed of proper methods for controlling infectious waste, including the disposal of such waste and the appropriate cleaning methods. Contaminated waste containers should be emptied daily using rubber gloves and the double-bag technique. Contaminated waste should be disposed of according to the procedures dictated by the county health department or by a licensed contractor.

TRAINING

All new employees should have already received an orientation on company benefits, service philosophy, employee policies, and work practices by the time they start working in their respective departments. At the very least, this should occur during their first week. Orientation to their specific job duties is critical to avoid potential communication problems and personal injury and to establish expectations for the job. Whenever possible, new employees should be paired with a senior housekeeper for at least one day to ensure that proper cleaning procedures, tasking, resident relations, and standards of cleanliness are thoroughly communicated and understood. In addition, the housekeeping supervisor should develop a departmental orientation checklist so that all aspects of the department's operation are covered in the orientation and documented. It is not enough simply to review a job description and have the new employee sign it as understood. There is no substitute for one-on-one time with the new employee or an employee with a performance problem to set him off on the right foot. Most people will want to do a good job, but may be uncertain of what a good job looks like. A thorough orientation and training program will help to bring clarity to the supervisor's expectations and better equip the staff to deliver. If the supervisor is unclear about his or her own expectations, the orientation and training plan should be reviewed by the executive director.

A well-conceived training plan should include coursework on cleaning procedures, tasking, mixing chemicals, safety, specific job duty orientation, relationships with other departments, sanitation, infection control, security, uniforms or dress codes, equipment handling, supplies, and, most importantly, resident communications. Nevertheless a good training plan is only effective if it is followed. The purpose of training is to educate and establish routine in accordance with defined standards. Not only should new employees be oriented, but long-term, experienced housekeepers can also benefit from a refresher course. The National Executive Housekeepers Association (NEHA) is a national organization of professional housekeepers that provides leadership and education and does research in the housekeeping field. They have a certification program and certify their professionals who meet all the educational requirements as registered executive housekeepers (REH).[4]

Other topics that should be routinely covered during in-service training include OSHA rules and guidelines, safety, new equipment and methods for cleaning, understanding the aging process, recognizing health problems in residents, motivation, and the importance of communication with fellow staff and supervisors. Because most laundry operations normally fall under the supervision of the housekeeping department, supervisors may want to consider including laundry employees in their training plans and weekly staff meetings.

PURCHASING

Supplies, service contracts, and equipment expenditures normally make up about 10 percent of the housekeeping department operations budget. For most communities, this combined cost should not exceed $6.00–$8.00 per month per apartment cleaned. Service contracts should be kept to a minimum due to the staffing overhead already in place. Copies of all contracts should be kept by the executive director and housekeeping supervisor. There should be at least two competitive bids on file, and all contracts should terminate annually to ensure competitiveness.

The housekeeping supervisor should also maintain a current ledger of all vendor accounts organized by service function. The ledger should include account and pricing information with cutsheets of frequently ordered or inventoried supplies. All vendor supply accounts should be put out to bid at least annually. Although some account service representatives will be friendlier and more attentive than others, price per unit should be the determining factor. Proper planning and monthly inventory will enable the supervisor to take advantage of bulk purchasing and the monthly special discounts offered by most vendors. Avoid buying premixed solutions (especially aerosols) as a time saver for staff. Modern dispensers make it safe and efficient to mix chemicals properly. Some mixing can even be done automatically, but be wary of automatic mixing systems, which normally do not save enough time to justify the additional chemical cost per unit. The supervisor should only consider cost per gallon, per use, or per application when evaluating chemical alternatives. Always be suspicious of vendor offers of "free" automated mixing equipment. Their cost is buried in the price of the chemicals or recovered through liberal mix settings.

All deliveries should be reviewed and inventoried by the housekeeping supervisor, who can check the purchase order against the packing slip and invoice to verify the order. Supplies should be kept in a secure location that is not accessible to residents or other staff. All supplies should be signed out from inventory by each housekeeper as they are used, for control and to facilitate reorder. Inventories of all supplies should be done at least monthly by the housekeeping supervisor with a copy to the executive director. Both managers should formally agree on the appropriate dollar amount of inventory for the community's size and historical consumption. This figure should not exceed 10 percent of the annual supply budget unless the supervisor and the executive director wish to avail themselves of some bulk purchasing discount.

All housekeeping and laundry equipment should be scheduled on a routine maintenance program. Much of this maintenance (e.g., cleaning and adjusting) can be performed by the housekeepers, leaving major maintenance and breakdown repairs to the community maintenance department. It is a good idea to keep a small supply of cords, belts, brushes, and other frequently replaced parts on hand. The housekeeping supervisor can be trained to make simple repairs to equipment that will keep the department running without going through the work-order process of the maintenance department.

All operating equipment manuals, including invoice receipts and warranty information, should be kept together on file by the housekeeping supervisor. All community tools and equipment should be inventoried by purchase date, purchase location, model number, and serial number and marked with the community's identification. Not only does this enable the supervisor to keep track of all equipment, it also provides useful information regarding the longevity and durability of equipment in use.

SAFETY

All housekeeping staff should be trained in the correct and safe procedure to follow when using a cleaning product, device, or appliance. Some common precautions follow.

All cleaning machines should be checked daily to make sure they are clean, operating correctly, and free of defects such as broken locks, switches, cords, and plugs. Employees should never operate power equipment with wet hands and should take care to keep cords out of the path of travel for residents or other staff. All cords should be plugged into the nearest outlets available with a minimal use of extension cords. Equipment should never be left unattended in a resident's apartment or corridor.

Employees should be trained to use scoops, measuring cups, or other containers to dispense soaps, detergents, bleaches, acids, or other cleaning solutions. They should *never* use their hands. Measure and pour accurately according to the directions on the package or dispenser. Ensure that there is adequate ventilation when mixing or using cleaning chemicals. Never smoke or light a flame near these chemicals, because many are quite flammable.

Employees should never pick up broken glass, china, or enamelware with their bare hands. They should also be trained as to the correct and safe way to empty trash receptacles, bags, or bins. They should never dig into any trash container with their hands, especially in health-care facilities.

Many communities have significantly reduced the incidence of lower back injuries by issuing back support belts to housekeeping and maintenance personnel. These devices are very lightweight and, when used properly, encourage proper body mechanics. Additional training can also be provided to improve employee awareness regarding proper lifting techniques and promote sensitivity toward the potential of back injury.

Regular safety classes or the development of a safety committee for the community can help to identify the potential vulnerabilities and serve to establish a plan for precautions. OSHA rules are very specific about the creation of a safe work environment and should be posted and reviewed with staff routinely. Be sure to obtain the non-English posting for employees who are bilingual. In addition, emergency procedures should be posted along with eyewash stations in areas where the mixing and storage of chemicals is handled.

All chemicals should be properly stored and labeled. Staff must be fully trained on safety and refilling self-dispensing chemicals. An inventory of and emergency procedures for each chemical should be kept on file and accessible. Material Safety Data Sheets (MSDS) must be on file for every product used, including products that have been discontinued. MSDS sheets should be kept on file and accessible indefinitely.

Housekeepers who work with contaminated wastes that could host bloodborne pathogens should be encouraged to consider a hepatitis series for their own protection. Federal regulations governing Occupational Safety and Health (OSHA) were amended on December 6, 1991, to encompass the management of employee exposure to bloodborne pathogens (Title 29 CFR 1910.1030). Compliance is mandatory for all those whose work involves potential exposure to blood or other infectious material. In senior housing, those positions could include housekeepers, laundry workers, nursing assistants, and other health-care workers. The regulations place on the employer the responsibility for the following:[5]

1. Developing an exposure control plan.
2. Offering hepatitis B vaccine to employees at risk for occupational exposure.
3. Recordkeeping and reporting of exposure incidents.
4. Staff training.

All employees who have potential exposure to blood or other infectious material should be trained in the *universal precautions* listed below:

1. Wash hands with soap and water or other antivirus or microbial cleaner before and after contact with any resident in the provision of patient care.
2. Under circumstances in which differentiation between body fluids is difficult or impossible, all body fluids shall be considered potentially infectious materials.
3. The anticipated contact with blood or other potentially infectious materials requires the employee to wear protective rubber gloves while engaged in this procedure.
4. Where it is not practical to anticipate contact with potentially infectious materials, protective rubber shall be worn.

All bins, pails, linen carts, or other types of receptacles intended for reuse should be inspected and decontaminated on a regularly scheduled basis, or immediately upon the observation of visible contamination. All spills or splashes of blood or other potentially hazardous materials should be cleaned only by properly trained employees, specifically instructed to deal with these special conditions. Mopheads or reusable towels should be prepared for laundering immediately after the spill is cleaned and the area is decontaminated.

UNIFORMS

The use of uniforms for housekeeping staff is normally at the discretion of the community's management. While many communities feel the lack of uniforms adds to the casual atmosphere of the community, there are many good reasons to justify their use. First, uniforms allow the employees to look and feel more professional while avoiding the continuous enforcement of community dress codes. When employees are in uniform, they are also more easily recognizable by the residents and their families as employees, which alleviates possible anxiety about strangers. In addition, uniforms provide for differentiation of community employees from private duty aids or personal attendants. Finally, proper-fitting uniforms can contribute to a safer working environment while allowing housekeepers freedom from worry about the effects that cleaning chemicals and crawling around on the floors can have on their personal clothes.

Always purchase a uniform that can be easily cleaned by either the housekeeper or the community, preferably one made from a polyester-cotton or wool blend that is wash and wear. Meta smocks can be ordered in 27 colors and are readily available from most uniform suppliers. All uniforms should be able to be laundered and stored at the community. Resist the temptation to allow employees to take uniforms home, as they will invariably be misplaced or forgotten.

Communities that require their employees to launder their own uniforms will normally issue to each five sets so that a midweek wash is avoided. Communities that launder their own uniforms need maintain only three sets for each employee.

NOTES

1. Rubbermaid # 6165 carts are large enough to facilitate laundry transport as well.
2. See Chapter 12 for more on key control.
3. See also Chapter 8 for detailed food-sanitation practices.
4. National Housekeepers Association, Inc., 1001 Eastwind Drive, Suite 301, Westerville, OH 43081, (800) 200-6342. Their trade publication is *Executive Housekeeping Today.*
5. Training materials are required and videos with sample exposure control plans are commercially available; references are listed in Further Reading at the back of this book.

Laundry

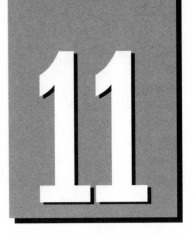

A community has many options to consider when evaluating its laundry service package. The decision to set up a laundry operation within the community or contract this service to an outside firm may be influenced by factors such as constraints of the water or sewer system, community water rationing (such as is common in California), shortage of space in the physical plant, and other mechanical barriers.

Commercial laundry services charge by the pound and will pick up and deliver. If the community contracts this service, it should use the laundry company's linen as well. Contract services can be very hard on linen because machine settings and chemicals may be designed to wash linen from a variety of sources, including nursing homes or hospitals, which have more stringent requirements. In addition, resident and community linen can easily become lost or mixed up with other customers' linen in a large commercial operation.

In circumstances where dining room linen is sent out, all items should be inventoried as they leave and again as they return. The contractor should be held accountable for any losses. When using an outside contractor, the linens are not the responsibility of the community to maintain, and typically are not sorted for quality or ragged-out by the service company. This can be easily accomplished by the housekeeping supervisor when receiving the delivery. It is a good idea to assign the responsibility for dealing with the outside contractor to one department head, who can keep track of residential as well as dining room and other linen.

In many areas of the country it can be very expensive to contract out laundry services owing to a lack of competition in the business, the fact that the contractor's operations may not be close to the community, and the risk that the community's linen will be priced at the nursing home or hospital rate per pound. Typically, it is much more economical to process laundry in-house than to contract for this service, allowing more control over the product, inventory, and costs. (See Table 11.1 for a comparative analysis.) Many planned communities will already have a laundry facility roughed-in during construction. This is especially true of communities that have a vertically integrated service package with several levels of care, such as continuing-care retirement communities. Phased communities, remodeled projects, or smaller communities may not have this provision. A laundry operation can normally be set up from scratch to service a 200-unit community for under $45,000 installed, assuming that a suitable location and electrical service are available. If a major plumbing or electrical modification is necessary, the costs can increase dramatically. In the following example, the conversion is not overly complicated and does not require any major reconstruction. Including the washers and dryers, an ironer, supplies, uniforms, tickets, mesh bags, and bins, the total conversion cost is $45,000. General operating supplies,

Table 11.1   Laundry Conversion Analysis

Salary/wages	$25,029
Employee benefits @ 20%	$ 5,006
General operating supplies	$ 1,000
Soap/detergent	$10,000
Repairs/maintenance	$ 1,000
Total annual operating expenses	$42,035
Contract service:	
Resident linens	$24,000
Food service/other	$50,000
Total annual contract	$74,000
Annual savings	$31,965
Conversion cost	$45,000
Payback period (yr)	1.4

soap and detergent, and repairs should run about $3.00 to $4.00 per month per resident. Assuming an hourly rate of $6.00 for two full-time laundry workers, the payback period of the conversion costs is an attractive 1.4 years.

Normally, the higher the level of care provided at the community, the more intensive the service that will be needed. In skilled-nursing facilities, state and federal regulations specifically govern the management of this function. For congregate communities, however, many options exist. These services can include flat linens only, both sheets and towels using resident-provided or community-purchased linen, and even residents' personal laundry. There are advantages and disadvantages to each of these options.

SERVICES

Items that are normally serviced by the laundry department can include:

- Resident flat linens and towels
- Resident personal laundry and coordinating dry cleaning (including pickup and delivery)
- Community and guest room linens, towels, and floormats
- Kitchen rags and uniforms
- Housekeeping mopheads, rags, uniforms, throw rugs
- Dining room table linen, cloth napkins, pillows, and uniforms
- Other uniforms (the service can coordinate certain dry cleaning for employees)

The laundry department can also make alterations and mend and hem clothing. A complete laundry orientation checklist is given in Exhibit 11.1.

RESIDENT LINENS AND PERSONAL LAUNDRY

Communities that purchase their own linen avoid the storage and the time-consuming sorting of the residents' personal linen. Computer software is available, however, for counting, sorting, and inventorying, which can cut down on paperwork and staff time. Any time a community accepts the responsibility for laundering residents' personal linen and clothing, it also accepts the problems associated with keeping it separated and, stored and the liability of washing it in accordance with the manufacturer's recommended

Exhibit 11.1   Laundry Orientation Checklist

___ Sorting
___ What to wear when sorting: apron, mask, gloves
___ Formulas for washers/operation instruction
___ Disinfecting procedures: carts and counters
___ Inventory procedures
___ Residential vs. health care
___ Proper folding
___ Separate containers used for transporting clean and dirty linen
___ Clean lint screens on dryers morning and afternoon daily
___ Supply inventory and control
___ Ironing: what is ironed and what is not
___ Drying: what is dried and what to avoid drying
___ Wrapping and storage procedures
___ Schedules
___ Health care inventory
___ General safety precautions
___ MSDS instruction
___ Handling isolation linens
___ Uniforms
___ Back support belts
___ Job description

Date: _____

Employee: _____

handling instructions. If the garment becomes lost or damaged in any way, it has a habit of immediately increasing in value! In addition, residents will misplace clothing, and employees may occasionally walk off with something for which management will be held responsible. Some communities launder only flat sheets and pillow cases, while others also include towels and washcloths in their service package.

If the community intends to provide personal linen service, there are ways to minimize such risk. Residents' laundry can be collected by housekeeping or janitorial staff, which will in turn issue a laundry ticket in triplicate that details the laundry accepted by the housekeeper. Whenever possible, the resident should complete the laundry slip and keep one copy. The second and third copies go with the dirty laundry, and one returns with the clean. The laundry can then be placed in separate washable nylon mesh bags fitted with an identification tag that corresponds to the laundry ticket. This way several residents' laundry can be washed in the same load and still be kept separate. Before residents send anything to the laundry, all items should be marked with an indelible laundry marker. Some communities prefer to use apartment numbers rather than residents' names.

Be sure to sort delicate or bleached items into separate mesh bags. Most modern commercial washers can be programmed to operate in a variety of different cycles and can even be custom programmed for special needs. Soiled laundry should be stored in covered containers for transport to the soiled-laundry storage area. Residents' soiled personal clothing should never be stored in laundry hampers or carts, or in the soiled-laundry room with the community's or service contractor's linen. For heavily soiled laundry, any loose material can be disposed of in the resident's toilet and the laundry placed in plastic bags to avoid cross-contamination. There are even plastic bags manufactured from a material that dissolves at high temperatures and is flushed out after the wash cycle. Latex or plastic gloves should be worn when handling laundry containing human waste. In some cases the double bag method may be appropriate when servicing residents who may be suffering from a contagious disease. In skilled-nursing centers with typically heavily soiled linen, the double bag method will significantly contain odors. High water temperature is very important. Temperatures greater than 180°F will kill most types of harmful bacteria and allow the fabrics to open up and expand for more efficient removal of soil. Cold water closes fabrics, and soaps will not work as effectively in temperatures of less than 140°F.

The housekeeper who cleans the isolation rooms or who handles contaminated linens should use the double bag method. The double-bagged linens should be brought directly to the laundry room and should not be stored with other dirty linens. The laundry worker should exercise care not to touch the contaminated linen and should wear rubber gloves, a mask, and an apron. The laundry worker should open the outer "clean" bag, then pick up the inner soiled bag and shake its contents directly into the washer without touching the inner bag or the soiled linen. In some circumstances a germicide can be added while the load is washed at the hottest setting.

Mopheads, cleaning cloths, and other housekeeping service linens should be washed separately. Soak kitchen linen, towels, aprons, and cleaning cloths in the machine or sink using a degreasing presoak or detergent for at least an hour to remove grease and stains before washing. Cloth hampers should be washed last, and cloth hampers from the isolation room or that are otherwise contaminated should be washed separately.

Conditions favorable for the growth of mold and mildew (temperatures of 70°–85°F under humid conditions with little air circulation) are typically found in most laundry operations. Mildew is not easily removed from fabrics. To clean mildew from hard surfaces, clean with chlorine bleach to whiten, then follow up with a disinfectant to kill the spores.

Never accept more laundry than can be reasonably processed during the day it was collected. This is especially true of nursing home linen. The longer the stain sets, the harder it will be to remove. Prespotting can be very effective. Dryers help to set stains, so be sure to check linens as they are removed from the washers. Perspiration stains can be removed with ammonia or alkaline products. Bleach will not remove perspiration stains and should *never* be mixed with ammonia, because this combination creates toxic vapors. Pretreat as soon as possible and avoid allowing soiled items to come into contact with other soiled pieces to avoid transferring stains.

Laundry should be picked up during the weekly or bimonthly housekeeping visit and returned clean to the resident at the next visit. Exhibit 11.2 can be

---

Exhibit 11.2   Linen Distribution Form

Apartment number _____

Linen type	Standard quantity	Quantity requested
Flat sheets / Sabanas		
Twin / Pequeñas		
Double / Doble		
Queen / Medianas		
King / Grandes		
Pillowcases / Almohadas		
Towels / Toallas		
Bath / Grandes		
Hand / Pequeñas		
Face cloths / Para la cara		
Bath mats / Para el piso		
Other / Otras _____		

---

used as a checklist for linen articles. Resist attempts by residents to persuade you to wash and return their linen the same day, for this is a very inefficient way to operate. The laundry can be folded and stored in a clean area near residential apartments where the housekeeper can pick it up at the beginning of each shift. Many communities have found that shrink-wrapping each order with the ticket on top can be a clever way to keep washed laundry clean and separate. This is a relatively inexpensive tool that can serve for other community laundry jobs as well.

In some smaller communities, housekeepers launder resident linens using washers located on the resident floors. This practice is not recommended, and it is even illegal in most health-care facilities. The washing machines in the residential areas are normally connected to the domestic hot water system. Water temperatures should not be set any higher in the domestic system than 110°F to avoid the possibility of scalding the residents. Because water temperatures of 180°F are required to kill most bacteria, a community laundry facility equipped with a booster heater will be required to protect the resident population from the

spread of disease. If operators choose this option, then chemical sanitizers should be added to the wash cycle as a minimum effort for infection control. Resident linens should be rotated rather than delaying remaking the bed until the linens are laundered. In other words, when the room is made up, clean linens should be immediately replaced on the bed, and the laundered linens should be dropped off when they are clean.

COMMUNITY-PROVIDED LINENS

There are many advantages to communities' choosing to provide their own flat linens and towels to their residents. The complications of sorting and separately storing the linens are eliminated, and in some circumstances it can be more cost-effective to contract this service. Community-provided linens will be more expensive to maintain. Except in skilled-nursing facilities, encourage or require residents to use their own linen. Residents will then have several sets of linen in a pattern they enjoy, which will make them feel more at home than the all-white institutional linens.

In communities where linens are provided, residents or housekeepers can simply fill out a linen request form to indicate the linen complement requested to be returned at the next housekeeping visit. (A bilingual sample of this can be found in Exhibit 11.2.) Housekeepers should be sure to double check that the dirty linen received matches the request in order to minimize loss. Three changes of linen per resident in assisted-living and nursing homes is usually adequate, including linen in use.

LAUNDRY LAYOUT

Dirty laundry should always be separated from clean to avoid cross-contamination. Hampers should be clearly labeled "Clean Linen" or "Soiled Linen." Dirty laundry should come into the laundry area through one set of doors, and clean laundry should exit through another. Ideally, the laundry flow should be set up in a circular pattern. A separate sorting room for receiving and sorting soiled laundry can help to keep the soiled laundry contained. Soiled linen should be transported in a closed container that does not permit airborne contamination of corridors and areas occupied by residents and clean linen.

When soiled laundry enters the laundry facility it can either be kept separate in mesh bags, or, if properly marked with the residents' identification, be sorted into tubs of like variety and temporarily stored in plastic bins. These bins can then be wheeled to the washers, where the laundry is washed, removed from the washers, and put into the dryers. Once the dirty/soiled bins are unloaded, they should be disinfected, then wheeled into the drying/folding area. It will normally take 15–20 minutes to complete a wash cycle, depending on the selection, and roughly double that time to dry. Therefore, the efficient laundry facility will provide more drying capacity than washing.

The drying/folding area is the clean side of the operation; here clean laundry is dried, ironed/steamed, folded, wrapped, and temporarily stored. To prevent infestation by rodents and insects, the laundry room door should never be left propped open. In addition, it is a good idea to provide air conditioning for employee comfort and to reduce the incidence of mildew, especially in warm climates. Ceiling fans to circulate the air continually are a must in humid climates.

Rubberized tile floors are easiest to clean and disinfect and provide the most standing comfort for employees. Laundry that comes into contact with cement floors is subject to increased stains and contamination. Cement is very porous, making it impossible to clean and disinfect properly.

Standard equipment will vary according to the community size and service package. It should include some combination of 50- to 75-pound washers, plus one or two apartment washers for delicate items and personal clothes, a gas-fired ironer, a steamer or steam cabinet for steaming uniforms and other items, irons, ironing boards, 75- to 110-pound commercial dryers, and folding tables. (The color scheme should be based on tan, which is easiest on the eyes; white can cause headaches.) Commercial washers are rated by maximum capacity in pounds of a single load. Most modern washers are capable of up to 30 programmable cycle formulas and come with 10 standard preprogrammed cycles. Machines with capacities larger than 50 pounds will normally have two motors: one wash motor and one extract motor, typically 1.5 horsepower. The smaller 35-pound washers will generally have only one two-speed motor. All washers should be capable of at least 500 RPM in extract speed in order to withdraw as much moisture as possible before the drying cycle. The more efficient the extract cycle in the washer, the less time in the dryer. The folding tables should be waist high to keep employees from bending over. Some

laundry bins can be fitted to rise as laundry is removed. Polyfilm wrap (36" wide) can be used to wrap the clean linen with heat-sealing hand irons. Commercial plastic wrappers are also available to automate this task. Clean linen should be stored in a clean, well-ventilated closet, room, or alcove used *only* for that purpose.

Pressing can be done with an electric presser capable of processing 40 pounds per hour, or with a gas-fired flatwork ironer. The Chicago Champ gas-fired ironer has a 60-inch usable ironing width and a 8 inch-diameter heated roll. These work the best for processing dining room and guest room linens (napkins should be spray-starched before ironing) and retail for about $4,500. Electric flatwork finishers will also get the job done but are somewhat expensive to operate. As a rule, most physical plants will operate equipment with gas because it is both more efficient and cheaper.

Steam cabinets can also be very cost effective for removing wrinkles from employee uniforms. The system uses a steam cabinet and a booster heater to generate the additional hot water requirement. Cissel's "Moist-Rite" finishing cabinet (model MR3FC) and Sussman's "Hot Shot" boiler (model ES30) are a good combination and can be purchased and installed for under $7,000. The steam cabinet can finish approximately 140 garments per hour versus 10 garments per hour in a hand-ironing production. Even wash-and-wear uniforms need to be touched up before use, and dining room uniforms should be pressed. The steam cabinet system can easily handle permanent press, woolens, loosely woven fabrics, flannels, tweeds, knit dresses and double knit suits as well as all poly blend uniforms. When compared with the cost of hand processing uniforms, the payback period to cover the capital expenditure is normally less than one year for retirement communities larger than 200 units.

Most communities also provide laundry rooms located throughout the building for residents' personal use. Washers and dryers are generally operated at no charge to the resident. Heavily soiled linens should be washed only in the central laundry facilities where proper operating temperatures can ensure infection control. Operating instructions for the washers and dryers should be posted in the laundry rooms. Also, large signs can be posted for visually impaired residents to denote common settings for machines. Laundry rooms should be open 24 hours a day, but residents should be encouraged to remove their clothing as soon as each cycle is completed. Because residents often forget their clothes in the machines, a plastic basket or wire mesh cart with rubberized corners should be made available so that other residents can unload idle machines. The residents should be reminded of their responsibility to clean the dryer lint traps after each use, and the laundry room should be fitted with an appropriate wastebasket for this purpose. Communities that provide ironing boards should also provide self-shut-off safety irons that can be checked out at the concierge desk. It is a good idea to keep several irons on hand and charge residents who fail to return them, inasmuch as they have a propensity to disappear. The laundry rooms should be cleaned and disinfected weekly, and a disinfectant-solution spray bottle and paper towels should be available in the room for resident use. Resident aides and family members should never be allowed to use the community laundry machines for their own purposes. This will lead to the introduction of pests into the community and resentment by the other residents when they are inconvenienced by busy machines. All resident laundry rooms should be fitted with a floor drain, especially if a laundry tub or sink is present.

CHEMICALS AND SAFETY

Dispensing chemicals into the laundry machines can be done either manually or automatically. Automatic dispensers have several compelling advantages over the manual system. They are fed by dispensing tubes that suction the chemicals from five-gallon buckets in preprogrammed amounts that can be stored in a secure location. This system virtually eliminates the need for employees to handle chemicals. The automatic dispensers are normally programmed to dispense chemicals for a *full* load, so some chemical waste is possible when processing partial loads. Manually dispensed chemicals are normally added to the top of the machines, generally at eye level. Employees should be instructed to use scoops, measuring cups, or other containers to dispense soaps, detergents, bleaches, or other chemicals. They should never use their hands. It is up to the employee to determine the correct amount of chemical used and to take appropriate precautionary measures when handling and dispensing the products.

There are five basic categories of chemical solutions used in the laundry operation:

- *Softeners* These soften terry and cotton, reducing static electricity in the dryer and wear of the dryer drum and the linen itself. They also freshen fabrics.
- *Sour* This reduces iron and brings down the pH of the water. It also neutralizes water and reduces alkalinity that causes stiffness in linen, which can contribute to skin breakdown and bedsores.
- *Destainer* This bleaching agent whitens and removes discoloration.
- *Emulsion detergent* This alkaline detergent with a wetting agent breaks up (emulsifies) and removes grease and heavy soil. It conditions water by suspending calcium and magnesium to keep stains down and grayness out. (XP is an additional wetting agent that is commonly used for restaurant linens. It penetrates the linen better to release food soils.)
- *Oxybrite* This is a concentrated, all-fabric liquid oxygen-bleach compound. It does not remove colors but removes stains, like chlorine bleach.

Material Safety Data Sheets (MSDS) must be kept on file and in an available location for employee access. They can be ordered from most manufacturers in several languages. It is the law the all chemicals used have MSDS sheets on file, even those products that have been discontinued. The MSDS contains information on each product, detailing hazardous components, first aid, handling data, protective measures, and storage recommendations. Employee orientation and training programs conducted upon hire should include chemical precautions and proper handling. (An orientation checklist is shown in Exhibit 11.1.) All MSDS sheets should be reviewed periodically and at least annually to insure that all employees are fully aware of the risks and first aid associated with exposure. OSHA requires eyewash stations capable of 8 to 10 minutes of continuous flow to be installed in chemical use and storage areas.

Biohazard waste receptacles are picked up and delivered by a specialized contractor with disposal authorization. The boxes should be used in laundries for the disposal of isolation bags and biohazard sharps that may have been accidentally thrown in with dirty laundry. Caution should be exercised by staff when sorting dirty laundry from health-care components of the community to avoid possible contamination. Gloves, masks, and vinyl aprons should be worn when handling soiled linen, which should be carefully sorted piece by piece. Back support belts are also recommended.

All spray bottles containing disinfectant, window cleaner, prespotter, or other chemical should be appropriately identified and labeled. Empty bottles should be triple rinsed and punctured before disposal.

Employees should never open a machine or touch its surfaces when it is operating. These machines run at very high temperatures, and workers can easily be scalded.

In health care communities, the linen and laundry services will be inspected and evaluated by the state health department or other regulatory agency. The evaluation will normally determine whether or not the community's laundry and linen services comply with state regulations and Federal Conditions of Participation pertaining to laundry services and infection control, which state: "The facility has available at all times a quantity of linen essential for proper care and comfort of the residents; and linens are handled, stored,

processed, and transported in such a manner as to prevent the spread of infection."

MAINTENANCE

The maintenance department should organize a preventive maintenance schedule for the laundry machinery. This should include routine oiling, balancing, gasket and belt replacement, and total lint trap and removal system cleaning. A washer that goes out of balance can excessively vibrate both the building and the internal workings of the washer. The cam shaft is susceptible to being bent under load and vibration, and it is very expensive to replace. Modern commercial washers are equipped with a vibration safety switch. Most small repairs and seals can be accomplished by the facility maintenance staff. Expensive maintenance service contracts can generally be avoided inasmuch as the machines are relatively easy to work on and parts are readily available. It is wise, however to stock a few more frequently used parts such as dryer door seals, washers, fuses, and belts so that down time can be minimized in the event of a breakdown.

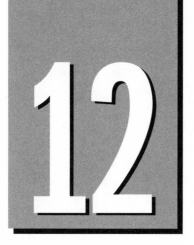

12 Maintenance

The maintenance department is primarily responsible for providing a safe environment for the residents and staff. The department is responsible for the long-term protection of the physical aspects of the building, including the equipment, furniture, and fixtures. The building systems are operated to provide a comfortable environment at a minimal cost. Finally, the department staff must demonstrate competence to the residents through resident satisfaction by maintaining public areas, occupied and vacant apartments, and ultimately ensuring quality and consistent response to resident requests. These essential functions of the department are performed best when standardized procedures and systems are established to accomplish these goals.

The objectives of the maintenance department normally fall into two basic categories: *maintenance* and *repair. Maintenance* is the day-to-day, periodic, or scheduled work required to preserve or restore community physical assets to an operable condition. It routinely includes work to prevent damage or deterioration that otherwise may be more costly to restore. Prompt maintenance is essential to facilitate peak operating efficiency. *Repair* is the restoration of a system to a condition that allows it to be used for its designed purpose. The repair may involve overhaul or replacing parts or materials that have deteriorated because of use or time and that have not been corrected through proper maintenance.

Minor repairs and maintenance of the building systems can be routine and part of the normal upkeep of the property. These routine repairs are normally handled through the annual budget process by estimating past expenditures to forecast future requirements. However, when major systems of the building begin to fail, the maintenance director will need to take a more detailed approach. The overall economy of the system, its cost of operation, and desired operational efficiency should be studied before a recommendation is made for major repairs. Factors for management to consider and evaluate on an ongoing basis can include:

- Replacement cost of the system in relation to the expected life span of the system, and to the cost of repairs.
- Operation and maintenance costs of the old system versus a new system.
- Possible obsolescence of the system and availability of parts.
- Present and future availability of maintenance funds.
- Operational hazards of down time on the resident population when major repair or replacement of the systems may be required due to failure.

The costs of some of these criteria are more easily quantified than others. The maintenance director can perform the basic financial evaluation, but it is up to the executive director and ultimately the owners to assess the long-term availability of capital for maintaining the building systems at their best and the possible risks to the residents and to investment of deferral. Many major system failures can be delayed or averted with an ounce of prevention.

PREVENTIVE MAINTENANCE

The primary objective for any preventive maintenance plan is to reduce the costs of operation and labor, and capital replacement expenses. When equipment and systems are properly maintained, they function more efficiently and are less expensive to operate. Clogged air-handler filters and heat exchangers operate at reduced capacity, which means they must work harder and will wear out sooner. Properties that have deferred maintenance over the years must invest large amounts of labor in repairs. It is much less expensive in the long run to make repairs as they are needed than to allow problems to accumulate. If the deferral is due to budget constraints, then the maintenance director should take these issues to the owners and have them resolved. Deferred maintenance will ultimately result in a decrease in the overall value of the property. It will cost much more to bring in contractors to complete the deferred projects than to have facility staff handle them.

Visual and mechanical checking of the condition of the building's major systems should be performed regularly on a scheduled basis. This way the maintenance director can keep a running status report of the extent of regular maintenance and repair work that is required to ensure proper operation of the systems. There are many ways to accomplish this. The process will vary according to personnel and skill levels.

Priorities should be established by the maintenance director and executive director so that the preventive maintenance plan can be focused. Of utmost priority is the equipment affecting the life and safety of the building's occupants. These systems include but are not limited to fire suppression and alarms, domestic hot water system, heating and air conditioning systems (HVAC), emergency power generators, emergency lighting, and emergency response systems. The temporary loss of any of these critical systems can have a significant impact on an aging population.

The second priority of the preventive maintenance program is the major cost equipment of the building. This includes the chillers, air handlers, recirculation pumps, major valves and shutoffs, boilers, and elevator equipment. This equipment, when properly maintained, should provide the community with many years of service.

Manufacturer operations manuals normally include recommended preventive maintenance schedules for each critical component of the equipment, and these manuals should be archived and used. In new buildings, these are available at the time of installation and should be kept in the maintenance office. Some general contractors or project managers will videotape the orientation and service recommendations from the installer immediately after installation before the manufacturer's representative leaves the job site. This way the current and future maintenance director can have a visual record of each of the building's major systems and can understand the components of the systems with actual footage of the equipment, rather than trying to decipher an owner's manual. Videotaping expensive maintenance and repair procedures performed by outside contractors or manufacturer's representatives can also help to minimize downtime in the future.

Building turnover from the general contractor to management should be coordinated to include information regarding all city permits and a description of the permitting process along with any sensitivities from the building inspector's or fire marshall's offices. Blueprints and "as-built" drawings detailing all of the building's utilities, including location in the building, and materials used for water, electric, gas, sewer, phone, and fire alarm systems are invaluable in the event of a major breakdown. All contractors (electrical, fire alarm, plumbing, mechanical, HVAC, painting, mill working, landscaping, flooring, and so on) should provide the following:

1. Specifications on materials used.
2. Where to purchase on a 24-hour notice.
3. How to properly operate all of the equipment.
4. How and when to do preventive maintenance on all equipment.
5. All warranty and guarantee information.
6. Complete walk through for all equipment installed.
7. Whom to call in an emergency and schedule of charges.

The third priority for a preventive maintenance program relates to equipment and finishes affecting the appearance of the building and ultimately resident satisfaction. The overall physical appearance of a community often can provide clues to its financial health and management competence. Normally operators will attend to the more visual deterioration of the common areas and the exterior of the building. These areas will receive more attention from the residents, their guests, and ownership representatives who tour the property as the building undergoes normal wear and tear. This attention to the "finish" of the building often comes at the expense of what should be the higher priorities of life safety and major cost equipment, which is typically located in secluded areas of the building. A strip of loose wallpaper will be noticed and repaired before anyone ever notices the badly worn bearings on a recirculation pump that distributes hot water throughout the building.

Finally, the fourth priority for the preventive maintenance plan is the identification and maintenance of equipment that promotes a more efficient operation. These systems are normally water or air handling and require frequent attention and cleaning to prevent breakdowns.

Preventive Maintenance Methods

The best way to organize an effective preventive maintenance system is through the use of a log system. This can all be kept in a looseleaf binder with sections for the major equipment serviced and a section for the apartments. The apartment log should include a single sheet for each apartment that serves as the basis for the history of all maintenance visits to each individual apartment. Information summarized on each apartment log sheet should include the date, description of service, any special comments about the job, and the initials of the person performing the service. Routine visits to the apartment for work orders as well as preventive maintenance should be documented. This way the maintenance director and executive director can keep a running history on each maintenance visit to each apartment. This information is very valuable as documentation for when the apartment was last painted, the carpet changed, the toilet serviced, and so on, so that management can identify and track such things as the life span of carpets and paint and the last preventive maintenance session, and use the information to estimate a replacement schedule for the unit's fixtures.

It is a good idea for the maintenance person to perform some routine preventive maintenance during short visits to the apartment. This way the department can maximize its time in each apartment, and the resident sees that the maintenance department is on top of its preventive maintenance program. As with any other department, maintenance needs to manage the residents' expectations, which ultimately translates to satisfaction. Routine preventive maintenance for each unit should include: running a short cycle of the washer and dishwasher and checking for leaks; verifying that the refrigerator doors are sealing when shut; checking the sink cabinet for insects; checking for odors such as mold and mildew; flushing toilets and checking the floor around the base for leaks; running all faucets; noting any water marks or leaks on exterior walls and around window casings; locking all windows; and checking seals. In addition, the apartment heating/cooling unit should have the cover removed for replacement of the air filter and a visual check of the condensate drain pan. These drain-pan tubes can build up with dust or algae, causing them to clog and back up, which in turn can cause significant water damage to the ceiling of the apartment or common area below.

A complete inspection of all public areas and exterior of the building should be conducted at least quarterly by the maintenance director, noting any servicing requirements that can be prioritized with the work order system. The maintenance director should also keep a set of blueprints of the building for use when bidding service work, with all valves, clean-outs, and major equipment locations highlighted.

Major system components such as pumps, motors, condensers and compressors, heat exchangers, boilers, rooftop air-handling units for public areas, instruments, and controls should be scheduled for routine maintenance according to the manufacturer's recommendations. The capital budgeting process will also depend on manufacturer specifications about the equipment, so be sure to collect and maintain all the relevant written material about each major system component.

It is also a good idea to maintain a filter log for all the filters in the building. Clogged or dirty filters can cause equipment to be overworked and can contribute to premature failure. The air filter log should include type of heating, cooling, and ventilation systems; type of filter(s) installed; manufacturer and manufacturer's instructions for cleaning and replacement; ASHRAE efficiency rating; manometer; and location of all the filters within the community.

WORK ORDER SYSTEM

Work orders are a key element of the maintenance department operation. They document necessary work and serve as a means for all departments and residents to communicate with maintenance and other departments. The system provides a unified method of handling requests for repairs and other community services. The functions of the maintenance request system are:

1. To provide a standard system for expediting the maintenance function.
2. To provide written records of maintenance requested, to whom assigned and by whom completed, along with the date and duration of the completion process.
3. To reduce oral communication and improve follow-through by providing a means whereby department heads and residents may originate written requests to be carried through to completion.
4. To provide a convenient means of screening and prioritizing maintenance requests by management.
5. To facilitate staffing assignments by providing a readily visual and traceable record of backlog work.
6. To provide a convenient means for providing backup for billable requests for services by residents to the accounting department.

Work order requests can be initiated by the reception desk, department heads, or by maintenance personnel. A work order request ticket should be developed in triplicate, allowing it to be routed to the appropriate personnel for completion. The reception desk and the resident should retain a copy, with the master going to the maintenance department. The maintenance director should then assess the priority given to the request and assign the request to a staff person for completion. If more than 30 minutes will be required to complete the work order, the resident should be called to schedule an appointment for completion of the work. Upon completion of the work, the completed work order ticket can be returned to the reception desk. The evening receptionist can then match the completed ticket to the original on file and enter the completed work into the work order log maintained at the front desk. The original can then be forwarded to the accounting department for billing (if appropriate) and filing. This system accomplishes the objectives outlined above while ensuring that resident and staff requests do not get lost in the shuffle. At any time, the resident or department head can check the status of their request at the front desk.

A work order board in the maintenance department is a convenient way to keep track of work order progress and assignment. The first step for the work order is the "Work to Be Completed" hook. The work order tickets can be sorted on this board according to who is assigned to do the work. This can be maintenance personnel, housekeeping staff, or an outside contractor. Occasionally parts will need to be ordered that are not in inventory. It is a good idea to keep a small inventory of frequently used parts so that work orders are not delayed. If parts are needed, the work order ticket can be put in a "Parts on Order" hook on the board. The director of maintenance should make sure that appropriate action has been taken to order the parts. The director should contact both the receptionist and the resident to inform them of the order and the expected delivery time. When the parts arrive, the work order ticket can be assigned to the appropriate person. Any work order that has been delayed due to the ordering of parts should be reassigned top priority once the parts have arrived. Once the work orders are completed and signed off on by the assigned staff and the resident, they can be transferred to a "Work Orders Completed" hook that can then be transferred to the evening receptionist and recorded as completed in the work order log book, completing the cycle.

The work order log can be used by all interested parties to monitor total requests, completion time frames, and requests that have stalled. It is also useful to illustrate patterns and abnormal numbers of maintenance issues that may require further investigation or different troubleshooting procedures to correct permanently. All turnover apartments (make-ready) should be given priority above all except emergency work orders to return the unit to move-in condition within 48 hours of moveout. Any painting and repair work should be scheduled in advance of the lease ending date. Be sure to obtain the resident's or responsible party's permission to enter the apartment for this purpose before the lease expiration date. The vacant apartment should be thoroughly cleaned immediately after maintenance is finished and should be left in a "showable" condition. The need to order parts or fixtures for the unit should be anticipated in advance. This is especially important when apartments turn over and need to be made rentable for the next tenant. Each day that the apartment remains unoccupied, the cost of completing the work order dramatically increases because of lost revenue potential.

CAPITAL IMPROVEMENTS

Fixed asset capitalization, also known as capital improvement, is a process of addressing the current and projected physical needs of a property, establishing the costs of maintaining or modernizing it, and creating a strategic plan for addressing those needs within financial constraints. The first step in developing such a plan is to establish a comprehensive inventory of the community's physical systems, both mechanical and aesthetic. The inventory should be as complete as possible. Managers have a tendency to focus on major systems such as the boilers, roof, in-unit components, and finishes. However, the little things that may be left neglected, such as a broken thermopane seal, window caulking, and upholstery, have a tendency to add up and to need attention all at once. With careful and comprehensive planning, community capital resources can be allocated in a deliberate fashion.

The inventory should also quantify things as specifically as possible. For example, the make, model, and size of mechanical equipment, square feet of paving, roof and common area carpets, and counts by type and size of windows and furniture should be noted precisely for easy reference later when bidding and budgeting repairs or replacements. Accurate quantity is essential in developing accurate cost estimates. Architectural plans will generally yield better information and can make this part of the job much easier than can hand measurements.[1]

The actual remaining life of any given system, fixture, or equipment will be a function of age, design, material type and quality, nature of use, maintenance, and environmental conditions. Determination of the estimated life for each item in the completed inventory can be derived from the manufacturer warranty, actual experience of subject site or other like site, industry standards, and firsthand estimates made by community maintenance staff and outside contractors. In some cases, actions may be prompted by changing market conditions or the development of a new community within the primary market area to keep the community looking fresh and competitive.

Cost estimates for repair and replacements can be accomplished with local contractors through a bidding process. In established communities, management will often have direct experience to rely on for such costs. If this information does not extend to larger mechanical systems, historic information may be available from other properties of similar design. There are a number of published cost-estimation sources, such as R.S. Means and Marshall and Swift, but these third-party sources should only be used as a general guideline, insofar as they will not account for the particularities of design and installation requirements in the existing facility. Third-party cost estimation sources normally deal with new construction and these costs normally differ substantially from rehabilitation of an existing facility. All cost estimates should include tax, freight, material, and labor costs. Typically tax and freight will be approximately 12–15 percent of the cost of goods. Should the project be underbudgeted initially, it may be possible to increase the budget by transferring funds from other projects or by canceling lower-priority projects. This reallocation of funds may be unavoidable when unexpected emergency capital needs become identified.

For projects involving contracted labor or construction, actual bids for the work completed, a signed standard construction contract for each company providing the labor, certificate of insurance, and a signed "General Waiver and Release of Lien Rights" should all be included in the submittal.

Having identified expected capital needs, ascribed costs to them, and projected when they are likely to occur, the next step is to project the impact of these costs on the bottom line. A 10-year capital spending plan should be prepared to estimate what total capital costs are likely to be in each given year. Spreadsheet programs permit this to be done quickly and accurately and also facilitate adjustments for future inflation of these costs. In this way it is possible to review the annual anticipated needs and appropriately allocate the resources evenly over time. In most cases, a capital reserve of 2 or 3 percent of gross revenue from opening should be more than adequate to keep the community in good repair and looking its best. For big projects, phasing the work over time may be necessary given limited resources. However, phasing may need to be judged against lost economies of scale.

The capital planning process should also identify the allocation of the resources by a priority system. The priority system should be defined to establish a comparative relationship between capital needs to facilitate informed decisions during the budgeting process. For example, those expenditures that are required for health and safety reasons normally would be assigned top priority. Second priority could be assigned to projects that facilitate a more efficient operation, thereby reducing the cost of operations. Third priority could be assigned to projects designed to meet company standards. Fourth priority could be reserved for major renovations, and fifth could be assigned to elective projects that may simply promote community enhancement or "wish list" items. Payback periods should be calculated on all items including installation that are intended to save operating money. The payback period is the time it takes for the cumulative operating savings to exceed initial total costs (calculate by dividing the initial cost by the annual operating savings).

Some financing vehicles require the maintenance of minimum replacement reserves. The adequacy of these funding levels should be reevaluated over time to identify the optimal reserve through an interactive process. These normally involve rather substantial amounts of capital that may not otherwise be required after the identification of need through the capital planning process.

▰▰▰ STAFFING

As a rule of thumb, one full-time maintenance person will be required for every 100 units of congregate or assisted living in good condition. If the property has a history of deferred maintenance, or it is new construction with extensive punch-list issues, more staffing may be required. Normally, new projects will be less demanding on maintenance staff due to the lack of residents, but as the population increases, the marketing department as well as new residents will place demands on the maintenance department. Continuing-care retirement communities will require at least one additional maintenance person to handle the rather specialized needs of the nursing home as they are subject to HCFA conditions of participation and state licensing requirements.

Generally speaking, most executive directors have little or limited knowledge of building systems and the appropriate expertise required to ensure proper management of those systems. Maintenance expertise tends to be very specialized. For example, one individual could be an excellent electrician but have limited knowledge of plumbing or HVAC. Conversely, a generalist who is capable of fixing just about everything may create a need for extensive work from outside contractors when major systems fail. The key is to find a generalist who can make most routine repairs and who knows when to call in the specialists and at what price.

Clearly, one must match the maintenance director's level of expertise with the complexity of the physical plant. Many large continuing-care retirement communities can afford to hire specialists such as plumbers, electricians, and HVAC technicians to maintain their extensive physical plants. Some communities with golf courses will need to hire specialized crews to keep their courses well groomed and looking their best.

Another key component of the successful maintenance director is the ability to deal with residents. Residents can be very demanding and unforgiving regarding their maintenance needs. Some can also be very lonely and will often look for excuses to interact with management staff or a favorite maintenance person. The skilled maintenance director will need to balance the needs of these residents and the attention they expect and deserve with the demands of maintaining their physical plant in top condition. This requires a commitment on behalf of the maintenance director to time management and clearly defined priorities. The better this individual can balance these often mutually conflicting goals, the more likely he will be successful in his job. As with other departments, resident perceptions can be a strong influence. The director must be able to demonstrate his compassion about the residents and competence in his role each and every day.

In some ways, resident perceptions about the maintenance department can be a bit of a popularity contest. Residents will compliment the department if they receive the attention they desire and conversely make the maintenance director's job stressful if they are not happy. The residents, of course only see a small portion of the maintenance director's job, as most of the equipment is located in the nonpublic areas in the back of the house. The successful director will learn to manage the residents' expectations and communicate maintenance priorities to them. Most residents will understand that the repair and maintenance of the major system components relating to their life safety have priority over their work order request. What they will not tolerate is attention to a vacant unit for marketing purposes at the expense of their personal requests. The maintenance director must reassure them of their importance and the estimated completion date for their request, in spite of the fact that vacant apartments mean lost revenue, and management may feel that marketing requests should receive priority over everything except emergency work orders.

For large communities (200+ units) it is a good idea to stagger maintenance shifts to provide evening and weekend coverage. These are times when apartment make-readys can be done with little interruption from the residents. Also, the maintenance director should outline a number of "typical" maintenance calls and provide simple instructions to be left at the concierge desk so that he can avoid being called for minor problems. The list should identify each maintenance problem, suggest a solution, and attempt to define what is considered an emergency that will require immediate attention and what can wait until the following day. For example, simple instructions on how to stop a toilet from overflowing and procedures to unclog it can be left with the concierge and accomplished by other management employees or housekeepers. Many times, quick action on the part of an informed nonmaintenance employee can avert considerable damage and save the maintenance director a trip back to the facility after hours.

■■■ KEY CONTROL

Key and lock control should be overseen by one central person. This is normally the responsibility of the maintenance director, with the approval of the executive director. The control of keys in the community is an essential element of building security: if left uncontrolled, it can expose the community to significant liability. Key control among employees is much easier to accomplish than with residents. Many residents will give their family members copies of their keys, which allows nearly unlimited access to the building.

There are two types of key systems: hard key traditional and electronic. Hard keys are more readily accepted and understood by residents, but electronic systems can be programmed to track each entry and can provide management some flexibility in monitoring both staff and residents. Electronic systems are normally much more expensive to install and maintain. Management will need to evaluate security needs against this added flexibility and cost.

Uncut and unissued keys should be kept in a locking key cabinet, with access limited to the maintenance director and executive director. Department operating keys can be kept in a locking box at the concierge's desk. All department keys should be signed out and in from the concierge.

Apartment keys are normally issued according to the following procedures:

1. Resident move-ins are confirmed via a notification of move-in from marketing. This notification is issued to all managers, and it states the date for move-in as well as other pertinent information.
2. The maintenance director, upon receipt of the notification from marketing, will prepare two apartment keys, one mailbox key (if different), and one exterior door key (when applicable) for the new resident. These keys will be attached to a key ring labeled with the new resident's name and apartment number and kept secure until one day before move-in.
3. One day before move-in, the maintenance director should hand deliver the new resident's keys to the office manager. The maintenance director must verify that he issued the keys to the office manager, and the office manager must initial the form to acknowledge that the keys were received.
4. The office manager must keep the new resident's keys secure until move-in. This policy is necessary to prevent unauthorized access to the community and to prevent unauthorized work on community apartments.

Only the following department heads should have a grand master key: executive director, maintenance director, marketing director, and director of housekeeping. Upon hiring, these managers will receive a grand master key, which must be noted on a personal property form. Upon termination, the employee must return the grand master key.

An Emergency "E" key should be kept at the Concierge Desk. The "E" key is a special master key that will operate all of the locks in a system at all times. There should only be four (4) "E" keys on the property: one should be on the executive director's key ring, one at the concierge desk, one in the emergency supply cabinet, and one available only to the fire department (to be kept in the "Knox Box" near the main entrance).

All departmental keys or locks should be issued according to the following procedures:

1. When locks or keys are needed, the requesting manager must complete a maintenance request form, expressing the reason for needing the lock or key.
2. The requesting manager must receive approval from the executive director by having the executive director sign the maintenance request.
3. The maintenance request is submitted to the maintenance director for processing.
4. When locks are installed a key is given to the department head, and a copy is kept in the maintenance director's key cabinet.

All departmental keys must be kept on the same ring, and that ring must be labeled according to the department (e.g., Food Service Keys).

- All departmental keys must be kept at the concierge desk. These keys must be signed out when taken, and signed in when they are returned. The date and time of day must be noted when these keys are signed out or in. Other vital information is the name and department of employee, purpose for key, and initials of concierge on duty. These keys are not to leave the property.
- Staff members who are authorized to sign for and hold keys may not, under any circumstances, pass their keys on to another employee.
- If keys must be passed from shift to shift, they must be signed in by the employee designated to have them, and then signed out by the next authorized employee. All keys must be returned and signed in to the concierge desk at the end of the staff member's shift.
- Under no circumstances will an employee have in her possession keys that have not been properly signed out. Any other keys found in the possession of an employee will be considered unauthorized.
- No person will use a key to enter an area that he or she is not authorized to enter.
- At no time, under any circumstance, will a person use a building key to enter an area other than the area designated in his work schedule. No employee will use her key to open an area for a person not authorized to be in the area.
- Any outside employee (from, e.g., the cable company or phone company) who requests building keys must obtain authorization from the maintenance director. These keys must be signed in and out by the outside employee using a key control log. This individual will be held accountable until the keys are returned and signed back in. "Extra" keys for this purpose will not be kept at the concierge desk.
- Any employee must bring to his or her supervisor's attention any incidents where keys are misplaced, lost, or misused. This notification must be accompanied by documentation, key logs, and the like. If the keys are not found, the supervisor must notify the executive director of the loss. The executive director will decide on the necessity of rekeying the lock.

SERVICE CONTRACTS

Service contracts on large and expensive equipment that normally requires specialized training for maintenance and repair are normally good insurance against the risk of a catastrophic breakdown. Equipment such as the elevators, fire suppression and alarm systems, emergency call system, and other critical systems that ultimately affect resident safety should be contracted out for routine maintenance and servicing. In urban areas, there will be a selection of vendors who have this expertise. It is a good idea to solicit bids from contractors who are dealers or service representatives for the specific type of equipment in the building. It is in their best interest to service their own equipment and to demonstrate to other clients how cost effective their equipment is to maintain.

As many vendors will deal in similar equipment, it is imperative to solicit at least two competitive bids for your major service contracts. In addition, these contracts should automatically *expire* rather than be renewed annually. This way, the community can evaluate the cost effectiveness of their contracts once each year. Most contractors will have an "evergreen" clause in their contracts so that they automatically renew at the end of the term. Arranging for the contracts to terminate each year will keep the contractors competitive with their prices. Whenever the prices are increased, so also should the contract be put out to multiple bid. Most service contracts and prices are negotiable. All you need to do is shop around and compare.

The maintenance director should keep a ledger book with a one-page summary of each of the community's service contracts. The summary should include

Exhibit 12.1   Emergency Procedures

Emergency number _____

Type of incident or emergency	Code	Reporting person will:	Concierge will:	Accounting director	Assistant director	Engineering	Director of engineering	Food and beverages	Executive director
Medical ■ Choking ■ Heart attack ■ Shock	1	Dial. Give name, dept., nature of incident and location. Speak clearly.	(A) Call to emergency designate and department heads. Give code and location. Repeat clearly.	Report to scene and assist. Obtain prompt medical attention. Administer first aid.	Report to scene and assist. Obtain prompt medical attention. Administer first aid. Document incident with all details.	Report to scene and assist. Obtain prompt medical attention. Administer first aid. Assist as needed.	Report to scene and assist. Obtain prompt medical attention.	Report to scene and assist. Obtain prompt medical attention. Administer first aid.	Report to scene and assist. Obtain prompt medical attention. Administer first aid.
Police ■ Robbery ■ Vandals ■ Terrorism ■ Threats	2	Dial. Give name, dept., nature of incident and location. Speak clearly.	(A) Call to emergency designate and department heads. Give code and location. Repeat clearly.	Report to scene if safe to do so. Assist as necessary. Set up command post if needed.	Report to scene and assist if safe to do so. Set up command post if needed.	Get details of incident. Respond to scene or command post. Assist as needed.	Stand by. Get details of incident. Respond to scene or command post. Assist as needed. Escort police.	Stand by. Get details of incident. Respond to scene or command post. Assist as needed.	Stand by. Get details of incident. Set up possible command post if necessary. Report to scene if safe to do so.
Fire ■ Extreme heat ■ Smoke ■ Large flames	3	Dial. Give name, dept., nature of incident and location. Speak clearly.	(A) Call to emergency designate and department heads. Give code and location. Repeat clearly.	Report to scene. Attempt to extinguish or contain fire. Assure guest and employee safety.	Report to scene. Attempt to extinguish or contain fire. Assure guest and employee safety. Follow fire marshall's instructions.	Report to scene. Attempt to extinguish or contain fire. Cut electrical systems and ventilation ducts as instructed by fire marshall. Assure guest and employee safety.	Report to scene. Attempt to extinguish or contain fire. Assure guest and employee safety. Follow fire marshall's instructions.	Report to scene. Attempt to extinguish or contain fire. Assure guest and employee safety.	Report to scene. Attempt to extinguish or contain fire. Assure guest and employee safety. Oversee and assist as necessary.
Engineering ■ Water main break ■ Sprinkler break ■ Structural disaster	4	Dial. Give name, dept., nature of incident and location. Speak clearly.	(A) Call to emergency designate and department heads. Give code and location. Repeat clearly.	Report to scene and assist. Minimize damage. Assure guest and employee safety.	Report to scene and assist. Minimize damage. Assure guest and employee safety. Communicate with or call necessary agency.	Report to scene. Handle corrective engineering-related action. Minimize damage while assuring guest and employee safety.	Report to scene. Make appropriate engineering decisions. Minimize damage while assuring overall safety.	Report to scene. Assist as needed. Assure guest and employee safety.	Report to scene after verifying details with maintenance director. Assist as needed.
Tornado Hurricane Earthquake ■ Flooding ■ Excessive damage	5	Dial. Give name, dept., nature of incident and location. Speak clearly.	(A) Call to emergency designate and department heads. Give code and location. Repeat clearly. Notify area of command post.	Set up command post in executive director's absence. Have call code with command post location. Delegate appropriate emergency action based on severity of damages or potential destruction.	Set up command post in executive director's absence. Have call code with command post location. Delegate appropriate emergency action based on severity of damages or potential destruction.	Respond to command post. Follow out safety and preventive destruction measures. Assure guest and employee safety.	Respond to command post. Follow out safety and preventive destruction measures. Assure guest and employee safety.	Respond to command post. Follow out safety and preventive destruction measures. Assure guest and employee safety.	Set up command post. Have call code with command post location. Delegate appropriate emergency action based on severity of damages or potential destruction.
Medical, not an emergency ■ Small cuts ■ Bruises ■ Hematomas	6	Dial. Give name, dept., nature of incident and location. Speak clearly.	(A) Call to emergency designate and department heads. Give code and location. Repeat clearly. Notify area of command post.		Report to scene and assist. Obtain prompt medical attention. Administer first aid.				

the contractor's name and address, contact name, home and work numbers, the essential elements of the contract and, if parts are included, a short description of when and when not to call. The service contractor will normally charge a premium for visiting the property on holidays and off hours, so it is important to have an idea of what constitutes an emergency and what can wait. This way *anyone* can locate help when a system fails and can quickly understand the key components of the service contracts. The ledger book should also include a list of all vendor accounts, technicians by service area, and contact persons.

Any time that an outside contractor is called to the community, a written statement should be collected from the service technician. This statement should include the date, the item serviced, and a detailed description of the work performed, the present operating condition of the building system serviced, and any additional repairs that may be required. Thorough documentation of each contractor visit can save considerable confusion as invoices are received and processed. Copies of all current service contracts should be kept on file and should have at least two competitive bids. Certificates of insurance naming the community as an additional insured should accompany these contracts and be updated as they expire.

TOOLS AND EQUIPMENT

Any well-equipped maintenance department will have its share of tools and equipment necessary to effect repairs and perform routine maintenance. Although some maintenance directors prefer to use their own tools, the community should stock some basics. Many maintenance directors possess unique skills such as those required to maintain and recharge air conditioning systems. These systems can be repaired and maintained by outside contractors, but in the long run, buildings in hot climates can greatly benefit from hiring someone with these skills. The cost of basic equipment to perform these functions is quickly amortized considering the cost differential between contract labor and in-house employees. When considering the purchase of major tools and equipment, the cost should be balanced against the expected usage and compared to the alternative cost of contracting the service. The payback period is the true test of the correct business decision.

However, in the end it is also important for the maintenance director to be able to keep his skills current, and employee satisfaction definitely plays a role in the decision.

The total cost to fully equip a new facility with basic tools should not exceed $1,000. The equipment can either be purchased at once using startup funds, or on an as-needed basis through the normal budget process. Regardless of the purchase timing, it is a good idea to mark the tools individually, using an electric pen, with the community's identification and to number them sequentially. This way the maintenance director can sign for them at his point of hire and an inventory can be done upon employment termination to protect the community's investment. Also, tools engraved with identification are less likely to disappear at the hands of other employees and are often returned when lost. This is especially true for large pieces of equipment such as lawnmowers and snowblowers.

EMERGENCY/DISASTER PLAN

All senior living communities should have an emergency and disaster plan. This plan outlines the order of communication in the unlikely event of a facility disaster. The plan should allow for medical emergencies such as choking, heart attack, and shock; police emergencies such as robbery and vandalism; fire emergencies; engineering emergencies such as a catastrophic building system failure; tornadoes, hurricanes, earthquakes, and other natural disasters; and medical contingencies that are not to be considered emergencies.

The reporting person will have the responsibility to dial the local emergency number and give the name, location, and nature of the incident. This person will stay on the line for instructions from the emergency dispatcher. The concierge should then initiate the communication plan and coordinate an emergency group call to the appropriate department heads. A sample emergency plan is detailed in Exhibit 12.1.

NOTE

1. T. E. Nutt-Powell and D. P. Whiston, "Capital Planning for Repair and Replacement," *Journal of Property Management* (September 1991): 48–50.

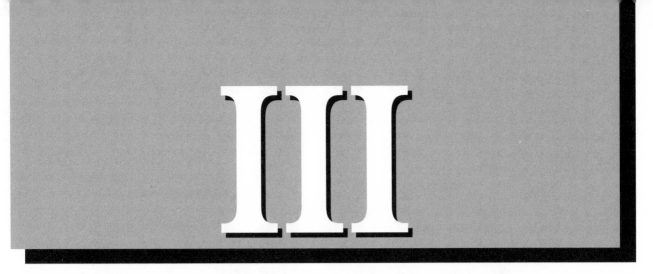

Marketing and Sales

Marketing

arketing comes first in our activities as managers. The marketing department must first attract and then convert prospects into residents. If a community is to be successful, residents and employees alike must all be marketers. The residents should be taught to recognize that a fully occupied community is a financially sound community and that their referrals are critical to their own stability. Employees on all levels need to be taught to acknowledge the importance of marketing to their own personal success; this applies equally to the housekeepers, the executive director, and even the president of the company. *Everyone* must adopt a marketing mindset.

Having the marketing mindset, though, is not enough. Employees on all levels need to be committed to delivering a quality product. If operations cannot deliver on the promises of the sales counselors, you will end up sabotaging your marketing success time and again. If you do not have a quality product, then you are wasting your marketing dollars attempting to create demand for something that people do not want.

Management must therefore convince employees that they are delivering a quality product. *Quality* is simply the difference between what people expect and what they get. If the employees are personally committed to exceeding the residents' expectations, then the community will be perceived as a quality operation. This commitment to service does not come easily. It is the result of painstaking training, motivation,

and employee recognition on a daily basis. (Refer to Chapter 3 for more on managing and motivating employees to promote the community.)

We will define *marketing* as the planning and processes designed to generate interest in and attract prospects to the community. We will define *sales* as the process of converting these prospects into tenants. The success or failure of this process will absolutely depend on a well-planned and well-executed marketing and sales strategy. Many well-conceived projects have collapsed under the weight of negative cash flow to the balance sheet resulting from too slow a fill-up. For every month that a community fails to reach cash flow, the more working capital must be borrowed to meet monthly obligations. Ultimately, this accumulation of debt will erode the return on invested equity and can, if left unchecked, jeopardize the community's ability to service the interest, especially if financed with an adjustable rate in an expanding economy.

FEASIBILITY

Feasibility analysis for senior-living communities is a two-step process. First and foremost, a financial analysis needs to determine the *minimum* absorption (fill-up) rate that will meet investment expectations for return, or break even for nonprofits. Second, it must be determined if sufficient demand exists in the marketplace with the demographic profile that the concept is intended to attract. This can be done by analyzing market penetration and market share. If competition allows, some flexibility in project concept and design may broaden appeal and facilitate a more successful absorption rate.

There is a direct relationship between the rate of fill-up of a community and its financial performance. Generally speaking, the quicker the fill-up, the better the return on invested capital. For example, an $11 million 100-unit community with a 75 percent loan to value ratio and a 20-year, 9 percent mortgage will require approximately $74,000 per month in amortizing payments. Let us assume that operational cash flow is 50 percent occupancy and that to service the debt will require 86 percent occupancy (86 units). At a net absorption rate of eight units per month it will take 11 months to reach cash flow (86 units ÷ 8 units per month). This means that for 11 months the project will need to borrow working capital to meet operational shortfalls. Interest will also accumulate on working-capital funds during this period. Normally, after this point is reached, the surplus balance will be used to pay down the more expensive working-capital loan. Only after this is completed will the project be able to realize any return on invested capital. Should the net absorption rate be actually only four units per month, then it will take approximately 21 months to reach cash flow after debt service.

To illustrate the financial impact of this, consider the $74,000 per month in debt service payments alone required for each and every month from month 11 to month 21, or the $750,000 plus interest that will need to be additionally financed due to the slower fill-up rate. This will add at least another $81,000 per year to the amortizing payment just using our 9 percent initial interest rate, and not including additional operational shortfalls incurred during this slower fill-up period, which could easily total $500,000 or more. The addition of $81,000 per year in debt service translates to $7,290 per month. At an average rent of $2,500 per month it will require 3 *more* occupied units to reach cash flow after debt service, or 89 units—89 percent (not including the additional cost per month to service these additional residents). Add in the debt service on the additional operational shortfalls of $3,750 per month and 1.5 *more* units to cover this and the figure rises to 90.5 units or 90 percent before the investor will see any return. This leaves only 4.5 units at 95 percent stabilized occupancy for return on investment, cap-

ital improvements, principal reduction, and coverage for unexpected contingencies. This small margin is further eroded if the inflated cost of operations each year cannot be passed on to the residents, who are normally on fixed incomes.

The larger the project, the faster the fill-up that will be necessary to achieve the same result. A 200-unit project may, for example, have $7 million more in debt service (100 additional units × $70,000 per unit project cost) than its 100-unit competitor. This project will need to fill at 8 net units per month in 20 months to reach the same 80 percent operations plus debt service cash flow threshold. The financial implications and risks of a slow fill-up are significantly amplified in larger projects.

The accumulation of operational shortfalls during the fill-up of projects is normally postponed by premarketing before or during construction. In fact, many states require presold thresholds of up to 70 percent to be met before construction begins on endowment life care projects. Prudent developers are now test-marketing concepts and proposed communities well before putting a shovel into the ground. This can be done through community focus groups, seminars, and mail surveys, and even by building a model and opening a local sales office.

Another factor affecting the financial feasibility is the effect of absorption on project financing. Construction loans normally bear a higher interest rate than the permanent loan that will replace them. The longer it remains outstanding, the greater the interest expense borne by the project. The permanent mortgage financing will normally replace the construction financing after the operating net income of the project is sufficient to cover the debt service of the permanent loan by about 10 percent to 20 percent. Therefore, for each month that the occupancy fails to reach this threshold and the construction loan remains in place, the project incurs a higher interest expense than was projected in the financial proforma, which in essence becomes a construction cost overrun.[1]

The absorption and continued occupancy is clearly the most critical factor affecting the financial feasibility of senior living (and other multifamily real estate) projects. The combined effect of the costs associated with a slower than projected fill-up or absorption rate of the project can quickly wipe out any contingency funds built into the proforma by the developer and can turn an otherwise well-conceived project into a financial disaster. The inability of developers to meet their projections has been the single greatest factor contributing to the preponderance of failed projects that were ultimately sold at a loss or foreclosed upon or that filed bankruptcy. These projects were then recapitalized by their new owners at the expense of their original mortgage holder and investor's equity. Not only does this have a hard dollar and reputation effect on the developer, but it can also have a devastating effect on the project's residents, who moved in based upon sales representatives' assurances and whose lives may now be inevitably tangled in the developers' problems.

◼ MARKET DEMAND

Before structuring a marketing plan and strategy, it is important to identify the demand for the project in the marketplace where it is being conceived. If the project already exists, the proper evaluation of market size and existing penetration will be instrumental in designing the marketing approach. In the early 1980s, burgeoning health-care costs associated with the growing baby boom generation generated considerable media coverage and served to overstate the anticipated growth of the 65-plus population. New developers in senior housing interpreted the fact that over 5,000 Americans turned 65 every day as a certainty that there would be unlimited growth in this apparently underserved market. This optimism spurred rapid development, mostly of rental communities. When these communities were completed, it quickly became evident that the profile of those who were actually attracted to their new projects differed considerably from demographic projections. Consequently, absorption fell significantly short of developers' (and bankers') expectations. We now know that seniors are not merely attracted to senior housing communities by their affinity to others of similar age. The market, in fact, is much more need-driven than developers anticipated. Even today, as health care and other services are more easily accessible to seniors in their homes, developers are even more cautious about their absorption projections.

There are many ways to estimate market demand, including absorption rates of existing communities, demographic statistics sorted by some age and income threshold, availability and cost of home health services, economics, lifestyles, and migration trends, to mention

a few. It is advisable to define demographically the target market for your community as specifically as possible. This should be done in terms of age, income, and anticipated level of care upon entry. The target can be upper income active, middle income frail, affordable housing, or some other demographic profile. The target market should also be identified by proximity to the community. For rural communities, the primary market may encompass a 15-mile radius; in a large urban setting it can be limited to a 10-block radius. The project should be at least 80 percent justifiable by the primary market area.

◼ RESIDENT PROFILES

There appears to be a clear distinction between projects constructed by for-profit providers and by non-profit providers, which has a definite impact on the kind of resident who is attracted to one or the other. For-profit developers have primarily concentrated on the construction and operation of rental communities that provide congregate services with or without assisted living. The rapid expansion of the industry during the 1980s by primarily for-profit developers was built around the independent-living congregate model. These communities were attractive to need-driven seniors seeking alternatives to costly nursing home placement within "institutional" settings. The average entry age of 80 years was in sharp contrast to the 70+ demographic projections of early developers. Providers are now marketing these projects to the 75+ demographic profile.

Children who anguish over sending aging parents to nursing homes play a major role in the decision. According to a recent national study of 4,800 older adults conducted by James R. Lumpkin of the University of Southwestern Louisiana, over half (53.6%) of those living in senior housing indicated that a daughter helped make the decision to move, followed by a son (47.9%), a spouse when present (34.2%), family doctor (17.1%), friend (17.0%), minister (12.2%), grandchild(ren) (10.5%), and/or sibling (10.0%).

Experience tells us now that prospective residents are not as attracted to the community itself as they are to the idea of nursing home avoidance. Nursing home scandals have fed these fears, but more often the core issue, as many seniors see it, is a life sentence to mental and physical imprisonment; the confinement to an institution in which they retain little control over their basic lifestyle routines represents for many their greatest fear. Lumpkin's qualitative focus-group research found that the senior housing industry "suffers an abysmal image" among the elderly owing in part to project failures, hardships created for existing or prospective residents, poor management of facilities, and lack of product affordability. Focus-group participants agreed that personal care and assistance in daily living were the most valued services a retirement housing project could offer.[2]

To qualify financially for rental communities, operators are looking for the prospect to apply no more than 60 to 70 percent of their monthly cash-flow disposable income to their monthly fees for independent living and 75 to 80 percent for assisted living. The lower the financial prequalification percentage at entry, the easier it will be for residents to absorb a series of rental or service fee increases during their stay. In some cases, residents can live five or more years in rental communities and incur annually 5 percent increases (Table 13.1).

There may be a substantial shortage for many homeowners who are expecting to finance their senior living with the proceeds of their home. The example below assumes $100,000 *net* proceeds invested at 7 percent interest; this will only cover about three months of service fees. Therefore, an additional annual income of $25,000 will be required to provide a safe margin for the new tenant. The income qualifier for the lowest rent at this project would be approximately $32,000–35,000. Sales and marketing personnel need to be well aware of the limitations of seniors on fixed incomes. The interest earned on cash or near-cash investments can drop significantly over the duration of the tenancy, even as operational costs continue to

escalate. Many residents routinely experience cash shortfalls of $400–$600 per month. During these times, residents are forced to finance their lifestyle by tapping their principal, which will in turn further erode their income-generating potential. Seniors do not relish the thought of outliving their savings. Some are even being forced to seek accommodations elsewhere, which can be a very unpleasant prospect for residents and providers alike.

The majority of nonprofit providers offer endowment or equity models that offer a full range of health-care services on a single site. As the senior market becomes more informed of retirement options, its constituents are turning in ever increasing numbers to this life-care concept of vertically integrated health care. Here they have access to progressive levels of care as they age in place and their lifestyle challenges become increasingly complex. Many now consider this the preferred choice among well-informed seniors, and it is increasingly being embraced by for-profit developers and their financial partners. This scenario is, in fact, confirmed by the reluctance of lending institutions to underwrite rental projects. Typically, life care attracts a younger entry-age prospect, averaging in the mid to upper 70s, as compared to the 80-year-old rental prospect. In endowment or entrance fee projects, operators usually require a prospective resident's net worth to exceed twice the amount of the accommodation or entrance fee and the prospect's guaranteed monthly income to be at least equal to the total monthly service fee plus $500 or 1.5 times the annualized monthly service fee, or to have 30–35 percent remaining assets after paying the one-time entrance fee. Some communities use a sliding scale for income qualification that becomes lower as the entry age of the applicant increases. Obviously, the amount of remaining assets required to service the monthly fee will depend on the amount of the monthly fee and can be affected by the prevailing return on the resident's investments. Occasionally residents do move into these communities and become financially insolvent. Normally this is handled either through a resident hardship fund established by nonprofit sponsors; or, in the case where a portion of the entrance fee may be refundable at termination of the resident's tenancy, operators have allowed residents to draw against this refund.

The extent to which a prospect relies on the selling price of a home to fund entrance fees carries a great

Table 13.1 Income Qualification

Income qualification	Independent	Assisted living
Lowest rent assumption	$1,600	$2,400
Percent of income for housing/meals	60%	80%
Annual income requirement	$32,000	$36,000
Home/condo proceeds	$100,000	$100,000
Assumed safe interest rate on principal	7%	7%
Additional income required from homeowner	**$25,000**	**$29,000**

deal of weight to communities who charge advance fees. Some residents may have sufficient financial resources to finance the entrance fee in advance without selling a home. It may be advantageous for them to transfer their assets to heirs who can inherit the home based on the stepped-up basis rather than sell the home now and pay the capital-gains taxes. On the average, fewer than 50 percent of prospective residents need to sell their homes to finance entrance fees.

ADMISSION POLICIES

Most providers establish medical criteria for admission to senior health-care communities. There have been several successful challenges to these types of policies in the courts on the basis of potential conflict with regulations outlined in recent legislation. The courts have found that providers cannot deny admission on the basis of disability. It has yet to be determined how the Americans with Disabilities Act (ADA) or the Fair Housing Amendments Act (FHAA) will affect retirement communities either upon the resident's admission or during subsequent operations. Some attorneys feel that the ADA will affect operators mainly in the area of employment, because retirement communities are not, in the meaning of the law, "public accommodations operated by private entities," except possibly for their health-care facilities, and some public areas, or communities that may lease out space to outside businesses.[3] The FHAA allows for the exemption of people with selected health problems from participating in the health-care benefits of a community, but admission cannot be denied unless these people have a contagious disease "which can pose a direct threat to others."[4] Renters can be allowed to modify their own living units at their own expense to accommodate their special needs. However, operators can require the tenant to restore the unit to its original condition upon the termination of their residency and can require the establishment of an escrow account to provide for such restoration. The FHAA also states that covered facilities cannot deny or limit services nor can their management assign residents to a special section or floor. In fact, both acts require that communities make *reasonable accommodations* of rules, policies, practices, or services when they may be needed to afford equal opportunity to use the dwelling, including public and common use areas. Most of the newer communities are residential models, as opposed to the old-style institutional types. They have been sold that way, and, in order to succeed, they must continue to be perceived as residential rather than "glorified nursing homes." Many life-care providers will offer amended residency agreements for frail prospects who may be attracted by affordable access to skilled nursing services. Normally, medical screening in senior-living communities is not challenged by unsuccessful applicants where operators have made the effort to find an alternate solution or a more appropriate setting elsewhere. The key to avoiding the legal arena is to position the sales counselors and management as problem solvers interested in finding the optimal level of care for prospective residents, with the appropriate support designed to allow them to maintain their independence and dignity. As advocates for the prospects, providers who take a genuine interest in their well-being are rarely criticized for leading inquiries to more "appropriate" settings.

Operators usually receive more resistance from existing residents who object to the frailty of new residents than from the prospects themselves. It is, however, usually acceptable for existing residents to become frail during their stay because they are part of the group and not viewed as outsiders. They may have come to a retirement community to have available additional care and support should they ever need it, but most believe that they will beat the odds of ever being admitted to the skilled-nursing component. Healthy residents may react negatively to the admission of frail prospects and are frightened by anything that reminds them of their own vulnerability. Residents will constantly remind management that they were attracted to the community because of its active, independent image and accuse the sales staff of a relaxation of standards to generate sales. They will ask, "How can you attract younger, active residents to the community if you let these people in with wheelchairs and walkers?" Salespeople will even complain to management at times that their prospects walk into the building, take one look at the frailty of the resident population, and tell them "I'm not ready for this yet." These are among the most challenging issues for providers to deal with on a daily basis.

Proactively manage your residents' and prospects' perceptions about the use of supportive devices. Do not allow them to set your admission standards. Not all people who use wheelchairs are unhealthy, and the law clearly protects their rights to be treated equally. The same principle applies to walkers. Explain to prospects that walkers are simply a supportive device to enable people who may be experiencing problems with their mobility to get back on their feet. Point out that the device does not define the person, but is just a tool designed to allow independence, not promote dependence.

The toughest sales job of all is to convince a long-term resident of a rental community to move to a higher level of care. The law is somewhat unclear in this area. Fortunately, most providers are able to handle these delicate issues with good family and physician counseling combined with naturally occurring peer pressure. Most people will understand and accept their deteriorating health status after first passing through the denial and bargaining stages. Providers must be proficient at managing these circumstances and anticipate problems well in advance of the expected discharge so that they can properly lay the groundwork with the family and physician. In most states, continuing-care retirement communities (CCRCs) require people to transfer to higher levels of care based upon their needs as perceived by management or the medical director, a policy that clearly violates the intent of the FHAA. It is not clear that there will ever be any hard and fast rules to govern these situations because of their political sensitivity and the need for case-by-case assessment. Communities will establish their own criteria, which may change over the life of the project, to manage these sensitive issues effectively. Any breakdown of communication can lead to conflict. Providers who can keep communication channels open will be most effective at avoiding having to hire legal experts to negotiate their policies for them, which could serve to set precedents and ultimately limit their options.

Normally, providers require that the applicant be capable of independent living based on the evaluation of the medical director, who uses a confidential medical application that has been completed by the applicant's attending physician. The application, together with a completed medical history, can be evaluated by a medical review committee for the final decision. Frequently the medical director will consult with the attending physician, or a personal interview will be conducted between the applicant and the executive director in order to assess the applicant's ability to live independently. Residents, physicians, and family members will willfully misrepresent the applicant's abilities, even with the best-intentioned medical screening. Be especially wary of family members who are in a hurry to make the placement on their relative's behalf, or who express an interest in signing an agreement *before* the applicant has even toured the community.

▪ MARKET PENETRATION AND ABSORPTION

The percentage of age- and income-qualified prospects in the primary market area needed to fill existing and proposed senior living communities to stabilized occupancy (95%), assuming that 80 percent of units are filled by prospects from the primary market area, is normally referred to as the *market penetration rate*. Statistics sorted by age and income qualifier and zip code are available from actuarial firms such as the National Data Planning Corporation or Claritas. This information is primarily derived from census information and can be projected based upon historical growth patterns in the area. These growth estimates can also be cross-checked for comparison with projections made by the local Chamber of Commerce. The number of gross households should then be reduced by the number of existing competitive units regardless of their relative occupancy. The number of households should also be adjusted for competitive units either planned or under construction. Planned units under construction can be discounted by the number of probable units that may actually be built. The *market* penetration rate is calculated by dividing the total number of stabilized units in the primary market area into the *gross* number of income qualified noninstitutional households.

The *project penetration rate* is the percentage of age- and income-qualified prospects in the primary market area needed to fill your senior living community to stabilized occupancy (95%), assuming that 80 percent of units are filled by prospects from the primary market area. This rate is calculated from the *net* number of qualified households after existing and planned competitive units have been deducted. Calculating the penetration rate helps to measure the degree to which the primary market is underserviced or saturated. The higher the penetration rate, the longer the potential expected time to fill the community. Penetration rates are not necessarily a wholly negative factor. They may indicate a well-educated and highly accepting market for senior-living projects, and despite a high rating, undeserved niches may still exist in certain market seg-

Table 13.2   Analyzing Penetration Rates

Penetration rate	Opinion
Below 5%	Good
5%–10%	Some concern
11%–15%	Significant concern
Above 15%	Material concern

Source: E.C. Merrigan, "Rating Guidelines for Nonprofit Continuing Care Retirement Communities." Fitch Health Care Special Report. Fitch Investor Services, Inc. June 1994.

ments. The guidelines in Table 13.2 are used by Fitch investor services for analyzing penetration rates.[5]

Penetration rate differs from the *market absorption rate,* which is the percentage of the existing supply of units in the primary market area that have become occupied over a specified period of time. A sample calculation of penetration rate is illustrated in Table 13.3.

The *project absorption rate* is generally defined as the total number of months it will take for a project to reach stabilized occupancy, beginning with the first month the project is offered to the marketplace. This period includes the preopening period and postopening period. The absorption could be equated to the occupancy only where there was no sales activity before the month that the project was actually ready for occupancy. As discussed earlier, an acceptable absorption rate for one project may be inadequate for another depending upon the community size, capitalization, premarketing, and a variety of other factors. Caution should therefore be exercised when comparing national absorption rates (which average 2.5 to 3.0 units per month[5]) to site-specific performance. Absorption in excess of double the national average could still fall considerably short of investment expectations.

The number of occupied units of a community expressed as a percentage of the total occupied units in the primary market area is referred to as the *market share.* This is simply a measure of strength by each provider participant in the primary market service area. It is interesting to note the trends in this figure over time. As additional participants enter the marketplace, the market share of the existing providers will decrease. Generally speaking, the greater the market share of an individual provider, the more opportunity to manage revenues and ultimately bottom-line profitability. Larger, well-established quality providers will

Table 13.3   Calculating Penetration Rates

DEMAND ANALYSIS
200 Planned units
Market area radius—10 miles sorted by Zip codes.

Age bracket		75+	70–74	65–69
Income qualifier		$35,000	$35,000	$35,000
Gross number qualified households		3,122	4,132	6,594
Percent absorbed by this age group		85%	10%	5%
Age and income qualified		2,653	413	330
Gross number of age and income qualified		3,396		
Less existing competitive units	450			
Less competitive units under construction	0			
Less planned competitive units	250			
Discount by		15%		
Anticipated number of planned units canceled		38		
Probable competitive units		212		
Net number of qualified households remaining		**2,734**		
Project planned units	200			
Stabilized occupancy	95%			
Percent units filled from primary market area		80%		
Number of units to be supported by PMA	152			
Penetration rate		**5.56%**		

be able to command a premium in a limited market-place with little competition. Many savvy owners watch market-share percentage closely. Downward trends of 10 percent or more can trigger a need for repositioning or remarketing to differentiate their product from the competition's.

■ COMPETITOR OVERVIEW

Comprehensive market and industry information is necessary in order to decide how to approach a specific market strategically, operationally, and organizationally to determine what levels of performance to expect. Collecting and summarizing information about your competitors in the primary market area can yield important clues about the relative strengths and weaknesses of each. All marketing staff should be keenly aware of the competitive advantages of the community they are marketing and be equipped with rehearsed answers to overcome objections about potential disadvantages that will surely be exposed by their competitors. Detailed and accurate competitor information enables you to identify the threats, opportunities, and likely future direction and responses of each of your key competitors. Armed with this intelligence, you will be in a position to improve your community's competitive advantage.

The competitor overview should include such information as location, year opened, percent occupancy, owner or management company, entrance fee, number of units, and floor plan. Pricing information should be gathered by unit type with a comparison to your own community by monthly fee per square foot. If an inventory of apartments by unit type and occupancy can be gathered, then market preferences can be assessed and strategies can be developed to market less desirable unit types. In some cases it may be possible to predict a competitor's financial performance and sensitivity to discounting prices.

Other useful information should include a comparison of each competitor's service package and amenities. The service package analysis should identify specifically which services are included in the monthly service fee and which may be billed separately. This enables the sales counselors to assist their prospects in understanding hidden costs and to analyze the value of each competitor's offering. The amenity comparison should itemize the community features (art studios, swimming pools, wellness center, beauty salon,

private dining, and the like) of each competitor in comparison to your own.

Another essential component of the competitor overview should be the collection of all collateral material and print media. This material can then be compared to your own in terms of message, ad type, size and location, presentation, and overall impression to strengthen your relative position. This information is most effectively gathered by a local clipping service. These services will perform searches of all or a select number of publications in your area or nationwide and are quite inexpensive for the valuable information collected. Community brochures and other promotional collateral material can be collected by employees, relatives, or even residents. In addition, it is a good idea to have a relative or friend attend your competitors' special events or seminars to evaluate their effectiveness and presentation.

The final component of the competitor overview should include an analysis of the sales presentation at each competing community as well as at your own. This can be accomplished through the use of a "mystery shop" visit. This not only provides a valuable assessment of the sales skills of your competitor's marketing counselors, but also can offer some insight into how they may be representing your property to their prospects. The mystery shop is best accomplished by someone with an eye for detail who has a basic understanding of the sales process. Real estate agents or professional shoppers are the most objective and will perform this service for a reasonable fee. In fact, some realtors will perform this service for you in exchange for home sale referrals from prospects who may need to sell their home before relocating to your community. Some knowing sales counselors will pick up on a mystery shopper early on in the information-gathering stage, but may not be aware if it is their own company's shopper or a competitor's. Whatever the case may be, it is generally understood among long-term professionals in the business that they will be mystery shopped from time to time. Information gathered during the mystery shop should include first impressions and greeting, information gathering, tour, close, confirmation, physical features, and overall impression. (Be sure to inquire how long the counselor has been employed at the community and to arrange the tour and presentation with a sales counselor, not the activity director or office assistant. It is also important to recognize that everyone can have a bad day; inform your sales representatives not to let down their guard in the event a competitor's sales presentation is not competitive.) The information gathered should be quantified for comparison to your community's performance, and strategies should be developed to strengthen your weak areas. A sample mystery shop analysis form is presented in Exhibit 13.1.

Many companies routinely mystery shop their own staff. This practice is employed both as a self-diagnosis tool to identify and solve problems, and also to keep salespeople on their toes. Often this tool is misused by management or ownership and can in some cases be demotivating and ineffective and cause distrust between sales staff and management. Will Nowell, president of ServiceCheck, Inc., a Scottsdale, Arizona, firm specializing in mystery shopping, claims that "if used properly, mystery shopping can be a very valuable tool and create a positive high-energy environment. If management can deliver consistent customer-oriented feedback that is specific to the issues the sales people control and is presented in a supportive nonthreatening manner, they will lift their levels of performance much higher than a manager can ever push them through fear, intimidation, or occasional constructive criticism." Salespeople should strive to do their very best on every presentation regardless of whether they anticipate an ultimate sale or performance evaluation.

After completing the collection of all pertinent information about the competitors in your primary market area, you should prepare a synopsis. This is a summary of all the strengths and weaknesses of your community against all others with whom you compete. A one-page spreadsheet can be prepared that lists all of the services, prices, and amenities across the top by competitor. This can be printed for distribution to prospects who intend to evaluate other projects. Specific strategies can then be developed to position your total marketing and sales plan as competitively as possible. In addition, sales and marketing issues and strategies should be developed to identify and address significant challenges that the department will be facing in the coming year. For example, if the department needs to increase phone-outs as an issue, then the strategy might be to establish a daily phone-out quota, review logs daily, offer small incentives, or initiate a contest. If the quality of leads is identified as an issue, then

the strategy may involve eliminating the ad coupon, and targeting the ad toward prospects rather than adult children. If the issue is to improve the quantity of leads, then the strategy might include developing a newspaper tabloid or increasing direct mail. The combined effect of issue identification and strategy development is designed to establish the primary and secondary goals that the marketing plan will need to address.

Market and industry intelligence on which you can act allows you to align your community's capabilities with the success factors of the primary market area to ensure proper levels of marketing funding, coherent strategic vision, and realistic performance expectations.

■ MARKETING PLANNING

The primary objective of any effective marketing planning approach should be designed around removing the guesswork out of what works and what does not. Many communities have spent considerable resources using the "shotgun" approach with only mixed results. This involves test-marketing a wide array of strategies, hoping that something will bring in prospects. Although a few marketing consultants still subscribe to this strategy, seasoned, results-oriented professionals prefer a more targeted, statistically based approach.

The statistical approach employs the use of the lead:lease conversion rate analysis for each media type and marketing strategy. The strategies with the highest lead:lease conversion rates are then allocated proportionally higher commitments of the overall marketing budget. This way the total marketing budget is allocated on the most efficient strategies first, with the remaining funds balanced between old standbys such as Yellow Pages advertising and new innovations that the marketing staff or management may consider to be effective. The lead:lease conversion rate is a combined measure of prospects' attraction to the media type and the perceived value of the service package, as well as the relative skill of the marketing staff to convert inquiries into sales. Therefore, if the conversion rate performance level seems low for the community, each of these separate components will need to be tested to determine areas of vulnerability and to implement strategic corrective measures.

The lead:lease conversion rate is simply calculated by dividing the average new leads per month generated

Text continues on page 209

Exhibit 13.1   Confidential "Mystery Shop" Analysis

Community shopped: _____

Date shopped: _____

Shopped by: _____

The following scoring key should be used for the shopping report:

Scale questions:	5 =	Excellent
	4 =	Above average
	3 =	Average; acceptable
	2 =	Below average
	1 =	Very poor; unacceptable
Yes/No questions:	5 =	Yes
	1 =	No

I. Greeting

A.	How would you rate the grounds surrounding the building?	5	4	3	2	1
B.	Were the signs identifying the building easy to read?	5	4	3	2	1
C.	How easy was it to find the correct entrance to the community?	5	4	3	2	1
D.	How well were you greeted when you entered the building?	5	4	3	2	1
E.	Were you kept waiting?	5				1
F.	How warm was the welcome extended to you by the marketing staff?	5	4	3	2	1
G.	How professionally dressed was the marketing representative?	5	4	3	2	1
H.	How clean/orderly was the waiting area?	5	4	3	2	1
I.	Were you offered refreshments?	5				1
J.	Were you offered a seat?	5				1
K.	Were you addressed by name?	5				1
L.	How effective was eye contact?	5	4	3	2	1
M.	Were you asked to complete prospect cards?	5				1

Comments: _____

_____

_____

Section I

Potential score   65

Actual score   _____

II. Gathering Information

A.	Were you asked how you heard about the community?	5				1
B.	Were common grounds identified between you and the marketing representative?	5	4	3	2	1
C.	How well were your needs established?	5	4	3	2	1
D.	Were you asked what prompted this visit?	5				1
E.	Were you asked about your current lifestyle?	5				1
F.	Were you asked about interests, hobbies, and pastimes?	5	4	3	2	1
G.	Were you asked who will be involved in making the decision?	5				1
H.	Were you asked about visiting our competitors?	5				1
I.	Were your "hot buttons" identified?	5	4	3	2	1
J.	Did the marketing representative take a personal interest in you?	5	4	3	2	1
K.	Were you asked whether you own or rent?	5				1

(continued)

Exhibit 13.1 Confidential "Mystery Shop" Analysis *(continued)*

Comments: _____
_____
_____

      Section II

      Potential score   55

      Actual score   _____

III. Presentation

A.	How effectively was the product described as a "lifestyle"?	5	4	3	2	1
B.	How did the presentation of features serve as a response to your specific needs?	5	4	3	2	1
C.	How effectively was the community product compared to competition?	5	4	3	2	1
D.	Were common areas toured?	5				1
E.	Were models toured?	5				1
F.	Were other staff introduced in the process of the tour?	5				1
G.	How did the tour presentation fit into your description of needs and interests?	5	4	3	2	1
H.	How knowledgeable was the staff on the general area and the community at large?	5	4	3	2	1
I.	How was the interaction between the staff and other residents?	5	4	3	2	1
J.	Was the "wellness" concept discussed?	5				1
K.	Was the continuum of care concept discussed?	5				1
L.	How understanding was staff of your objections?	5	4	3	2	1
M.	How factually did staff answer your questions?	5	4	3	2	1
N.	How sensitively did staff answer your questions?	5	4	3	2	1
O.	How valuable was the amount of information provided?	5	4	3	2	1
P.	How neat and clean were the models?	5	4	3	2	1
Q.	How neat and clean were the common areas of the building?	5	4	3	2	1
R.	Were you made to feel that you would "fit" into the community?	5	4	3	2	1
S.	How well was the value of the complete package explained to you?	5	4	3	2	1
T.	Was the staff able to turn negatives into positives?	5	4	3	2	1

Comments: _____
_____
_____

      Section III

      Potential score   100

      Actual score   _____

IV. Closing

A.	How direct were staff questions to you?	5	4	3	2	1
B.	How effectively were objections dealt with?	5	4	3	2	1
C.	Did staff attempt a trial closing with you?	5				1
D.	Did staff ask you for a deposit?	5				1
E.	Was collateral provided to you?	5				1
F.	Was the collateral informative and easy to understand?	5	4	3	2	1
G.	Did staff promise to make a follow-up contact with you?	5	4	3	2	1

(continued)

Exhibit 13.1 Confidential "Mystery Shop" Analysis *(continued)*

H.	In attempting the closing, how effectively did staff deal with your "hot buttons"?	5	4	3	2	1
I.	How effectively was the issue of value addressed?	5	4	3	2	1
J.	Did staff compare costs at the community to your current costs?	5	4	3	2	1

Comments: _____

_____

_____

Section IV

Potential score   55

Actual score   _____

V . Follow-up

A.	Was a follow-up time set?	5	1
B.	Was the follow-up time commitment kept?	5	1
C.	Did you receive correspondence following your visit?	5	1
D.	Did you receive a follow-up phone call after your visit?	5	1
E.	Did you receive additional literature (sales material) if requested?	5	1

Comments: _____

_____

_____

Section V

Potential score   25

Actual score   _____

Staff shopped: _____

_____

_____

_____

Recap:

Section	Potential	Actual	%
I	65	_____	_____
II	55	_____	_____
III	100	_____	_____
IV	55	_____	_____
V	25	_____	_____
TOTAL	**300**	_____	_____

Table 13.4   Marketing Conversion Ratios

Lead:lease conversion rate	Lease:lead conversion rate	Performance level
10:1	10%	Excellent
15:1	6.67%	Very good
20:1	5%	Good
25:1	4%	Fair
30:1	3.33%	Poor

from each marketing strategy by the average gross leases/sales from those strategies. For example, a community with an average of 200 new leads per month from media placements with an average of 10 gross leases per month from those placements will have a lead:lease conversion ratio of 20:1. In other words, the community can expect one lease or sale for every 20 new leads. *It is important to note that sales will also be generated from the site, resident referrals, and nonresident referrals. Each of these lead sources will also have their own conversion rate, and should be considered separately when allocating marketing dollars. The inclusion of these other lead sources when calculating the community's conversion rate will over inflate true marketing results.* To calculate the lead:lease conversion percentage rate, simply divide the lead:lease figure into 1 and multiply by 100 (in our example $1 \div 20 = 0.05 \times 100 = 5\%$). Table 13.4 details this relationship for a number of scenarios.

The lead:lease conversion rates can then be calculated on each individual marketing strategy to determine which strategies are the most effective for that marketplace. At a minimum the community should track the conversion rates for its collateral advertising, direct mail, newspaper, and Yellow Pages appearances, both by the month and by the piece. In addition, other useful applications of these conversion rates can also help to evaluate walk-in, phone-in, mail-in, and phone-out effectiveness. Generally speaking, walk-in or referral conversion rates will be the highest as they indicate someone who may be either an interested party or a prospect who is "shopping" and may already be convinced of the advantages that senior housing has to offer.

Equipped with these tools, the marketing planner is then able to custom-design a marketing plan for an individual community that is justified on proven results with statistical backup. The marketing planner should not build the entire marketing plan upon a single strategy, inasmuch as conditions may change throughout the year; a well-balanced approach that distributes the marketing budget among a variety of proven strategies will be less risky. The statistical approach is more clearly defined each year as more information about the market is gathered and new strategies are refined. Ultimately, the marketing planner can become very skilled at predicting the response to and conversion rates for each strategy. This will enable the community to forecast more accurately marketing budget requirements as the project matures.

ANNUAL FORECASTS

Before developing any specific strategies to market the community, the marketing planner needs to determine the number of units that must be leased and the corresponding volume of leads and leases required to meet the annual forecast. The projected net occupancy for year-end of the current year, based on current trends, needs to be estimated. The projected year-end occupancy for the following year will normally be established by the owners. The difference between year-end occupancy next year and year-end occupancy during the planning years will yield the unadjusted gross leases required during the year. The next step will be to review the year-to-date move-out activity and project this trend at an estimated number of units per month for next year. The resulting figure is added as the first adjustment. Next, any outstanding sales pending move-in should be subtracted, and finally projected cancellations should be added to yield the total gross leases required. Table 13.5 details an example of the *annual unit sales forecast* calculation.

Table 13.5   Annual Unit Sales Forecast

Projected occupancy year-end planning year	250 Units
Projected occupancy year-end current year	150 Units
Gross unadjusted sales	100 Units
Plus projected move-outs at __2__ per month = __24__	124 Units
Minus outstanding sales pending move-in __15__	109 Units
Plus projected cancellations at __1__ per month = __12__	121 Units
Total annual gross sales required in the planning year	**121 Units**
Units to lease/sell per month	**10 Units**

Table 13.6　Annual Lead Forecast

Total annual gross leases/sales required in the planning year	121
Lease:lead conversion rate	4%
Gross leads required in the planning year	3,025 Leads
Minus existing active leads in lead bank	1,000 Leads
Plus lead deletions of __75__ per month or __900__ per year	900 Leads
Total annual new leads required	**2,925 Leads**
Total monthly new leads required	**244 Leads**

It is important to note that a specific budgeted occupancy for the month implies that the budgeted number of units will be generating full revenue for the entire number of days in the month. In other words, additional sales may be required per month to offset revenue losses from prorated move-outs and move-ins that may occur other than on the last or first day of the month, respectively.

The *annual lead forecast* calculates the number of new leads required in the planning year to achieve the forecasted gross leases/sales. Review the lead:lease conversion rate for the current year to determine if it is realistic to forecast into the planning year. To obtain gross leads needed in the planning year, simply divide the gross leases required calculated from Table 13.6 by the lead:lease conversion rate. For example, 121 gross leases required in the planning year ÷ 4% lead:lease conversion rate = 3,025 gross leads. Subtract from this number the existing active leads in the lead bank and add lead deletions to yield the total new leads required in the planning year. Table 13.6 details a sample annual lead forecast.

The marketing planner can now begin to construct the specific marketing plan strategies that will be designed to generate these leads. Sharon Brooks, president of a Virginia-based marketing, advertising, and public relations firm, believes that "proper market positioning of effective collateral material should be designed to inform, create an image, be a tangible representation of the community and the owner, shape expectations, remind the prospect and to ultimately create a dream." The development of effective marketing materials will require extensive insight into the value systems and sensitivities of today's wary

senior. For the message to be fully effective, it must be delivered in a manner that will strike a familiar chord with seniors.

■■■■ UNDERSTANDING THE MARKET

The decision to move into a senior living community can involve the psyches of many people (spouse, daughter, son, grandchildren, friends), and it is normally emotionally charged and personal. Residents as well as decision influencers will have their own perspective and biases about senior living according to their experience or knowledge of the business, views that are all filtered through their personal value system. It is critical to target the market as specifically as possible, but marketers need also to be aware of these filters and deliver messages that are creative, memorable, penetrating, clever, persuasive, and sensitive to the emotional forces that motivate their audience.

To succeed with any target market, market planners must show that their community and its services reflect the values of the seniors targeted. Considering the demographics, it is not surprising that there has been a tremendous amount of research into the lifestyles and values of older adults. Although opinions differ, some general conclusions can be drawn. Seniors are interested in being depicted as active, interested, and involved, and they see themselves as at least 10 years younger then their true chronological age. In fact, seniors' anxiety about their age is more closely associated with an aversion to the health complications associated with growing old, which will eventually place restrictions on their personal freedom. They are in fact looking for empowerment so that they can live fuller lives and stay in control longer. They are generally private people, especially about their finances, are comfortable with themselves, and are more experiential and less materialistic than their children. They see themselves as morally conservative and intellectually liberal; they are more aware and educated and consider learning to be a lifelong experience. It is also a time in their lives when they experience a growth in their own spirituality and altruism toward their fellow humans. They are among the greatest givers of time to volunteer causes. They are particularly interested in helping other, less active seniors. They are spouse- and family-oriented, proud, and independent.

As a market segment, seniors control more than 50 percent of the nation's discretionary income while composing only 26 percent of the population. It is important to remember that even though they have significant buying power, they are by nature very reluctant to exercise it. These are people who lived through the Depression years, when they worked very hard for very little. They were thankful for what they had and know the meaning of a dollar. They are particularly interested in preserving their estate for their heirs so that their descendants will not face deprivation. And they live off of the interest generated by their investments.

The typical prospect is over the age of 80, female (10% are men or couples), and need assistance with two or more activities of daily living (ADLs). They generally live within ten miles of the community or have family who do; 50 percent are homeowners, and 83 percent of those homes are owned free and clear of any mortgage. They may be slightly confused, but they are clear about outliving their funds and about the escalating costs of health care and services. Most inquiries can be categorized into a desire for services, need for companionship and security, and access to health care as their lifestyle needs change. Above all, they are interested in options and value. Seniors may want a high-priced item, but they want to pay as little as possible to get it. They want a deal.

Normally, the decision to inquire about one's senior-living alternatives is precipitated by a change in health or lifestyle—for instance, loss of a driver's license due to failing eyesight, the death of a spouse or friend, or the onset of a degenerative medical condition. Prospects are typically enduring a stressful time in their lives. Seniors generally need the services and conveniences that a senior-living environment has to offer long before they acknowledge that need. Due to denial, the decision to move into a senior-living community can be a long process. The earlier the prospect is contacted, the better, but frequent contact will be important to the relationship-building process (this will be discussed at length in Chapter 14).

The average woman in America today will spend more time caring for her parents than for her children. Children may recognize the need for an assisted-living environment long before the senior acknowledges that need. Unlike the senior, they will probably accept the marketing messages much more willingly. Family members can quickly see the inherent benefits and value associated with the product and tend to focus themselves on the stability, reputation, and management of the

community in order to avoid the potential difficulties associated with influencing their parent to make a decision that may not work out. Adult children want to free themselves of the guilt surrounding their inability to be the primary caregiver in their parents' time of need and will turn to the senior-living arena for relief. The ultimate decision to move into a senior-living community is generally made by the senior, but in 80 percent of the cases it is strongly influenced by children and in-laws, most particularly women. The decision among family members is rarely unanimous.

The decision-influencing adult child is typically a 45- to 65-year-old married female who lives and works in the area. She normally has children living at home, in college, or with families of their own; she thus can feel herself sandwiched between two generations. Such women are prone to guilt, sensitive to their own aging, and concerned with preserving their parents' estate or conserving their own funds.

When developing advertising and collateral materials designed to attract seniors, marketers need to keep in mind that they are selling a lifestyle, not real estate. Ads need to show things that attract seniors' attention with pictures of people that tell a story, "real" people who are active and involved, people whom they might like to meet. Always state the benefit in the headline and use the copy to demonstrate value. Do not use too much copy or provide too little information. Learn to anticipate questions and answer them in advance. Hard-hitting is good; mystical or hidden implications will fall flat. Clever is good; contrived is not. Fluff will hurt your credibility.[6] Seniors sense that if it looks too good to be true, it probably isn't. The single most important question for most seniors is whether the community will enable them to maintain their independence, privacy, and control in their lives. They will reject media attempts at communicating a catered lifestyle. The very idea of being catered to implies a loss of control. Seniors are interested in fact-oriented collateral that shows they will participate in planning and choosing activities and lifestyle options.

Before designing the individual marketing strategies it is important to gain some insight into the target market's awareness or understanding of your community. In spite of the massive amounts of advertising you may have already done in the market, seniors may still be unaware of exactly who you are and what services you provide. Or they may be aware of the community's existence but remain unconvinced that your community will benefit them directly. In senior housing, there is also a great potential for public misunderstanding of the product. Seniors may still think your community is some type of "old folks' home" where demented people are put away. Finally, the project, former management, or owners may have had an image problem. This is common in financially distressed situations. Whatever the case may be, the informed marketer is the targeted marketer. The better job the marketers can do at identifying the market sensitivities and awareness levels, the better equipped they will be to design their strategies to address them.

The best way to accomplish this is through research. This can be done through direct mail surveys or telemarketing or by using focus groups.

■ Focus Groups

A focus group is a small gathering of people in your target market who meet for an informal discussion about the likes, dislikes, fears, and motivations with which they approach your community. The focus groups should be made up of current leads, age- and income-qualified prospects, decision influencers, family members, residents, and even employees. Each group should be interviewed separately so that specific conclusions can be drawn from each target audience. Often it is better to conduct focus groups with an outside consultant, inasmuch as people like to be helpful and will tend to tell you what they think you want to hear. Conversely, they may be reluctant to confess their concerns to management for fear of misinterpretation or retaliation.

It is a good idea to prepare a thorough list of the information that you are seeking so that the discussion leader will be sure to cover all your questions during the session. Start with an icebreaker discussion about senior-living communities. Next, probe for the group's awareness of each senior-living community in your primary market area. Next, an initial perceived-value testing will be helpful to gauge the group's awareness of their own costs of living in comparison with what they think is offered at your community. Describe the services and amenities of your community in detail and solicit specific reactions to each. Before a discussion of the pricing, a slide show or tour of the community and models may be appropriate to set the stage for the associated costs. After the tour ask the

group to estimate the cost to live at the community. Most will overestimate, having just completed the exercise to determine their own "real" cost of living. At this point the group has a solid appreciation for benefits, services, and amenities you offer and is primed to discuss the general pricing. They will then be prepared to discuss issues such as the entrance fee, price comparison with the competition, fee increases, security deposits, nursing home deductibles, and so on. Solicit specific reaction to each and every aspect of your financial package. Then discuss the positive features and opportunities as well as the challenges to marketing that you may consider eliminating or neutralizing. You might also choose to engage in a discussion on the continuum of care and how the community offers many choices as the residents' lifestyle needs become increasingly complex. For example, discuss their concerns about health-care accessibility and reactions to assisted living, home health care, and long-term care coverages. The final rating of the community in terms of location, physical features, ownership and management, services and amenities, and overall perceived value should be done by each privately (on paper), then as a group. Finally, the discussion leader may choose to do a "trial close," asking under what circumstances the individuals would consider a move to the community and in what time frame. Also ask them if their perceptions of the community changed as a result of the focus group, what would they tell others to convince them to move into the community, and what it would take to convince them. If the discussion group takes off in an unexpected direction, pay attention. They may be expressing some concerns and motivations that may not have occurred to you. Videotaping the sessions can provide management with documentation of the meetings and some clues as to the emotional response to the questions. Reviewing each session with the discussion leader as they are completed can serve as a basis for exploring sidetracks and refocusing to refine subsequent sessions.

The discussion agenda can be tailored differently for the decision influencers, lead bank, residents, and staff. The idea remains the same. The discussion should begin with an icebreaker, then proceed from general to specific issues. Solicit feedback on each key attribute of the community while communicating the benefits and demonstrating value. Not only will a well-planned and focused discussion provide you with critical information about the perceptions of the market, it can also be a powerful selling tool. Many participants have been converted to residents through this process. Even after opening, focus groups should be conducted annually to gauge continued reactions to the community and its overall operations.

Surveys

When researching the target audience by survey, you can reach a much larger group to verify the accuracy of your focus group results. Many of the same general questions from the focus group should be incorporated into the survey. Any good survey should open with a screening question that will eliminate wasting time with people who are not your target audience. This should be followed with a simple but interesting question to get the respondent "hooked" on completing the survey. Start with easy questions that can be answered quickly and suggest that the survey will be quick and easy to complete. Group like questions together in a logical manner so that you can give proper instructions on how to answer each group once. Save psychographic and demographic questions for last, inasmuch as many reluctant seniors will provide this information only after they have already gone to the trouble of completing the entire survey. The income question should be dead last.[7]

STRATEGIES

Newspaper Advertisement

Advertising in local or regional newspapers is by far the most economical method to reach the greatest number of seniors. Seniors as a group generally read the daily paper cover to cover, especially the midweek coupon inserts. With advertising, you control not only the message but also the level of exposure. Advertising's biggest drawback is that it costs money to reach the exposure level at which the target market becomes familiar with your message and the results begin to materialize. New projects can normally expect about 50 percent of their leads from referrals and 50 percent from print media advertising. Of the print media leads, they should expect to close about 20 percent.

Advertising works by the following process: capturing attention, holding interest, luring the reader, prompting action, and leaving a lasting impression. Effective marketing materials should include three main elements:

1. Thorough description of the product/service and the benefits related.
2. Testimonials from the residents validating your claims.
3. Third-party reinforcement of your message.

Develop a few good concepts and stick with them. Resist the temptation to abandon a campaign if at first it does not succeed. It may take some time for your message to become absorbed by the market. There are not normally any significant incremental results along the way. Only until your message has had enough exposure to break through the results threshold will the responses start coming in numbers. Give your advertising and promotional campaigns the chance to take hold and grow. Repeated exposure to the same message minimizes the efforts to interpret it. Frequent changes in the message or "look" of your ads will only confuse your market. Marketing through newspaper advertisement is a cumulative process, and results don't always kick in until well into the fill-up. When you shake things up by changing too often or too soon, you are wasting your budget on each successive effort before your first impression has a chance to grab hold. This does not imply that if results are totally flat you should not do some more research and testing on senior prospects.

Plan the ad around one idea. It is vital in advertising to seniors that each ad should have a single message. Know exactly what you wish a particular ad to accomplish. If the message needs reinforcing with other ideas, keep them in the background. If you have several important things to say, use a different ad for each one and run the ad on succeeding weeks or months.

Never assume that you know what will appeal to seniors. Each age group cohort in this country grew up in a different socioeconomic era that contributed to the formulation of our individual value systems. You can only see the world as a result of the world you have seen. Develop your advertising according to the strengths of your service package and competitive advantages in your marketplace, then *test them* on actual age- and income-qualified prospects. Identify the *differences* of your community and talk about them. Although this process does not necessarily guarantee success, you might be able to influence your results significantly by eliminating concepts and layouts that turn off your market. Seniors are normally quite clear about what they like and what they do not. Without first testing your ideas on your readers, your investment is a gamble.

Ads should be placed in the lifestyle or health sections, never in the real estate section. Consider purchasing placement of the ad. The location of your ad in the paper or on the page can significantly affect your results. Keeping your ads near the edge of the paper and out of the "gutter" near the fold can make your ad easier to spot and your coupon easier to clip. Generally ads are more effective if they appear in the front of the newspaper than the back. Most direct response advertisers prefer right-hand pages. Avoid the placement of your ads in the obituary section or adjacent to ads for cancer or alcohol-treatment centers, and avoid placement on the same or opposite page with a competitor. The placement of an ad adjacent to a feature article on one of your residents or programs is particularly effective in humanizing your community. Studies have shown that the retirement housing prospect or decision influencer is primarily female, so placement of the ad in the women's section should yield the best overall results.

Using photos and testimonials of actual residents will project the image that will encourage prospects. Research has shown a 28 percent increase in readership when quotes are used in the headline because people want to read about what other seniors are saying.

All capitals in reverse white with a black background are harder to read for aging eyes. The body of the ad should be at least 12 point type and include ample white space. Seniors need high contrast to absorb printed media visually. Unlike other parts of the body, the lens of the eye does not shed old cells when new ones are added, and over time the retina of the eye becomes somewhat thickened and increasingly rigid and opaque, and it acquires a yellowish tint, making it more difficult for older persons to distinguish between greens, blues, and violet. It is much easier to see orange, yellows, and reds.[8] Understand the relevant regulatory requirements such as Equal Housing Opportunity (EHO) specifications and incorporate the appropriate minority mix into the models or resident subjects. There is not a discernible negative effect on the responses from ads that properly comply.

Using clip art or some other creative memory aid can help to link subsequent ad placements. Many people will see an ad or commercial several times before they will respond. Ads that carry the same theme or recurrent art work will complement each other and maximize retention value.

Timing of newspaper advertising is also important. The effects of seasonal insertions can have a tendency to overwhelm the reader. Most people will skim the ads during seasons such as Christmas and back-to-school. There is no question that newspapers are an integral part of practically everyone's daily life. Although magazines may be set aside for reading at a convenient time, newspapers are read the day they are delivered or purchased or not read at all. Many advertisers prefer Monday through Thursday, but judiciously avoid the weekday issue containing grocery advertising. You can obtain circulation statistics from the newspaper to determine if any particular day has the highest readership, but according to an Audits and Surveys Study, the percentage of people opening an average ad page on any weekday varies less than 3 percent. You might want to compress the frequency of your ads by running them closer together in terms of time frame. "Flighting" of ads rather than spreading them out over time will produce more leads per ad. This practice works best for established communities. I will cover marketing strategy in detail later.[9]

Circulation tallies the daily number of newspapers that are sold. Most newspapers do extensive research on their readership and can give you a breakdown on the relative proportion of their circulation that fits your target audience. You can use this information to determine which of the available newspapers that you are considering will be the most cost-effective. This is accomplished by determining the cost to reach 1,000 people in each specific newspaper. Simply divide the readership or circulation for your target audience into the cost of your ad (number of column inches × cost per inch) and multiply by 1,000. This tells you how much it will cost you to reach 1,000 members of your target audience. Compare this figure with other newspapers. The best dollar figure will be your most efficient use of your advertising budget. Bear in mind that some papers will produce better results than others, and that the cost per lead or sale is the true test.

Few professionals will dispute the claim that a larger advertisement generally will get more attention than a smaller one. But whether a full-page ad gets twice the attention as a half-page ad or four times the attention of the quarter-page ad is debatable. It is cost per response that counts. Smaller ads can work just as effectively as larger ads in some markets. Constant testing of ad sizes will establish the proper size to produce the most efficient cost per response.

Consideration should be given to the inclusion of a coupon in newspaper advertising. Coupons will facilitate the ease of response and therefore will generate a higher number of responses than ads without a coupon. However, many people will not include their telephone number, making it difficult for the staff to prequalify the prospect. Ads without coupons will require the prospect to walk in or call in, which generally will separate the serious prospects from the "tire kickers." In other words, coupons will produce quantity, and ads without coupons will produce more quality responses. In addition, the inclusion of a map will help increase drive-by and walk-in traffic. This is particularly important in new developments or when attracting prospects to a sales office or model during construction.

In your ad copy, keep sentences and descriptions short, and provide the "facts." Avoid the use of "catered," "quality," and "caring." Everyone else has worn out these terms, and even marginal operators will claim they stand for quality. Avoid criticizing the competition. It only draws attention to them, and seniors may infer that you are threatened by a competitor. You will run the risk of offending seniors with comparative statements such as "sit back and enjoy your retirement" or "retirement at its best."

Newspaper display ads are generally sold in one of two ways: by the column inch or by the agate line. A column inch is one inch deep by one column wide. How much space this amounts to in real terms is determined by the format of the newspaper. Some newspapers use eight-column format, so the actual width of the column will be about 1.5 inches. Column width in papers using a six-column format is about 2 inches. This information is usually included on the newspaper's rate card. To determine the number of column inches in an ad, multiply its height in inches by its width in columns. An ad that is two inches high and three columns wide equals six column inches. Some newspapers sell ad space by the agate line. There are 14 agate lines to a column inch, so an ad two inches high by one column wide would be 28 agate lines. Simply multiply the number of column inches by 14.

Many suburban areas issue weekly newspapers devoted primarily to local news. The rates for advertising in these are much lower than the daily newspapers because the circulation is smaller. These should not be overlooked because the primary market for the community may fit very well with the circulation boundaries of the weekly. Therefore, if you have some budgetary constraints, the weekly can afford you the opportunity to purchase large ads at a reasonable rate. Some weekly papers that are distributed free of charge will not be able to give you accurate estimates of the size of readership, and therefore no way for you to determine if the rates you are being charged are cost effective considering your exposure. Its best to experiment with weeklies with a proven ad to determine if this medium will produce for you.

Newspaper Tabloids

Newspaper tabloids, sometimes known as "advertorials," are very effective in producing a high quantity of responses in a short time frame. Tabloids have been known to produce 300 inquiries in the period of one week and then a trickle over one or several years. These are generally designed as an advertising supplement piece in black and white and two or four colors and are made to appear like a special real estate section produced as a feature by the newspaper itself. In fact the newspaper can produce your supplement in-house with their own graphics and typeface, which will make your piece look like the paper is endorsing your community, save you shipping costs, and even offer a 10 percent discount on insertions. The decision to use a "broadsheet" or "tabloid" format that matches the format of the newspaper in which you plan to place your insert will also make it appear as though it was generated by the newspaper. It is a good idea to print overruns of your insert to use for brochure stuffers and direct mail.

These supplements normally consist of four pages printed on a single 24" × 28" newsprint paper with a fold in the middle. The front page should provide a full description of the community, its benefits, a third party endorsement by the mayor or some other local conservative celebrity, and a resident testimonial to validate your claims. A supplement entitled "Narrows Glen Redefines Senior Living" with a photo of the community and a food layout on the first page was very successful. The second and third pages inside should include articles and photos that paint a picture of the benefits and value associated with the community. A comparison of all the services included in the monthly fee with the costs associated in purchasing the same or similar services out of the home is also very effective in communicating value. Seniors typically underestimate the cost of their monthly living expenses by $300–$500, and this worksheet will help them discover their "hidden" costs and help them over the "sticker shock" hurdle faced by many who first learn about the cost of senior housing. The back page of the tabloid should include several residents' testimonials detailing their initial fears and subsequent satisfaction with the community along with pictures of real people participating in some activity. Finally, a map to the community along with a coupon, can be helpful. Remember to position the coupon so that when it is removed it does not also destroy the cost comparison on the opposite side of the page. Layout of the piece can easily be accomplished with a computer desktop publishing program that can quickly be learned by community or corporate staff.

According to a Bureau of Advertising study using 100 top markets as a group, two-color publication will cost 17 percent more than the same full page in black and white. Four-color publication will cost 29 percent more. To keep your costs down, use color sparingly for only the front or back pages. Use only the highest quality photographs, inasmuch as even the best photos will lose some of their sharpness when reproduced and color separated.

Placing the supplement should take into consideration the timing considerations discussed earlier. Normally these supplements have a considerable shelf life because they are easy to remove from the newspaper and file or mail to a relative. I have even received yellowed coupons three years after the insertion date from someone who saved the piece until they were ready. In markets where major syndicated newspapers control smaller newspapers in a large metro area, the low cost and high impact in blanketing the region can be very attractive.

Magazine Advertisement

Magazines are the most psychographically targeted of all media. There are numerous magazines such as

Modern Maturity, published by the American Association of Retired Persons, targeted specifically to seniors with very large readerships. In fact, *Modern Maturity* boasts a readership that exceeds *Time, Newsweek,* and *U.S. News and World Report* combined! Unfortunately, their rates can be a bit out of reach for the typical retirement community. Other local senior publications, church bulletins, newsletters, and financial or real estate magazines can all be producers. As with newspapers, most magazines will know exactly the profile of their readership, so just compare what publications have the greatest circulation to your target audience.

The reproduction capabilities of most magazines are quite high. The layout or picture that disappointed you in the newspaper will look better here than in any other media. Detailed photographs of the community interiors or exterior lend themselves quite nicely to the reproduction capabilities of the magazine.

Magazine ads that are placed in a local tourist publication can effectively target the out-of-town decision influencer who is in town for a local convention. A good example of this is the annual convention of the Church of Latter Day Saints in Salt Lake City, where Mormons from all over the country converge. Other events that attract decision influencers and seniors are golf tournaments and estate and Medicaid planning seminars.

In contrast to newspaper advertisements, which can tolerate a lead time of up to 48 hours, magazines typically require the material to be prepared and ready for press months ahead of time. Planning is thus critical. Production costs can also be expensive; whereas newspapers will generally provide some assistance in putting your ad together, magazines require camera-ready artwork, which means that some artwork and printing may need to be done well in advance.

Periodical space is normally sold in fraction-of-page units such as full page, half page, quarter page, half column, and quarter column. Most rate cards will translate the page unit sizes into actual ad size. Discounts may be available based on the season, frequency of insertion, or whether the ad is a two-page spread. Some media buying services establish "umbrella" contracts where they reserve space with given publications and can offer discounts even for one-time ads. Your local library will have reference books entitled *Standard Rate and Data Service* (SRDS) that cover radio, television, direct mail, advertising and magazine rates, circulation figures, and general coverages. The SRDS publishes a directory of magazines that provides information on over 1,200 consumer magazines in 67 different classifications. You will also be able to determine if special geographic inserts or customization is available. Some magazines feature a classified section with their own rate structure for advertisers with a little creativity.

Although magazines can be expensive, they can also be one of the best ways to reach a highly selective target market. As a general rule you can expect to receive 90 percent of your total responses within three weeks when advertising in monthlies.

Magazine ad placement also mirrors newspaper advertising. The closer to the front of the magazine and the more visible the position the better. Research has showed that a position in the first seven pages of the magazine will produce a significantly better response than the same insertion in the back half of the same issue, the only exception being the back cover. Insert cards follow the same rule: the best position for an insert card is closest to the front. "The pull of position is as inexorable as the pull of gravity."[10]

Telephone Directory Advertisement

The need-driven senior or decision influencer with an immediate problem to solve will almost always turn first to the Yellow Pages. Leads from this source generally tend to produce conversion ratios second only to walk-in traffic. Directories are used by people who have already made up their mind regarding the benefits of retirement housing and are psychologically ready to be sold.

The challenge, then, is to purchase an ad that is larger or more attractive than a competitor's ad but not larger than you need. The ad should cover just the facts, preferably in bullet format. The retirement housing industry lends itself very well to larger display ads, which are competitive, attention grabbing, and aimed directly at the needs and questions of the potential resident and his or her family. A bold listing or a space listing that gives you extra lines within your regular listing surrounded by a border may be all that is required to differentiate you from the competition.

Choosing a listing category can sometimes play an important role. Check to see where competitors have placed their ads. They will normally be listed under "Retirement." Rather than listing your community in other categories, such as nursing or health care, you might be able to get a cross-reference in each and thus avoid paying for three separate ads.

It is important to remember that these directories are only published annually and will have a closing date beyond which they will not accept any changes or additions. Regional directories in a metropolitan area will all have different closing dates, so be sure to contact them all and incorporate these deadlines into your planning calendar in order to complete production on your ads with plenty of lead time.

In addition to the local city directory, the community might also benefit from exposure in several outlying areas. The National Yellow Page Service Association (NYPSA) publishes a rate and data publication that covers more than 5,800 telephone directories in the country and that helps to identify the areas that may be beneficial. Be sure to check that directories for small towns are not already duplicated in the larger metropolitan directory. The Donnelley directory, although not as widely distributed as the Yellow Pages, is gaining in popularity and can even be the preferred directory in some areas. Specialty directories such as *The Source Health Care Directory*, published by Data National Corporation, lists local health-care resources intended for use by physicians and therapists. These are normally inexpensive to advertise in and allow exposure to potential professional referral sources.[11] Professions, associations, and special interest groups also publish directories for their members, who can be highly targeted. Many will accept only standard listings, but some will allow display ads. Check rates and circulation to determine cost effectiveness.

Radio/Television Advertisement

Radio and television advertising can be used to promote interest in senior living, as long as the market that you are trying to reach matches up with the demographic profile reached by a specific radio or television station in your area. There are usually two or more stations in each market that appeal to senior audiences and can include nostalgic/standard, news, news/talk, business news, easy listening, full service, and classical. You must have a large enough budget, however, to be able to expose your message to your target audience at least three times within a one-week period to expect any response. Some communities have successfully used this medium to advertise the opening of new developments or additions to currently established communities.

Seniors will generally find one or two stations in the area that provide the type of programming they enjoy and will stick with them for years. Compared to other alternatives, radio is relatively inexpensive considering the cost per 1,000 listeners reached. Most radio stations will also provide assistance with production and offer suggestions about copy and content of the ads. In addition, they can provide information on specific time slots when your target audience is more likely to be listening. The major disadvantage to radio is that it does not have a shelf life; listeners are not afforded the opportunity to sit back and evaluate the details. Radio also tends to be regarded as a background medium. Listeners generally do not give it their undivided attention, as they would a direct mail piece or newspaper insert.

Radio is normally sold in spots, with a premium for selective time slots. The SRDS, mentioned earlier, has separate books for radio and television that describe the area of coverage, format of each station, and rates. Drive time during rush hours twice per day is normally the most expensive time to advertise, followed in order by daytime, evening, and overnight. Most seniors are early risers and will typically listen to their radio in the kitchen over breakfast and lunch. Breakfast falls within the most expensive drive time category. Advertising during lunch may thus prove to be the most cost-effective. In addition, female adult children may also hear the ads while listening at their desks. Be sure to check the availability of seasonal and frequency discounts that the station may offer. It is best to determine the time of day that attracts most of your target audience and concentrate your spots there. This way you are likely to hit the same individuals each time rather than a new set of ears during various times of the day.

Many radio stations will offer sponsorships for specific program features such as the weather, news, health watch, and the like, which for a slightly higher rate will cause people to stop and listen to your message. Sponsorships of National Public Radio programs such as "Talk of the Nation" or "All Things Considered" have been especially productive. There is also a psychological benefit of goodwill from people who may appreciate the value of the program you have sponsored.

As we age, the body experiences a normal degradation in hearing acuity. These deficits tend to be minimal in early adult years but then tend to accelerate rapidly after the age of 40. "The most limiting result of hearing deficits is increased difficulty in understanding speech. Research has shown that when speech is clear, undistorted, and presented without competing noise, older people suffer very little loss in ability to understand. Auditory deficits in the elderly become especially pronounced with adverse listening conditions. Interruptions to speech signals and increased rate of presentation both result in reduced sentence understanding."[12] When developing spots for radio, avoid the use of background music or special effects audio, which can be an obstacle to the communication of your message.

Many of these same suggestions apply to television as well. Television differs from radio in that it is a prestige medium. Television advertisers are viewed as a major concern when their spots are seen on the screen. Although seniors tend to be frequent TV watchers and may schedule their meals around favorite programs, the total production costs and rates will be affordable by only the largest of senior-living communities, and then only to advertise new developments or grand openings. Some cable stations offering programming that may be specifically targeted to seniors may be the exception. The reason television is so expensive is that the audience is very large. Smaller cable stations that cater to a more specific audience that may fit your psychographic profile might have more reasonable rates.

As with the other media types, keep the message short, sticking to the facts. Show the community interior and exteriors, particularly garden areas, and real people who look like they might be fun to get to know. Resist the temptation to allow radio and television advisers to get carried away with creating special effects. Seniors do not respond well to cute or clever messages. Stick with what you know will work, or, better yet, test your spots out on your market audience to confirm that they will be well received.

It is important to pick one audio and video format and stick to it. Using the same typeface or the same audio format for radio or television helps people to recognize your ads quickly. A very effective radio campaign was once launched that featured a 10-year-old boy who described his frequent visits to his great-grandfather in a retirement community. The spots were unique in that they were aired on a news/talk radio station where most people would not expect to hear a young voice. It was a real attention grabber and triggered numerous inquiries each time it ran. The ad featured a "real-life" situation at the community and told a continuing story, much the same as the successful Tasters Choice ads on television. The campaign was so well thought out that it actually inspired a small following among the listeners.

Direct Mail

Direct mail is considered by many to be the best lead generator of all the various strategies. With the advertising discussed so far, the costs are largely controlled by the media. Using direct mail, you control the expense by designing the mailing and deciding on the size and frequency of the distribution.

The greatest advantage of direct mail is that it is the most directly targeted of all advertising media. You can tailor your mailings to a very specific age- and income-qualified audience. With direct mail you also get direct feedback from your advertising message. The main disadvantage is the average cost per thousand. The better the mailing list, the greater the expected response. A high cost per thousand to reach the qualified target market will be justified if the responses are converted into sales at a higher rate than an alternative, less expensive strategy with a lower conversion rate.

There are essentially three types of lists that can be used to conduct a direct mail campaign. House lists are the marketer's own leads and represent the community's most valuable asset, although they will never be represented on the company's balance sheet. These individuals are presumably already age-and income-qualified and likely categorized by interest level. People in your lead bank are often neglected as many marketing representatives look for "fresh" leads to work. It is important to remember that these leads have been bought and paid for at the average cost per lead and can represent an investment of $100–$300 each. Responses from the lead bank or house list will generally be more qualified and generate higher conversion ratios. Direct mail is also a good vehicle to resurrect old leads that were deleted by the marketing staff. A high response may indicate that the sales staff is deleting leads too quickly.

Next in importance to those who have responded to your own promotional efforts are those who have responded to someone else's targeted efforts. These are the house lists of other companies or organizations such as the local Retired Senior Volunteer Program (RSVP), a hospital mail list to senior consumers, a list of patients who may frequent an optometrist or gerontologist, or even a list of seniors from the department of motor vehicles. These may all be sources of individuals who can match your psychographic criteria.

Many of these lists can be printed on address labels through a laser printer to avoid hand addressing. In addition, thousands of mail-order lists are available from firms targeting senior hobbyists and their adult children. These lists are commonly rented through mailing list brokers. Normally the persons on the list have a history of responding to direct mail appeals. List brokers do not own these lists; rather, they act as agents for many companies who will rent their list for a fee. These lists cannot be photocopied or used more than once without extra payment.

The third source of names is generally the poorest producer of responses, but the best for potential volume. Compiled lists come in a great variety and are generally developed from several sources. They can be sorted by zip code, age, income qualification, and other demographics. Sometimes large lists are merged from a number of sources and can contain duplicate appearances, so the sophistication of the list developer is very important. Information gathered from such lists is reliable most of the time. However, many nuances will exist such as widows who may continue to use their deceased husbands' name to protect their anonymity. Others still may be offended by mail addressed in this manner.

With the rising cost of postage, it is increasingly important to target the direct mail piece to the most qualified prospects that you can find. Although many communities will normally drop to their own lead banks, few take the initiative to investigate thoroughly the option of using the house lists of others and will drop their mailings to a compiled list instead. Planning the timing of the direct mail campaign to allow for the use of bulk mail and designing the size of the piece in conformance to post office standards can also help you avoid paying postage premiums. Check with the post office for insertion of the appropriate barcodes in the address fields, and make sure that your address panel is positioned for proper insertion into post office optical reading equipment. If the piece is upside down, it may get jammed in the reader, requiring the use of a wafer seal to close the piece. The wafer seal and the cost of labor to apply it will be charged to you.

Direct mail pieces range from postcards to multi-piece packages. Postcards can be very effective and are very low in cost. They can be of high quality and can include a response coupon. Response rates can be increased by offering a low-cost fulfillment piece to those who return the coupon. This can be, for instance, a guide to planning your move or selling your home or conducting a yard or tag sale. Seniors like to send away for free information, particularly if it may directly apply to their personal situation. Be sure that the fulfillment piece is of a quality nature, printed and accessorized with clip art, as it will be a direct reflection on the image of your community. Postcards can also be used as a coupon where the prospect is asked to bring the card to the community to receive a free gift or handout—along with a tour, of course. It is a good idea to put an expiration date on the offer to prompt a response. Postcards are relatively inexpensive to produce and mail, and can be used to mail to a larger audience such as a compiled list. The inclusion of a fulfillment piece will serve to identify the more interested prospects within the list. Do not use postcards to communicate complicated information. When announcing a grand opening, special event, or seminar, however, they can't be beat.

A self-mailer is a brochure (normally number 10 size) that is folded so that one portion of the back can be used for the address of the recipient, thereby eliminating the need for an envelope. Folding can be done by machine, which eliminates costly labor. Self-mailers can be multicolored or one colored and can be designed as a trifold to include reply cards or other inserts. Single-sheet flyers designed on the computer with a desktop publishing program are also an effective and cost-saving alternative to the more elaborate professionally printed brochures.

Always follow up your direct mail drop with telemarketing to improve the response rate and generate appointments. Consider seeding your direct mail list with staff or corporate addresses to trace delivery time frames or to track the mailings of those with whom you may have shared your list, or who "borrowed" it from you. Finally, it is a good idea to send each direct mail piece to your home address to track delivery time. Bulk rate postage can legally sit in each postal office for up to three days, and this can be an important consideration for time-sensitive material.

Special Media

Other nontraditional forms of advertising, such as outdoor advertising, transit advertising, posters and displays, community vehicles, and even business cards and letterhead should be carefully considered. These media types are typically extremely visual. They will create a graphic image of your community and establish your logo and colors in the minds of the general public. These media forms normally can be done well at minimal cost and provide a wide degree of flexibility.

People are rarely prompted to buy from these media sources; rather, these sources provide the community exposure and familiarize the general public with your existence. They are the least demographically targeted, and can for some environmentalists be a turnoff.

The entrance sign to the community is for most a very important investment. It is your property's own business card. A classic and elegant sign that is easy to read by day and by night can speak volumes about what may be inside. You can tell a lot about communities that have signs at their entrances that are ill-repaired, dirty, full of bird nests, or covered with weeds. The look of your sign gives the general public clues about your standards and can even speak to the financial stability of the organization. The colors used in a sign should complement your business colors, logo, and even interior design. Remember to include the Equal Housing Opportunity designation somewhere on your sign as required by law. Temporary sign or "A" boards that invite passersby for a tour of the community can do a lot to boost your walk-in traffic, particularly in new developments where the locals have watched the community being built in their neighborhood over time and may be curious with the end result. You may get a lot of "tire kickers," but often it takes only one referral to make a sale.

Marketing Events and Seminars

Most active seniors are seminar junkies, and they love a good party. Many newly opened communities will organize frequent marketing events to attract their prospects to the community in hopes of generating some real interest or even converting a sale or two. These grand events can be quite expensive to produce. By the time the cost of equipment rental, decorations, tables, additional silverware and china and food cost is figured in, the total production can easily top $15,000. Marketing events can be useful to introduce the community or to celebrate anniversaries or reaching occupancy thresholds, but sales are rarely made during such events. Normally the marketing staff is so preoccupied with producing a flawless event that there is little time to visit with and prequalify the guests. In addition, oftentimes the sales staff is involved with planning these events, which takes them away from valuable sales time. All major event parties (other than the grand opening) should be limited to the top 50 prospects in terms of motivation. This will minimize the disturbance to the current residents, keep freeloaders out, and allow salespeople at least some opportunity to mingle with the guests. Although some parties may be necessary or expected, residents can sometimes feel as though their activity budget is being spent for marketing purposes rather than for their entertainment or programming. In the end, it is important to preplan these events and develop an appropriate budget in order to compare the value and cost-effectiveness of this strategy with alternatives.

Seminars, on the other hand, are very inexpensive to produce and can be designed to attract a specific audience. Seminar curriculum can be developed by the executive director and marketing staff to encourage prospects from the lead bank to visit the community and meet existing residents. Existing residents will welcome the opportunity to "host" these events and will be receptive to the concept. They will see value in these seminars for themselves and will often invite friends living outside the community to attend. To promote public awareness of the facility and educate the elderly and their families to key health-related topics, monthly seminars throughout the year can be conducted, covering such subjects as

1. Senior nutrition
2. Senior fitness and exercise
3. Podiatry and foot care
4. Long-term care insurance
5. Understanding and managing your cholesterol
6. You and your aging parents
7. Skin cancer awareness
8. Wills and estate planning
9. Medicare eligibility and coverage
10. Medicaid planning
11. Women's or men's issues
12. Trust planning

Guest speakers can be engaged to deliver these talks on a pro bono basis. They may be local professionals interested in developing business with the resident population. Light refreshments should be served. Attendees can be encouraged to tour the community and interact with the residents. Programs such as these can draw very large crowds, especially if premarketed with a direct mail flyer, and the cost is minimal. The general effect is to position the community as the hub of senior activity and education in the geographic community.

Resident Referrals

In the end, resident referrals are your greatest endorsement. There is nothing more reliable than a candid representation from someone satisfied with your community and its services. Residents and their families will represent your community favorably to their friends if the following conditions are generally met with some consistency: (1) The service package must match their expectations and the promises of the sales representatives. Never overpromise and underdeliver. (2) Management is consistently fair in its treatment of residents and employees. (3) The owners are viewed as stable and fiscally responsible. (4) Fee increases are generally in line with the health-care cost of living and/or competing communities. (5) The food is good. Residents will tolerate reasonable swings in most of these categories and will generally give management the benefit of the doubt. However, if you miss the mark on any one of these consistently or if residents begin to identify a negative pattern, referrals will come to an abrupt end. Herein lies the symbiotic relationship of operations and marketing. Operations depend on marketing to fill the building and cover attrition, which can be accomplished only if operations are able to deliver on the promises made, either real or implied. To that end, management should remind all employees that marketing is ongoing and that every time they provide a service to a resident, they are in effect making a sales presentation.

The typical senior-living community evolves through several stages from first opening to stabilized occupancy, starting with blind optimism on the part of the developer through to the euphoria of the grand opening, then on to operational "can do," followed by marketing panic, investor panic, and finally the reality of balancing everyone's objectives. The number of resident-referred leads should increase as the community reaches stabilized occupancy, then stabilize or even fall off. During the fill-up stage of the project, there is usually a lot of excitement and energy generated by the marketing department that infiltrates the entire community. Residents see their community promoted in the media and may even be the subject of a feature article. During this period residents will usually encourage their friends and acquaintances to visit the community. Management needs to learn to anticipate residents' needs and grow their variable expenses slightly ahead of new resident demand. Resist the temptation to shower the first move-ins with attention, inasmuch as that attention will surely be divided among many as the community fills, leaving the early residents feeling as though their influence has been diluted. If management is able consistently to deliver the quality service package that residents expect, referrals should continue to grow with occupancy. Resident referrals may fall off in mature communities with a very old or frail population due to resident apathy or lack of friends outside the community. Ultimately, a well-run, stabilized community should be able to rely on 15–20 percent of its new leads coming from referrals (for assisted living this number should be closer to 50 percent). Many communities offer financial incentives to encourage residents to recommend their friends. Small rewards for referrals may be appropriate, but large incentives may serve to diminish value of your services or cause alarm. Although this strategy has been known to be effective, it can also backfire on the resident who may have encouraged a friend to move into a community that subsequently suffers from operational or financial difficulties. If you do offer financial incentives to your residents for their referrals, be sure to include a message on their monthly statement to remind them.

Assuming that the resident satisfaction with the overall community and services is maintained, there are many ways to market to your residents internally with little or no cost to the community: Test resident satisfaction with surveys of the operations, referral surveys, and resident focus groups.[13] Establish resident referral goals at your community and spread the responsibility for their solicitation to the executive director, resident relations staff, and other employees.

Offer guest passes for residents to bring their friends to lunch or to a coffee klatsch, or allow them to use meal credits for "qualified" guests. Form a resident marketing committee to test marketing concepts and solicit advice on how referrals can be generated. Develop contests and incentives between salespersons and other company communities. Develop doorhangers to kick off resident-referral contests or raffles. Develop your own change-of-address cards for new move-ins to send to their friends with an attractive postcard. Communicate to the residents about how they benefit from referring their friends to the community through companionship, increased occupancy, and financial stability using flyers and monthly reminders in the newsletter or activity calendar. Be sure to let them know that resident referrals are the least expensive way to market the community, and that all the expenses are ultimately borne by them. Offer special distinction to residents who have given referrals, such as special meals or wine with dinner, a corsage or lapel pin, personalized note cards, or small donation to their favorite charity, or use their photo and testimonial in your ads or direct mail pieces if appropriate. Another great source of resident referrals is direct mail to their membership directories or to a directory from their former apartment building. Many senior apartment buildings have evolved into naturally occurring retirement centers (NORCs) and can be a virtual bonanza of new leads.

Most importantly, simply ask the residents for their referrals or what you can do to earn them. Many residents do not see themselves as a potential referral source. Teach them to recognize their "sphere of influence."

Public Relations

Establishing a symbiotic relationship with the local press is the first step in earning publicity. Most editors are looking for newsworthy stories as well as headlines. Your public relations program should be designed to disseminate information primarily through the news media to increase public awareness to the existence and benefits of the community.

There are many naturally occurring publicity opportunities. Employee stories featuring a new hire, promotion, an accomplishment, or an act of valor in saving a resident's life are always worth notifying the press about.

Resident marriages and anniversaries are popular, as are stories about a resident's accomplishments or continued contributions later in life. Generally, anything out of the ordinary that promotes that senior capabilities are ageless makes for good reading for other seniors and their concerned relatives. Organize a panel discussion with the National Council on Aging and invite residents or local spokespeople to participate. Involve the local media when residents receive a special award or recognition for their contributions to local service organizations or charities. Or organize your own Senior Hall of Fame awards program and seek nominations from senior groups or organizations who would like to honor seniors for contributions they have made to the community at large.

Changes such as a new wing or added services—home health, long-term care, the opening of a specialty store or delicatessen—will help to freshen the image of your community.

Create your own news by hosting special events. One community in Dallas hosts an annual gingerbread-house competition through the local chefs' association each year. The houses are auctioned off and the proceeds go to needy seniors in shared housing. Tap into the creativity of the activity program to promote intergenerational programs, senior fitness clubs, aqua aerobics, volunteer programs, or programs that coincide with hot topics such as recycling and nutrition. You might also want to consider a joint project with nonprofit groups such as Senior Olympics or host a senior beauty contest. Nonprofit groups normally attract more attention in the media than for-profit groups.

The best publicity comes from events that offer something particularly visual. The newspaper may not have a lot of space available or want to waste a reporter's time writing an article, but they will often send a photographer if there is something worth seeing.

The best way to pitch your story to the press is through the editor who normally handles the type of story that you propose. You should have already laid the groundwork with this person, but if not, simply call the switchboard and ask for the appropriate editor. Summarize your story or idea in a fact sheet or press release and review it briefly with the editor over the phone. Always follow up in writing and check in by phone just before the event. The fact sheet should cover just the facts—the who, what, why, where, and when

of your story. Always include you name and phone number for further information.

A survey of newspaper editors identified seven factors that most often prevented them from using material from press releases: the information is not newsworthy, the release contains too much advertising fluff, the information is not localized, the release arrived too late to be used, the release is too long and cumbersome, the release is poorly written, or the contact listed is not accessible. A little insight into the needs of the editor can go a long way toward getting your ideas in print. Regional or national stories that are released in "mat release format" may increase their likelihood of being picked up by smaller community newspapers. This standardized, camera-ready, tabloid format is utilized by thousands of community newspapers across the country who do not have large enough editorial staffs to produce in-house materials.

If you have an employee who writes well, take advantage of the press release to explain your story in detail. Do not be overly concerned about the journalistic style, inasmuch as most press releases are rewritten by reporters anyway. It is a good idea to ask for the opportunity to review the final copy for accuracy and presentation so that it conveys your real intention behind the story. Essentially the press release paints a portrait of your fact sheet, providing clarity and an image supported by the facts.

Your press release should have a professional format if you want to improve your chances of its use. Be sure to include your name and phone number (upper right-hand corner) as well as the name and title of the editor (upper left-hand corner). Always give your story a short title in all caps and include a release date. The story should be double spaced with one-inch margins at the top and "-more-" on the bottom if the story is more than one page. You might want to follow up with a different angle if at first the story is rejected. Press releases should be designed to stimulate motivation by interest and generate inquiries.

Newspapers prepare editorial calendars that plan feature articles well in advance. Be sure to ask for a copy early in the year so that you can offer timely and appropriately targeted submissions.

Community Outreach

No retirement community is an island. It is an integral part of the neighborhood and depends on the support of local businesses and professionals to communicate its reputation. The community outreach program should be designed to generate a continuous referral base from the various interest groups and agencies who have regular contact with the facility's primary and secondary market targets.

Community outreach is often a two-way street. Not only will you be attempting to influence the information flow in the local service area, but you will also want to identify local resources who can provide superior service to the elderly and refer your residents to them. One of the best ways to accomplish this is through the development of a directory of senior services in your community. This way you can systematically contact either in person or by phone all the potential senior resources in your community and invite them to be a part of your research. Most will willingly cooperate and even offer to help sponsor the program by purchasing an ad. By developing this resource directory, you will gain great insight into the business and professional community, provide a reliable source of information about senior services that are available in the community to both seniors and their relatives inquiring on their behalf, and generate inquiries that can reasonably be funneled into your community.

Any community outreach effort should be organized and thorough. Start by researching the phone directory in your area for senior adult services organizations and inquire about a list of services available in your community. Next categorize your research into the various service groups. A complete listing of community outreach targets can be found in Exhibit 13.2. Then organize a fact sheet for each referral source to determine the description and costs of the services available. As you phone or personally visit your sources, tell them what you are organizing and ask them for a few minutes of their time to help you collect information about their services. As you compile the information during your personal interviews, always follow up your factfinding visit with a letter addressed to the owners or managers of the services thanking them for their time and interest and informing them that they have been selected as a referral source for your residents due to their quality of service and commitment to the elderly in your community. When referring residents to fee-for-service sources, always give them a choice of at least two different contact groups to limit your liability for inappropriate direction or advice.

Over time you will be able to focus your follow-up with those sources that reward you with the most referrals. The disadvantage with developing a directory is that it can become quickly outdated, so if you choose this strategy, you might want to limit the scope.

Another important component of the community outreach program may involve inviting professionals into your community to conduct seminars and presentations. This can normally be arranged pro bono on an individual basis. Some communities have even sponsored senior fairs at which a variety of businesses are invited to set up booths or displays or deliver a lecture. The end result you are seeking is exposure to the vast network of word-of-mouth advertising. The more organized and professional that you appear to be, the more likely someone will take a chance and refer to you.

Collateral Materials

The information packet should be an attractive brochure containing all of the information necessary for a prospect to evaluate the community. If the prospect calls in advance to make an appointment, the marketing department should take the time to personalize the information packet with his or her name printed on the outside cover or on a personalized letter inside. The inquiry thank-you letter can provide a nice introduction to the services and amenities of the community, thanking the prospect for his or her interest and highlighting the most positive reasons why your residents are happy living there. It is a good idea to itemize all the materials that have been included in the packet. Invite the prospect to call and ask questions on any of the materials or information that you have sent.

The rate sheet should include all possible community charges—the basic charge and what is included, plus any optional services and their charges. If the community offers several financial options, it is best to describe each in chart form so that the differences are easy to compare.

If the community distributes a monthly newsletter, bulletin, or activity calendar to the residents and it is well printed and speaks to the quality of the community, then it should be included. Never include an unprofessional in-house communiqué in a finely printed brochure packet. The differences in the two pieces may communicate to the prospect that marketing

Exhibit 13.2   Categories of Community Outreach Service

1. **Advocacy**

   Programs designed to be the advocate or liaison for seniors with concerns or problems:

   A. County ombudsman
   B. Disability advocacy services
   C. Alzheimer's and related disorders group
   D. Senior citizens coalition
   E. State department of aging and adult services

2. **Consumer/health education**

   Health or nonhealth related education or materials:

   A. County assessor
   B. Adult learning centers
   C. American Association of Retired Persons
   D. American Cancer Society
   E. American Diabetes Association
   F. Arthritis Foundation
   G. Council on Aging
   H. Public library home services
   I. Senior centers
   J. Financial services
   K. Seniors in Action
   L. Stroke support groups

3. **Employment/volunteer opportunities**

   Employment referrals or volunteer work opportunities:

   A. Retired Senior Volunteer Program (RSVP)
   B. United Way service groups
   C. Foster grandparent programs
   D. Green Thumb—gardening, park services

4. **Equipment/assistance services**

   A. Arthritis Foundation
   B. Medical supply companies
   C. Surgical/prosthetic supply companies

5. **Financial**

   A. American Cancer Society—financial assistance
   B. American Diabetes Association
   C. State emergency financial assistance
   D. Health and welfare—Food Stamps
   E. Estate planners, brokers
   F. Medicaid eligibility—state health and welfare
   G. Veterans services division
   H. Social Security Administration

6. **Health screening**

   A. American Diabetes Association
   B. Medical clinics
   C. Home assessment services
   D. Hospitals

7. **Home health**

   Services of skilled professionals, such as registered nurses, physical therapists, social workers; occupational therapy; personal care:

   A. Dial-a-nurse organizations
   B. Continuing care programs
   C. Home health care

8. **Hospitals and medical centers**

   A. Major hospitals
   B. Clinics
   C. Medical centers
   D. Pharmacy services

9. **Housing**

   Residential care in service centers, i.e., retirement centers:

   A. Your retirement center
   B. Adult rehabilitation program—Salvation Army
   C. Local reliable realtors
   D. Local reliable moving company

10. **Legal services**

    Planning for estates, wills, guardianship, power of attorney, conservatorship:

    A. State legal aid services
    B. Local attorney referral service
    C. State bar pro bono program
    D. Senior citizen—legal/tax counseling

(continued)

Exhibit 13.2 Categories of Community Outreach Service (continued)

11. Meals

In home or at service centers:

A. Rescue mission
B. Food banks
C. Meals-on-wheels programs
D. Senior citizen center
E. Senior nutrition programs

12. Miscellaneous human services

A. County medical society
B. Continuing care planning
C. Discharge planning (medical centers)
D. Family service planning
E. Home hair care
F. Salvation Army
G. Association of realtors
H. United Way
I. Veterans Administration
J. State health and welfare community services

13. Nursing homes

A. Local nursing homes
B. Outpatient therapy
C. Veterans homes
D. Alzheimer's special care units

14. Physicians/specialists

A. American Medical Association
B. American Optometry Association
C. American Dental Association
D. Physician referral services

15. Rehabilitation services

Inpatient and in-home services designed to assist client to regain/maintain maximum physical ability:

A. Adult rehabilitation program
B. Arthritis Foundation
C. Physical therapy services
D. Discharge planning (medical centers)
E. Outpatient therapy groups

16. Socialization/recreation

A. Local council on aging
B. Local YMCA
C. Senior centers
D. Senior exercise programs
E. Golf clubs/courses
F. City parks and recreation programs

17. Support groups

A. Alzheimer's Disease and Related Disorders Association
B. American Cancer Society
C. American Diabetes Association
D. Arthritis Foundation
E. Cardiovascular support groups
F. Diabetes support group
G. Pain management program
H. Stroke support groups
I. United Ostomy Association
J. Outreach ministries and major religious groups
K. Catholic community services

18. Transportation

A. Local metro bus/van services
B. Senior services
C. Cab companies
D. Dial-a-ride programs
E. Hospital/medical centers

and operational materials serve two different purposes depending on who is on the receiving end.

Reprints of any favorable articles or press releases published in the local media about the community or its residents help to validate the claims outlined in the brochures. Newspaper supplements or tabloids can also give prospects the impression that people are talking about the community and that it is attracting attention. Mentions of any national awards received by the community or company help to demonstrate industry leadership. Finally, reprints of articles from local and national media giving positive information on the methods of choosing a quality senior living community and the benefits of the lifestyle can be very convincing.

The information packet can be designed with a cut-out pocket in the back to allow the sales representative to customize the packet with floor plans, information on the nursing component or wellness center, and other selective material that may apply to the prospect's particular needs. This can also be a cost-effective alternative to reprinting the entire brochure in the event management changes the service package or price structures.

MEDIA SCHEDULES

The media schedule and calendar are the final planning tools that combine all advertising marketing strategies, establish their frequency, assign their relative priority, and allocate the budget. Essentially they are a summary of where and how you will advertise for the year, broken down by month.

There are three main scheduling strategies to consider, depending on the stage of occupancy, turnover, and budget availability for the community.

New developments that need to generate a general awareness of their community and a large volume of leads will commonly use a tactic called *continuous advertising*. Their media schedule is always full and they will advertise every week using a variety of media. This type of strategy tends to be very expensive and is generally not practical or necessary for more established communities. In fact, new competing communities frequently overestimate the price that their units will command due to optimistic pro forma projections during development. They will generally enter the marketplace with a big splash in the media, attracting considerable attention to senior living in general. Research has showed that many retirement housing prospects will comparatively shop the market before making their final decision. The established community that has successfully built a reputation for quality and value can expect to benefit from the awareness created at the expense of the new development, provided its prices are competitive. Communities in some markets have on occasion been pushed to stabilized occupancy riding in on the wave of awareness created by the new community.

The hybrid of continuous advertising is the planning strategy called *pulsing*. This is when a community runs a small base of continuous advertising but accelerates in pulses during peak seasonal periods or before significant events. This strategy works best for the community that is in the fill-up stage and has a continuing need for a large volume of new leads each month. Communities in the fill-up stage will generally experience an ebb and flow of activity in their marketing departments. Sometimes this is related to external factors such as holidays, the economy, elections, or something else in the marketplace, but often is linked to internal factors such as employee morale, management, departmental politics, financial thresholds, employee productivity, and especially move-outs. Any of these factors can trigger an acceleration or pulse in marketing activity.

The third strategy is normally practiced by established communities at or near stabilized occupancy that are already well recognized in their primary market area. This strategy is called *flighting,* where the marketer will concentrate the frequency and maximize the impact of the marketing exposure with a minimal investment. Using this strategy, the advertising is in for short periods at a high frequency, then off, then on again. The determining factor that turns the media placements on and off will be the size and quality of the lead bank combined with move-out projections. Wary marketers learn to anticipate swings in their lead bank status and understand that at a minimum it may take 60 days to convert new leads to sales with another 60 days before move-in. Therefore, by flighting media placements 60–90 days before the hot and warm leads are converted or receiving news of pending move-outs, they can maximize every budget dollar. This practice works very well when complemented by established lead generation from resident and professional referrals. Flighting is even more cost-effective when media purchases are concentrated to qualify for bulk discounts.

All effective media plans should be based on four concepts: reach, frequency, cost per thousand, and lease:lead conversion rates. *Reach* is the average number of people who are exposed to your advertising message at least once. Reach helps to develop awareness and understanding of your community. *Frequency* is the number of times the average person in your target audience is exposed to your message. Reach advertising, also known as attitude or image-building advertising, is harder to measure in terms of response because you cannot always attribute a specific sale to it. There is a lead time relationship in such advertising, and sales are usually created long after the ad has appeared. Reach-advertising messages linger in the minds of those who have some contact with the ad if it is of interest to them. These messages will be acted on sooner or later when people decide that they are ready to inquire.

The frequency of your ads will generally motivate prospects and interested parties to inquire once they have become aware of your community. New developments that blanket the media are trying to reach out into the marketplace to create awareness. Established communities are generally interested in prompting qualified inquiries and will normally focus their media with frequency. The media mix is the combination of media types that will provide a balance between reach and frequency at the statistically most cost-effective rate governed by the lease:lead conversion ratio. Exhibit 13.3 will help you build a media schedule that will maximize the results from your media choices.

Fine-tune your media schedule by developing a calendar for media placement. This calendar should also schedule major projects that will feed into your placements, such as a photo shoot or production of ads and direct mail pieces. The media calendar should itemize all activities in each strategy for each month, broken down by the percentage of the total budget that will be allocated to each for the month. This way you will know what percentage of your total budget for each month will be earmarked for each strategy. The calendar should also be marked with dates of special events and production deadlines. As you progress through the months and develop statistics on responses, you can adjust your ad size, placements, or frequency to meet your needs. Always save some funds for contingencies so that the marketing budget will last throughout the year. There is nothing more embarrassing than asking the owners for additional funds midyear, which implies that your planning process may have been flawed.

The media schedule provides management and owners statistically based, by-the-numbers justification for the amount and allocation of the marketing budget. Although the plan still only represents your best guess of what will work, it is weighted by historical cost-effective producers. The statistical approach depends on the collection and analysis of accurate lead response statistics and conversion ratios. This is not an exact science inasmuch as the prospect response may be the result of a number of media placements through a variety of vehicles. It is important to remain flexible with the marketing plan throughout the year. Anticipating changes in turnover and staffing productivity can and will have an impact on your lead generation strategies. The conversion rates will grow

---

Exhibit 13.3   Developing the Media Plan

1. Collect all the media information that you have researched.
2. Prioritize each strategy according to cost per thousand.
3. Prioritize historical producers by lease:lead conversion rate.
4. Choose the medium that has the highest conversion rate for the dollars invested.
5. Choose the second and third best that will coordinate well with your top producers.
6. Assign a percentage of your total advertising budget to each according to results.
7. Determine which strategy to maximize: continuous, pulse, or flighting, according to occupancy projections.
8. Schedule the media placements each month on a calendar according to your strategy.
9. Estimate the number of leads that will be generated from each strategy/month based on historic results.
10. Allocate the specific dollar amounts to each placement by media type each month (be sure to include production costs).
11. Calculate the cost per lead.
12. Multiply the cost per lead by the appropriate closing ratio to get cost per sale.
13. Summarize the total leads, cost per lead, total leads, and projected conversions by month, by year, and by media type.
14. Include lead and sale estimates from special media, seminars, resident referrals, etc.
15. Refer back to the annual unit sales forecast and annual lead forecast to determine the leads and sales required each month or for the year and compare to your summary. Adjust if necessary.

with the refinement of each strategy and as sales skills improve.

The entire planning process is only as good as the sales representatives who will convert the leads into sales. Good salespeople can convert your plan into reality and represent the foundation on which the success or failure of the community rests. We will explore the management of the sales function in the next chapter.

NOTES

1. A. J. Mullen, D. Cwi, and D. Yulish, "An Analysis of Nationwide Absorption Rates: The Critical Element in the Feasibility of Senior Living Projects," p. 2.

2. Copies of the study, "Retirement Housing and Long-Term Health Care Choices of the Elderly," are available from Dr. Lumpkin by calling (318) 231-5882.

3. C. H. A. Hoskins, "The ADA and Retirement Communities: Time to Be Proactive," *Retirement Housing Business Report* (1993): 6–10.

4. This would also apply to those individuals whose behavior is chemically managed. See pp. 99–100 for medication red flags.

    The FHAA allows for the establishment of "housing for older persons," defined in the act as intended for, and solely occupied by, persons 62 years of age or older; or intended and operated for occupancy by at least one person 55 years of age or older per unit. If the operator chooses to impose these restrictions on their establishment, then the publication of, and adherence to, policies and procedures that demonstrate an intent by the owner or manager to provide housing for persons 55 years of age or older must be in place. See 42 U.S.C. § 45 (1994) or visit *www.efn.org//fairhouse/usc4245.html*. This means that admission can be denied on the basis of creating "housing for older adults" as long as this designation for the project is supported in writing through policy statements, and consistently applied.

5. E. C. Merrigan, "Rating Guidelines for Nonprofit Continuing Care Retirement Communities," Fitch Health Care Special Report, Fitch Investor Services, Inc., June 1994.

6. S. Brooks, "Who Is Our Senior Housing Client? Marketing and Public Relations Ideas That Hit the Target," presentation to the National Association for Senior Living Industries, Dec. 1994.

7. C. W. Wallace, *Great Ad! Low Cost Do-It-Yourself Advertising for Small Business* (Blue Ridge Summit, Pa.: Liberty Hall, 1990).

8. F. B. Colavita, *Sensory Changes in the Elderly* (Springfield, Ill.: Charles C Thomas, 1973).

9. M. G. Leary, "Maximize Your Investment: Lead Generation for Tough Times," presentation to the National Association for Senior Living Industries, May 1992.

10. B. Stone, *Successful Direct Marketing Methods* (Chicago: Crain, 1979).

11. Copies may be obtained by phoning the corporate headquarters at (800) 544-0516 or writing to National Data Corporation, Corporate Headquarters, 925 Chestnut Street, Philadelphia, PA 19107.

12. C. D. Schewe, "Marketing to Our Aging Population: Responding to Physiological Changes," *Journal of Consumer Marketing* 5(3) (Summer 1988): 67.

13. See Chapter 5 for more information on developing, conducting, and interpreting resident surveys.

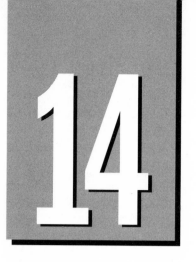

Sales

Selling retirement housing is very different from selling anything else. You sell not only the actual apartment, but also the services and intangibles that go with it. Often the buyer is there out of need rather than choice, and the decision is almost always emotional. An effective sales program must be designed around the process of building relationships and trust in an environment of change. Salespersons must be able to establish rapport with prospects and their families while developing a familiarity with the assets of the community.

It is widely held in the retirement-community industry that sophisticated marketing and community outreach plans, excellent collateral materials, and targeted advertising are the essential elements to ensure a rapid fill-up of a project. But in reality, its relationships between people fill a community.

A top sales director was asked by the sponsoring board of directors how she filled her building. Her response was "one person at a time." Although it is important to have a plan of and strategy for marketing the community, there are no shortcuts to building trust and inspiring confidence in people that you (and your community) will be able ultimately to meet their complex needs. The process takes a lot of work: commitment to building relationships and overcoming barriers, and reassurance, repeated in its entirety for each and every prospect and family member that comes along.

PROSPECT CLASSIFICATION

Prospect classification is a system that rates each prospect in terms of urgency and desire to buy. Prospect-classification systems allow the sales counselors to prioritize leads for effective follow-up. For example, *hot* leads who may decide to purchase within 30 days will require more frequent contact than *warm* leads who may be ready to purchase within 31–90 days. Prioritized by urgency, these leads can be scheduled for the appropriate frequency of contact. The sales counselors can then spend more time working leads who are likely to sign a residency agreement sooner, thereby maximizing their productivity. Other leads classes can include *active,* for those leads who are expected to sign within 90–180 days; *unclassified* leads who may have sent in a request for information without including a phone number, or who have replied to a mailing and have not yet been called and classified. *Inactive* status can be assigned to leads who may not be ready yet but still want to remain on the community's mailing list. *Deleted* leads can include those prospects who have been deleted by the sales counselor or who may have requested deletion for a variety of reasons.

Prospects will be classified either by telephone or personal visit. The sales counselor will typically explore what may have prompted the inquiry and attempt to determine the prospect's motivations and current status. This is part of the qualification process and will establish the initial level of urgency. During the course of the sales process, it is the sales counselor's main job to move prospects from a lower level of urgency to a higher level.

Salespersons have been known to inactivate or delete prematurely leads who have later become residents somewhere else. Due to the acquisition cost of the leads in the lead bank, the marketing director should approve all lead deletions.

The classification of prospects also provides a way to track the efficiency of various marketing strategies according to the level of interest that each generates. For example, a newspaper ad campaign may need to be revised if it is found to be only attracting *active* level leads after the responses have been called for qualification and classification. Conversely a direct mailer may be a big hit if several of the responses generated are determined to be *warm* or *hot* prospects.

LEAD MANAGEMENT

Management of contact frequency in the lead bank is the single most important controllable aspect of the sales program. Too-frequent contact will risk alienating the prospect, and too-seldom contact may leave the prospect feeling neglected or allow the leads to become stale. Marketing strategies are designed to attract prospects to the community. The marketing process can involve investments of hundreds of thousands of dollars to generate targeted, qualified prospects. This money is all wasted if the inquiries are not appropriately contacted. Time is of the essence because the personal status of each individual in the lead bank will be changing continuously. Prospects expect to be contacted after making an inquiry, and it can be a very poor reflection on the entire operation if they are neglected. Commissioned sales counselors tend primarily to work hot and warm leads and to ignore the rest of the lead bank.

For any sales program to be successful there must be a failsafe system to ensure that all leads are appropriately directed toward closing. It is important to control the advertising and other lead-generation strategies so that the lead bank can be properly managed by the sales counselors without losing track of any qualified leads. There are many good systems available on the marketplace to automate this task, but, as with any system, they require daily management and supervision to be effective.

All hot, warm, and active leads should be scheduled for monthly contact. Hot leads should be contacted weekly, warm leads three times per month, and active leads twice per month. You should try to classify all unclassified leads. Unclassified leads that are generated by a coupon or mail-in without a phone number should receive an "unable to reach you" letter to prompt a phone-in confirmation. It is also possible to track leads down using the reverse directory, which lists names by address.

Contacts should be alternated between personal phone contacts designed to close on an appointment and relationship-building calls. Contact type should include phone calls, personal letters, and newsletter or article mailings. This does not include routine or scheduled direct mail contacts to the lead bank. The approach should be designed to build relationships, not just to schedule appointments. This way the prospect will learn that the sales counselor has a genuine interest and is not merely pestering him or her to visit the community. Scheduling all leads for monthly contact will assure management that its marketing investment to generate responses will be maximized so that no one falls between the cracks.

The lead management analysis in Table 14.1 schedules lead contact frequency based on level of urgency. All leads are contacted at least monthly to ensure that the lead bank is properly maintained and the leads are kept current. The mail-out contacts can alternate between event flyers, personal letters, and the monthly newsletter. For all active leads, including hot, warm, and active classifications, the total numbers of contacts are split evenly between phone-outs and mailings. Inactive leads are routinely contacted by direct mail and perhaps telemarketed quarterly to attempt to upgrade.

This system is simply an example to illustrate how the entire lead bank can be scheduled for monthly contact. Monthly contact will keep the leads fresh and create an understanding among the sales staff of the mechanics behind their performance expectations. The point to stress here is that it is important to have a system—any system that ensures that all leads are contacted at least monthly and appropriately directed toward closing. Systems may vary, but if the marketing director leaves the lead follow-up scheduling to the discretion of the sales counselors, he runs the risk of neglecting leads that may have cost him thousands of dollars to attract.

Table 14.1   Lead Management Analysis

Lead urgency classification	Total leads	Monthly contact frequency	Total personal contacts
Hot	8	4	32
Warm	32	3	96
Active	1,310	2	2,620
Unclassified	181	1	181
Inactive	1,368	0	0
TOTALS	**2,899**	**10**	**2,929**

Productivity	Annual	Monthly	Weekly
Phone-outs	17,574	1,465	366
Time/call: @ 10 min	0.17	0.17	0.17
Total phone time	**2,929**	**244**	**61**
Mail-outs and letters	17,574	1,465	366
Time/letter: @ 5 min	0.08	0.08	0.08
Total mail-out time	**1,465**	**122**	**31**
Closing time			
Visits/sale	5		
Avg. hours/visit	2		
Time/sale: @ 10 hr	10	10	10
Sales budgeted	108	9	2
Total closing time	**1,080**	**90**	**23**
TOTAL SALES TIME REQUIRED	**5,474**	**456**	**114**
Sales time available			
Hours per week	40		
Weeks per year	48		
Total	**1,920**		

Selling time		Hours
Selling time	85%	1,632
Nonselling time	10%	192
Miscellaneous	5%	96
Total	**100%**	**1,920**

TOTAL STAFF REQUIREMENT	**3.4**

Size of the Sales Force

The size of the sales force is a function of the size of the lead bank, the classification of the leads, the urgency level, and the frequency of contact desired. The sales counselors will assign the lead classification category as they work with the prospect. Rarely do prospects enter the system as hots; most are progressively upgraded from a lower classification. The urgency level will then determine the follow-up frequency. The sales director averages the amount of time generally required for each activity, whether it is the phone-out, mail-out, or closing time. The next step is to calculate the number of hours annually required to work the lead bank properly. Because not all of the sales counselors' time is spent in the selling process, the available hours per sales counselor need to be adjusted. The sales director's objective is obviously to maximize the time spent selling. In fact, the sales director should also have leads assigned to him to work just like everyone else. The number of staff required to work the lead bank is then calculated by dividing the annual hourly requirement to work the lead bank by the total available of sales time per year (see Table 14.1). As the size of the lead bank fluctuates, management can estimate the work force required to service all leads weighted by classification.

Another method to calculate manpower requirements is to compare the contact frequency and time requirements to an average productive work week. Total monthly contacts for each lead classification are calculated, then divided among the sales counselors. This number is then divided by an average of 22 working days per month to calculate the daily productivity of each person. Time requirements for each activity are factored in and the total hours per week to service the lead bank are calculated. This way the marketing director can evaluate the overall workload. If the total amount of time required by the formula exceeds 40 hours per week, then the number of full-time equivalents may need to be increased incrementally (see Table 14.2).

Sales Productivity

Staff productivity expectations should be established and managed through the lead management system. This lead management analysis determines the total number of personal contacts required for the entire department. Each sales counselor should be able to make a minimum of 20 phone contacts and 20 mail-outs each business day. Assuming 22 average working days per month, this totals 880 contacts per month. Higher expectations may result in a pressured environment that can be sensed by the prospects. The marketing/sales director wants to create a sense of

Table 14.2 **Work Week Allocation**

	Total contacts	2,929		
	FTEs	3.5		
	Monthly contacts / FTE	837		
	Daily contacts / FTE	38		

Productivity per person	Monthly	Weekly	Daily
Phone calls	418	105	21
Time/call: @ 10 min	0.17	0.17	0.17
Weekly time: hours	70	17	3
Letters	418	105	21
Time/letter: @ 5 min	0.08	0.08	0.08
Weekly time: hours	35	9	2
Closing time			
Hours/sale		6	1
Total hours/wk		32.6	6.5

urgency among the sales staff without burning anyone out. At the same time, clearly stated productivity expectations should leave little time for wasting on activities that will not yield sales. (See the section on sales analysis for more on productivity targets.)

Contacts are equally split between phone-outs and mail-outs. Phone-outs assume approximately 10 minutes per call; mail-outs assume 5 minutes per letter. Clearly some will take more and some less, but these averages have withstood the test of time and can be used for planning purposes. Each sales counselor's day leaves little time for nonselling activities—three hours of phoning, two hours of mailings, and an average of one hour per day of closing time amounts to 6 hours of selling per day. In our earlier lead bank example, each of the three sales counselors plus the sales director (part time) will need to spend approximately 33 hours each week working their leads. The balance of the work week can be used for training, meetings, home visits, and the closing process. In short, sales staff should be managed so that their time is spent almost entirely on sales activities, not on paperwork or planning.

Normally, a slowdown in sales results can be usually traced to insufficient phone-out productivity. As a rule of thumb, each sales counselor should be able successfully to complete the 20 phone-outs per day mentioned earlier. (These are phone-outs where they actually *talked* to someone.) If the sales counselor falls short of this goal, management needs to intervene to determine the cause of the problem. For example, if the sales counselors are spending too much time organizing events, then management should consider reassigning the responsibility to operations staff.

Residents can be another common distraction. They will often visit the marketing department during the day to maintain their relationship with the sales counselors. Although these relationships can often yield important referrals, these activities should not interfere with phone-out goals. Marketing directors must protect their sales counselors' valuable time.

It is a good idea to incorporate weekly phone-out goals into the sales counselors' team incentive plans and chart their progress each day. In extreme cases, the marketing director might consider establishing phone-out quotas to ensure that all leads receive the appropriate attention.

The marketing director should organize the sales department so that all staff time is scheduled as either "floor time," where a single sales counselor handles all incoming walk-ins or phone-ins on a rotating basis, or as "sales time," where the sales counselor makes phone-outs and mail-outs, schedules appointments, or conducts tours. Only specific marketing events should require sales staff to be in attendance.

Operations should be responsible for planning and coordinating all major events to allow the marketing department to spend its valuable time on selling. This can be accomplished using function sheets that fully describe the function and the associated costs of producing it. Normally the resident relations or activity department initiates the process, which typically culminates with food and beverage.

The closing process will vary greatly by individual. Some will sign early, after only a few contacts, whereas others will require 10 or more contacts over an extended period to confirm their decision. The example in Table 14.1 assumes five personal visits per sale at two hours per visit for a total of ten hours closing time. Although each prospect will be different, this is a good average for planning purposes.

Computerized Lead Management

The decision to computerize the lead management system is normally predicated on the size of the community, occupancy, volume of inquiries, and the level of detail required in analyzing results. Small or even mid-sized communities have effectively managed their lead banks manually with a tickler card box system, whereas others have chosen an integrated contact management system with a computer on each sales counselor's desk. There are several good contact-management software packages that can be purchased off the shelf, but some may be limited in their ability to generate custom reports for tracking advertising results. Still other communities develop their own system using templates created from database programs.

There are numerous lead-management software packages on the market today that were specifically designed for the senior-living business. A good program should contain two main components: lead tracking and lead analysis. These two components should be designed to provide the marketing director with information about the sales and marketing program efficiency. Equipped with this information, the director can quickly identify weakness in the responses from individual marketing strategies or problems in their conversion to sales.

Lead Tracking

The lead tracking component should serve as a contact manager that will automatically schedule contact frequency of all leads according to classification. The sales director should be able to generate a daily or weekly contact schedule that sorts each lead by classification, last contact, phone number, "hot button," "obstacle," and unit type desired. The lead tracking component should also be able to generate traffic reports such as number of walk-ins, phone-ins, coupons, or "be backs." Production statistics such as phone-outs, appointments made/kept, and conversion ratios by sales counselor should also be collected. The system should also produce a current status report on all move-ins sorted by sale date and move-in date in order to track the first inquiry to lease and lease to move-in time frames.

A snapshot of the lead tracking for one month will only yield the profile of the lead bank today, but when it is compared with historical results in the same format, important trends may materialize. Monitoring the number of leads by classification along with the total leads (including new and deleted leads) can provide important clues to project short-term performance. For example, if the hot and warm lead classifications begin to fall, more of the sales will need to be generated from the active classification, which

may take longer to convert. Over time the director may notice that the overall size of the lead bank is shrinking, which could mean that there are more monthly deletions than new leads, triggering a need to boost media placements.

Finally a cancellation report that details which leads or sales were canceled or rejected and their reason can be very useful to identify problems in the offering, or weak follow-up by the sales staff or move-in coordinator. This can also focus sales staff on the importance of *net* sales and appropriately place an emphasis on follow-through. A sale is not complete until the prospect has been converted to a resident.

Lead Analysis

The lead analysis component should itemize each lead by classification and demographics and detail how each was attracted to the community. For example, the leads may have originated from a coupon, a call from the Yellow Pages, walk-in, radio message, and so on. This information is normally collected and entered on a lead card by the person taking the call or the prospect when he or she comes for a tour. It is essential to create a profile of each prospect to determine which marketing strategies are working.

The lead analysis component should also be structured to provide an advertising summary that details the date, location, cost, size, day of week, coupon, and the like and response by prospect classification for every media placement. This information enables the marketing director to evaluate quickly the effectiveness of each ad in pulling prospects from the various media types. Sorting the responses from each ad by urgency classification will further help the director separate what placements will generally yield quality leads from those that produce a high quantity. This way minor adjustments can be made to manage one or the other. For example, if you are interested in producing more quality leads, the advertising summary may indicate that the quarter-column coupon "services" ad was the most productive. If quantity is what you are after, the summary might indicate a large response to the "decision influencer" ad that you ran in the local weekly. Armed with these response statistics, the marketing director can begin to recognize patterns that over time may deliver predictable results.

Some communities employ a marketing assistant who updates the database daily; inputs daily sales activity logs, new leads by source and media type, and ad responses; and produces a weekly contact list for each sales person generated from the automated tickler system. This person can also be trained to assist with events, tours, and recordkeeping. Many marketing assistants who have learned the sales process go on to become sales counselors and even marketing directors. As the community reaches full occupancy, the marketing assistant should also be able to perform the essential functions of the move-in coordinator. The ability to perform these additional duties will of course depend on the size of the community and the amount of turnover that it routinely experiences.

The purpose of these reporting systems is to identify strengths and areas of vulnerability of the combined sales and marketing efforts so that adjustments and corrections can be made each month to keep things on track. The following worksheet details some useful statistics collected from a sample community. Important trends and meaningful statistics can be used by the marketing director to identify results from the marketing plan and media schedule. In addition, potential problem areas in sales or leasing activities can be recognized when evaluating monthly trends.

◼◼◼ LEAD BANK

Communities in the active fill-up mode should as a rule of thumb have approximately 20 times as many leads in their lead bank as the number of apartments in the community. For example, a 100-unit community should have 2,000 leads (20 × 100 units). At least half of these leads should be classified as *active* status—hot, warm, or active.

Communities that have reached stabilized occupancy may be able to maintain their occupancy and cover attrition with a lead bank that is 10 times the apartment count. Established communities that rely on resident and nonresident referrals may even be able to get by with less. However, referrals can fluctuate widely, so marketing directors are well advised to keep a healthy number of qualified leads in their lead bank at all times.

Trends in the overall size of the lead bank are important to watch. A continual shrinkage in the number of leads over time may indicate problems in response rates to media placements or a media calendar that may need a higher frequency of placements. Shrinking lead banks can also indicate an imbalance

between new leads and deleted leads. Leads can be very expensive to generate; therefore the marketing director should approve all deletions. Conversely, lead banks that exhibit excessive growth may make it difficult to schedule appropriate follow-up and strain staff resources.

The marketing director should carefully evaluate the trends and composition of each classification. Obviously, the higher the percentage of strongly motivated leads the better. A healthy yet realistic lead breakdown should run about 0.5 percent hots, 1.5 percent warms, 55 percent active, 10 percent unclassified, and 33 percent inactive. Lead banks with too few hot leads can indicate a need to improve the quality of leads. They can also indicate that leads are not being progressively upgraded to higher-motivated lead categories. Lead banks with greater than 10 percent of their leads unclassified may need to reevaluate their coupon design, or may have an excessive amount of phone-ins that have not been followed up. Lead banks with greater than 50 percent of the leads designated as inactive or unclassified might indicate a need for stepped-up media placements to generate fresh new leads.

It is important to remember that a shrinking lead bank, left unnoticed, can create significant delays in sales as new leads will take some time to be generated and then to convert. When you first notice that your lead bank is inadequate, it may already be too late to cover vacancies as they occur.

The completion of the marketing plan will have established specific goals for the number of new leads and leases or sales required each month to meet the financial projections of ownership. Other very useful goals to consider establishing might include average new walk-ins per month, average new resident-referral leads per month, and site leads. Strategies can be developed to maximize lead generation from these types of mechanisms that will not involve significant investment from the marketing budget.

Many times the differences between results from one community to the next amount to attitude. It is not that the quality of leads is necessarily better at other properties, but that the sales staff is more likely to classify leads as "warmer," even if prospects say they are "not ready yet." The warmer the lead status, the more frequent the contact with the prospect. The quality of contact is normally better because there is a higher expectation on the part of the sales counselor. To improve your lead split, you might want to consider the following suggestions:

- Be optimistic when initially classifying a lead. This will optimize quantity and quality of follow-up.

- Do not automatically downgrade a lead just because the last contact with the prospect was not encouraging. Give your leads adequate time to adjust to the idea of retirement living and try several attempts to close them on an appointment before you downgrade them.

- Implement a system whereby any inactive lead who is logged into the system and has not been verbally contacted within the previous 60 days is "up for grabs" and can be worked by another sales counselor. This will direct attention to inactive leads and encourage sales counselors to upgrade them if there is a chance of closing.

LEAD SOURCES

Any effective marketing effort will be defined by the quality and quantity of responses from the target market. It is important to distinguish between the lead source and the sales source. The lead source is where the leads originated, and the sales source is where the sales originated. Marketing efforts may generate a large quantity of leads from a single strategy that has a dismal closing percentage. It is therefore important to focus attention on strategies producing leads that ultimately convert to sales. Although sales can sometimes be difficult to track to a particular marketing strategy, the objective of marketing is to allocate the marketing budget according to the best conversion rate of the lead responses to sales. It is important to note that sales will also be generated from the site, resident referrals, and nonresident referrals. Each of these lead sources will also have its own conversion rate, and should be considered *separately* when allocating marketing dollars. The inclusion of these other lead sources when calculating the community's conversion rate will overinflate true marketing results. Tracking these responses in detail will yield important information about the lead location, method of inquiry, and source. Trends in this information are then evaluated from month to month so that vulnerabilities can be identified and adjustments can be made in media planning and marketing. Lead location is generally categorized by *primary market, secondary market, tertiary market, rest-of-state,* and *out-of-state.*

Primary Market

The *primary market* is normally defined as the geographic location where 80 percent of the age- and income-qualified leads required to fill the community will be generated. This can be defined as a specified radius in miles, Zip code, or county in the immediate vicinity of the community. Normally the boundaries of the primary market area are established relative to the size of the market in the area and their relative distance from the community. For example, in urban areas where there are typically high concentrations of people, the community may be able to reach this 80 percent threshold within even a 10-block radius of the community. Conversely, a community in the suburbs may need to expand its primary market definition to a 10- to 15-mile radius from the project. In extreme cases rural communities have been known to define their primary market to encompass a three-county area.

Clearly, the more concentrated the target market, the easier it will be to reach it and schedule appointments. Communities that are unable to attract 80 percent of their leads from within their primary market may cause serious concern for management, for the marketing effort will need to be expanded to cover other, less attractive markets with consequently lower lead:lease conversion ratios. Most seniors prefer to move into a senior-living property that is situated within their community circle of friends and business acquaintances.

Shortages in leads generated within the primary market may also indicate that the penetration rate analysis, as discussed in Chapter 13, could have been flawed. In any event, the average cost per sale will tend to increase with the relative distance from the property. Marketing directors should keep a close eye on the percentage of leads from the primary market location and adjust media placement frequency and location to attract more local responses.

Secondary Market

The *secondary market* is normally defined as the geographic area outside the boundaries of the primary market, but still considered local. Typically, up to 10 percent of the total lead bank should originate within this market. For example, the secondary market could include the areas beyond the five-mile radius from the community, but still within the major metropolitan area reached by most major media. It is important to remember that your secondary market may also be a competitor's primary market. Media placements within the secondary market should be designed to improve your community's *reach* rather than its *frequency.*[1] The competition will surely be budgeting more dollars within the boundaries of its own primary market, and it is not normally worthwhile to attempt to match the competition's exposure. In addition, it will be more difficult to schedule appointments with prospects who live a distance from the community primarily due to transportation constraints.

Tertiary Market

The *tertiary market* is very loosely defined in the industry. It normally includes family members who are interested parties actively involved as decision influencers. They can live locally or out of state. Some marketers also include rest-of-state and out-of-state markets in this category. The ratio of prospects to interested parties in the initial contact will generally run about 3:1. However, among the 75 percent prospects, 80 percent of those will have some family involvement in their decision making process. As explained in Chapter 13, family members will generally recognize a need for retirement housing long before the prospect will even admit that there may be an issue. Marketing efforts that target lead-generation activities to age- and income-qualified prospects and use the family to assist in confirming the decision will convert more leads. Prospects to interested party ratios that fall to 2.5:1 or lower may indicate a potential problem with the entry level of care. These ratios will naturally fluctuate by level of care. As a rule, the percentage of interested parties as the initial contact will run approximately 5–10 percent for continuing-care retirement communities, 25–50 percent for congregate communities, and 80–95 percent for assisted-living or skilled-nursing communities. Many interested parties will not only be first to inquire on behalf of a reluctant relative, but they may also be gathering information because their family member is *unable* to do it. Be especially cautious about family members who indicate an interest in arranging a placement or signing a lease without their relative or friend having visited the community personally.

The *rest-of-state (ROS)* and *out-of-state (OOS)* markets are the most costly to reach, considering their corresponding conversion rates. Communities in destination retirement locations such as Florida or Arizona

may rely heavily on leads generated from these markets. However, retirees will normally relocate to the destination area while they are still relatively active and independent. Most out-of-state transplants are admitted to the senior living community after first living several years in a local apartment or condominium.

Many destination retirement communities have successfully marketed before and during the summer months to "snowbirds" in colder climates. This can be done in the same manner as a second market, but should always include an 800 number to facilitate easy response. Many seniors will reserve an apartment for four to six months sight unseen. It is important to note here that some existing residents may resent the short-term snowbirds living in their community each year. In any event, the marketing director will need to evaluate the cost of marketing these units against the total revenue collected over the short length of stay to determine if this strategy is financially feasible. As a rule of thumb, the average cost per sales should not exceed two months' rent for short-term residents and three months' rent for long-term residents.

As people age, their lifestyle challenges become increasingly complex. Normally they will look to family and close friends for support. As many families become geographically diverse they may experience a sense of frustration about their limitations to provide assistance to an ailing parent. Therefore, many ROS and OOS inquires will be triggered by families seeking to move closer together. This is normally accomplished by the prospect's moving closer to her immediate family members.

Methods of Inquiry

Methods of inquiry to retirement communities are normally categorized as *walk-in, phone-in, phone-out,* or *mail-in.* Prospects who inquire at the community as walk-ins circumvent the need for sales counselors to schedule an appointment. Generally speaking, walk-in conversion rates will be the highest because they indicate someone who may be either an interested party or a prospect who is "shopping" and who may already be convinced of the advantages that senior housing has to offer. In fact, walk-in conversion rates can be as high as 15 percent, which underscores the importance of creating a positive first impression at the reception desk.[2] Walk-in traffic will normally be the highest shortly after opening. This statistic may be a bit misleading, inasmuch as the community may be visited by people from the local neighborhood who have taken an interest in the project during the construction stage and are eager to have a look inside. Although few of these visitors will ever be serious prospects, they do represent a significant referral base. The smart manager will recognize the importance of local support of the community in the primary market area and tap into the vast word-of-mouth network for promotion.

Phone-in inquiries are normally the result of an ad in the media or telephone directory, or are prompted by a referral. Like walk-ins, these responses are also highly motivated. Many such calls are received by the receptionist who is responsible for collecting the appropriate data to allow the sales counselors to respond. It is best to designate the sales counselors to rotate through "floor time" when they are available to handle these calls and any unannounced walk-ins who may drop by. If the sales counselor is busy with another inquiry, the marketing director can designate who is next up. Because these leads are normally very motivated, some fair system of equal rotation for sales counselors who are paid on commission is advisable.

Leads generated by the sales counselors through the course of their phone-out activity can be substantial. During the sales call, the counselor should always ask prospects for referrals to their friends and acquaintances. Many active seniors who may not be ready yet for the community will have friends who may qualify. These are a very inexpensive and often prequalified source of leads and should not be overlooked.

Finally mail-in leads can normally be traced back to a newspaper or magazine coupon or direct mailing. These leads may not always include their phone numbers and may be difficult to qualify. Mail-in leads are often only looking for information and may be seeking to avoid the sales pitch. Mail-ins who include their telephone number invite a follow-up call, which could demonstrate a higher level of motivation. Although walk-ins and phone-ins can sometimes be difficult to associate with a specific lead source, mail-ins can be traced directly. Because of this characteristic they will represent the truest translation of the lead:lease relationship.

When evaluating leads from the various marketing media placements, it is important to recognize that some placements will yield a higher volume of leads, whereas others may yield higher-quality responses. Generally

the cost per lead and cost per lease or sale are measured against the lead:lease conversion rate of each to determine the success of each strategy. This is covered in detail in Chapter 13.

Not all leads and ultimately sales will cost money to generate. Sales generated from resident and nonresident referrals and from the site itself can represent a considerable component of the overall lead bank. For example, if the community is situated in a good location with high visibility and has good curb appeal, it should generate as much as 10 percent of the total leads collected at the senior-living community. Curb appeal can be enhanced with attention to the planting beds, landscaping, exterior finish of the community, and neatness. There is nothing more telling about the quality inside a property than how it appears outside. Seniors are particularly attentive to their own homes after retirement, and many believe that their yards are a personal reflection of their own standards and pride in their home. Quality signage offering information about the availability of apartments and directions on how to inquire can also help to invite passersby into the building.

Resident and nonresident referrals can also represent a considerable component of new leads. The percentage of referral leads will be greater as the level of care increases. For example, the marketing department should expect 70 percent of its leads to assisted living to come from mostly professional referrals. Continuing-care retirement communities should expect about 50 percent of their leads from referrals, primarily coming from satisfied, active residents. Finally, congregate communities should expect about 30 percent, 10 percent from residents and 20 percent from nonresidents. Effective internal marketing to residents by delivering on the promises made by the sales counselors and a commitment to service on the part of all employees can save thousands of dollars in advertising otherwise spent on lead-generation strategies. External marketing to professionals and senior advocacy groups in the area can also be a big producer if handled well. See Chapter 13 for more on developing an effective community outreach program and ideas for improving resident referrals.

SALES PROCESS

Selling retirement housing is more than just leasing apartments. You are selling a lifestyle. Many inquiries to retirement housing projects are prompted by individuals who may be looking for solutions to their problems. Few seniors research their local retirement housing community because it looks like a nice place to live. Although some prospects may recognize the inherent value of the lifestyle and convenient services or may be planning for their future needs, most inquiries are triggered by a problem—for example, they may have lost their spouse, their ability to drive, or the ability to manage their household. When this occurs, they may experience feelings of helplessness and despair. Most seniors figure that they will beat the odds of ever having to live in a retirement center or nursing home, preferring to live out their days in their own homes. At best, the sales counselor is dealing with a reluctant buyer whose life may be in upheaval and who may grasp at straws to avoid the move-in decision.

The successful retirement-housing sales counselor, then, must wear the hat of the social worker as well as the real estate and services salesperson. The traditional sales model simply will not work on this type of client. The sales process must be designed around problem-solving and trust. Many of these issues can be very personal, and the sales counselor will need to build a relationship with the prospect based upon trust and patience to allow the prospect's interest level to mature.

Table 14.3 compares the traditional sales process with relationship selling. The phases of the sales process in both models involve information gathering, presentation, affirmation, and follow-through. In the traditional model, little time is spent fact-finding, and the salesperson will normally concentrate her efforts on features and benefits during the sales pitch and then on overcoming objections. Many times this high-pressure environment will require the process to reverse itself and the salesperson will need to resell the client on the features and benefits.

Contrary to popular belief, the top persuaders in the country say that the most important aspect of influence is not closing, but rapport. Trust between the sales counselor and the prospect is the single most important element that will influence the success or failure of a particular sales interview. People often buy products they do not need from salespeople whom they really like. If they believe in you and are on the edge of making a decision, the savvy sales counselor can influence them to buy.[3] The number-one aspect of persuasion is to align with someone and redirect him. The only way this is going to happen is to have first earned his trust and confidence.

Relationship selling first involves a rapport-building process wherein sales counselors use social workers' skills to thoroughly identify the prospect's needs. The counselor then proposes how those needs can best be served by the community, and confirms the proposal by familiarizing the prospect with the many amenities and services the community has to offer. At this point, the counselor provides reassurances that the prospect is making the right decision. In contrast to the traditional sales model, where the emphasis is placed on the sales pitch and overcoming objections, relationship selling focuses on the development of trust between two (or more) people who are both looking for solutions and options. Let us explore the process in detail.

Information Gathering

The manner in which the prospect is initially received often plays a large part in the success of the overall relationship-building process. The lobby or reception area should be a bright, cheerful room, with an atmosphere that is warm and friendly. The room should be furnished with a comfortable seating area with community photo albums, newsletters, tabloids, brochures,

Table 14.3   Traditional versus Relationship Selling

Phases of the sales process	Traditional selling techniques	Relationship selling
Information gathering	Prospecting	Preparation
Presentation	Conversation and fact-finding	Rapport building
Affirmation	Pitching	Needs assessment
Follow-through	Closing and overcoming objections	Proposing
	Reselling	Confirming
		Assuring

and any awards within easy reach so that prospects can browse through them and become familiar with the community before they even meet the retirement counselor. It is a good idea to have two scrapbooks: one filled with photos of special events at the community (Oktoberfest, birthdays, food displays, and parties), the other filled with letters, cards, and news items sent by residents, families, and community leaders commending the community or its employees for their high-quality service.

The receptionist (as well as front office personnel) should always give prospects her immediate attention, trying her best to make them feel comfortable and relaxed. The first impression of the community will often establish the attitude of the prospects toward the entire visit. In extreme cases, the sales counselor may never be able to overcome a bad first impression created by the front desk. The operation of the reception area is detailed in Chapter 4. Some communities will ask prospects to fill out lead cards while they wait, but this can make for a cold reception. It is better to have the sales counselor collect the information during a personal interview.

The sales counselor should lead the prospect(s) to a quiet and private area that will allow an uninterrupted conversation. This could be a back office, a private sitting room, or a conference room where comfortable seating is available.

The initial few minutes of conversation are critical for both the prospect and the sales counselor. They will give each an opportunity to evaluate the other. The prospect will be looking this person over carefully to determine if the sales counselor represents the kind of staff person who will be responsive, caring, and professional. The sales counselor will use this time to discover a number of qualifying criteria (income, age, medical condition) and to begin to evaluate the needs and wants that the community will be required to fill for this prospect in order to convert him to a resident. The sales counselor will also use this time to establish a friendly relationship with the prospect and to demonstrate that she is particularly interested in finding a fulfillment of the prospect's needs rather than making a sale. The axiom "make a friend, then make a sale" is particularly valid in the senior-living industry.

During the information-gathering stage the sales counselor will begin to formulate a profile of the prospect. This is accomplished by asking key questions about the decision time frame, who will be involved in the decision process, where he is in his search, what prompted his visit to the community, and so on. Most of all, the sales counselor will need to practice active listening skills. Many salespeople become so involved in what they have to say about the community that they inadvertently leave prospects feeling that the sales counselor knows what is best for them. In selling, the sales counselor will want to learn as much about the prospect as possible during the valuable time she has to spend with the prospect. She will then use this information to relate the community's services and amenities to the prospect's needs. Here are some tips for improving listening skills.

- Successful salespeople are great listeners. They will ask questions and hear the prospect out. Sometimes it is effective to use silence to control the flow of conversation and draw out the prospect. Most salespeople feel uncomfortable during moments of silence, but silence can be a sales ally.

- Avoid situations that may subject the conversation to interruptions, and never interrupt the prospect. If you think of something during the conversation, jot it down and wait until the prospect has finished her thought. Ask prospects if they mind if you take notes. This will help to keep the focus on the prospects and demonstrate a sincere interest in them.

- Concentrate on the topic at hand and avoid the temptation to let the discussion wander. Listening speed is faster than talking speed, so make a conscious effort to keep the concentration on the prospect. Cultivate the ability to stick with the topic.

- Listen for everything you see as well. Reading nonverbal cues and using them yourself can be a powerful influencing tool. Look for conflicts between the spoken word and the prospect's body language. Nearly everything we do is a form of communication—posture, eye movements, speech patterns, even skin tone. Communications experts say that over 90 percent of our messages are interpreted based on how we deliver them. A message is interpreted in this way: 7 percent is based on the words, 33 percent is based on how the words are said (pitch, tone, volume, rate of speed, and inflection), and 60 percent is based on body language. Tune into the nonverbal cues of your prospects and learn to mirror them. It subconsciously tells the prospect that she can trust you.

- Listen to all the information offered, even details that may not interest you. Skilled listeners do not discard information that can be useful later.

Ask probing questions to help clarify information and keep the prospect talking. Probing questions help the sales counselor get below the surface and define motivation. There are five types of probes: open-ended, closed-ended, operant-word, clarifying, and testing.

The *open-ended* probe is a question or statement that invites a wide-ranging response, and that often asks for ideas, opinions, or views. It is used to open up a discussion, invite the prospect to offer comprehensive responses, and give the prospect the freedom to say what is on his mind. Such questions cannot be answered with a yes or no. They often start with "What," "Why," "Tell me about," or "What do you think of." For example, "Tell me about what prompted your visit today."

The *closed-ended* probe is a question that limits the answer by asking for specific facts or a yes or no response. These are useful to discover specific details, test understanding, direct the discussion, or get the prospect to take a position on something. They often start with "Which," "Who," "When," "Where," or "How many." For example, "Do you think that you will be able to move in next month?"

The *operant-word* probe involves taking a key word from a prospect's previous statement and using it to create the sales counselor's next sentence. This method is useful to check the sales counselor's understanding or prove that she is listening. It increases the quality of information being gathered and builds rapport. It can be a restatement of an essential idea and be used to clarify wants and needs. For example, Statement: "One of the things I'm concerned about is security." Response: "Security is important to you. What security concerns do you have?"

Clarifying a question is a type of feedback that asks the prospect for more information about a specific aspect of an earlier response. It shows that the sales counselor understands and prompts the prospect to provide additional information. It is also useful to refocus the prospect's thought direction. For example, "What exactly do you mean when you say that you are not

ready yet?" This provides an opportunity to explore the subject in more detail so that the sales counselor can tailor a response or buy some time to think.

A *testing* question asks where the prospect stands on a particular issue. It can be useful to determine the relative value of something to the prospect and helps the sales counselor determine what to stress during the presentation. For example, "How does the continuum of care provided here match up with your wife's needs?"

Experienced sales counselors use probing questions to gain insight into the prospect's needs and feelings. They can also be used to help the prospect to clarify his own thinking. Many prospects are unsure about what retirement communities offer and how they would fit in. The right questions can both clarify needs and create awareness.

It is important for the sales counselor to be polite, courteous, and respectful to prospects at all times. They may not seem to appreciate a sales counselor's time and effort at the interview, but when their decision-making time arrives, they will remember the help and kindness. This residual effect will be a favorable reflection on the entire operation and will help to paint a picture of their upcoming move-in experience.

People can spot a phony from a mile away. Senior consumers are especially knowledgeable and shrewd. If the sales counselor does not believe wholeheartedly in what she is selling, the prospect will sense it immediately. If the sales counselor's primary concern is in making the sale or earning an incentive, the prospect will sense that immediately, too. The prospect should feel the sales counselor's enthusiasm. It should shine forth in the way the counselor expresses herself verbally, in her body language, and in the light of her eyes when she talks about the community.

The retirement counselor's appearance is also extremely important. It plays an important part in forming the prospect's initial and lasting impressions of the community. Dress and grooming should always be professional and tasteful, and never flashy.

The sales counselor will be expected to know practically everything about the community. She should understand the service limits of each department so that promises are not made that operations cannot fulfill. The cardinal rule is, never overpromise and underdeliver. If the sales counselor is asked a question she is unsure of, she should tell the prospect that she would like to consult with the appropriate person regarding that issue before she answers. If it is handled in a factual manner, the prospect will appreciate the honesty.

Sales counselors should resist the temptation to try to accommodate all the prospect's wishes. They should not try to paint too rosy a picture. Seniors have been around a long time and do not expect anything to fit perfectly.

Presentation

Some prospects do not consider retirement living until they are ready or forced to make an immediate decision. Others spend months shopping and gathering information before making their choice. Many will appear on the hot lead lists of every competitor in town. When prospects initiate contact with a community, they have reached an important level in their decision-making. They will be looking to maintain independence and control, but in reality, they are taking a big step toward declaring their own dependence. They recognize that they are in need of something that the community may have to offer. They may be looking for something to enhance their current lifestyle or to protect them from their declining ability to handle all of the pressures of daily living. Whichever the prospect is seeking, enhancement or protection, he is really looking for someone to give him a compelling enough reason to make a decision.

It is not only the content of the presentation that is important, but also the method of presentation. The sales counselor's style should be friendly, concerned, but professional. The presentation should be relaxed and avoid the appearance of being canned. The sales counselor should use positive phrases in the current and absolute tense when describing common features. For example, "When you are living with us, your meals are always served at your table. We have a 'restaurant-style' dining room that serves our residents their choice of entrees. We listen to our residents and design the food service around their likes and needs."

Consider where the presentation is given (the surroundings) and where it begins and ends. The sales counselor should avoid giving the prospect an information packet before the tour; it could be a distraction from the presentation of the community. It is important that the sales counselor use every means available to focus the prospect's attention on the messages she is attempting to communicate.

The sales counselor should always make a dry run to check out the condition of the models or other apartments that the prospect may be showed. This takes only a few minutes and can save the sales counselor considerable embarrassment in the event an apartment is dirty or has a big bug in the middle of the carpet. She should check to see that all fixtures are in place and in good working order and should show only apartments that are clean and fresh. The models should be *detailed daily,* and all other vacant apartments should be on the weekly housekeeping cleaning schedule. Maintenance staff should also be held responsible for cleaning up their own messes and should only disassemble equipment when they have parts to make the repairs. If parts are not available, the fixtures or equipment should be reassembled and the marketing department notified of all apartments that are not in showable condition. The models should have the lights on, the blinds or window coverings open, and even some soft music playing.

Be aware of the possibility of interruptions during the presentation and tour of the community. If interrupted by a resident, and this interruption can be used as a positive example, by all means encourage the encounter. If this particular resident is known to be positive, he or she can be introduced with a positive statement such as, "I was just telling Mrs. Cameron about our beautiful apartments. Don't you agree, Mrs. Jones?" A happy resident will agree, and may even offer to show her apartment. Such arrangements can be made in advance with residents who have nicely decorated apartments that they are proud to show off. Most occupied apartments are more "homey" than the models. If the resident is known to be negative in attitude, gently but firmly refer her to another staff member to deal with the problem or concern and avoid any introductions or involvement with the prospect.

The presentation and tour should be customized to the characteristics and needs of the prospect. The sales counselor should anticipate the prospect's questions after the information-gathering interview and be prepared to make immediate adjustments to the presentation based on new information that arises out of the tour. The presentation should stress the areas of the community, and its amenities, services, and residents that will be the most beneficial to the prospect's needs.

Leave the discussion of the costs of the program until the end of the tour, if possible. The sales counselor should not bring up the subject of fees until the prospect has seen the entire community and heard about the spectrum of services and amenities. If the prospect brings up the subject earlier in the presentation, the sales counselor can respond with something like, "Well, our apartments begin at $1,600 per month and go up from there depending on the size of the apartment you choose. The cost is relevant only when you consider the benefits of the additional services and amenities that go with it. Let me explain." Then proceed with the tour and presentation and offer an additional feature that has not been covered. If the presentation successfully builds a desire to become a part of this lifestyle, then the question of cost will be a barrier only to those whose incomes truly cannot support residency at the community. This should have already been determined during the information-gathering stage when qualifying the prospect. When discussing rates, all charges the resident or responsible party can expect and when they are due should be made clear. *Be sure to define what services are included in the monthly fee and what additional services are available at additional cost.*

Many prospects may experience "sticker shock" when they become aware of the cost of senior living. After all, many of them will be living in their own home free and clear of any mortgage. Suggest that they do a cost comparison of what it costs them to provide all of these services for themselves. Many seniors underestimate their cost of living by as much as $300 per month. All things considered, it is much more cost-efficient to provide services to many seniors living in a community together with mutual needs than it would be for them to purchase similar services individually. It is simply an economy of scale that our residents have recognized and taken advantage of.

Overcoming Objections and Confirming the Sale

The best salespeople in the world make their sales after overcoming a minimum of five objections. They see objections as something to be welcomed. It helps them gather more information and clarify needs. Overcoming objections is part of the confirmation process. In a traditional sales approach this is part of the closing process. In relationship selling, the sales counselor is helping the prospect to confirm his decision which will be followed by assuring that the best decision has been made for him.

"I'm not ready yet." Translation: I'm afraid of giving up my home, independence, and lifestyle for an unknown. What if I don't like it? What if they don't like me? What if they raise the rents and I can't afford to live here anymore? Prospects will look for ways to avoid making the final decision, often out of fear or an unwillingness to commit. If an objection can be found they will usually find it. When someone says she is not ready yet, what it really means is that perhaps your client is afraid or does not understand all the benefits and value retirement living has to offer. In any sales program, the better the job the marketing counselor can do at communicating the benefits and overcoming any objections as he relates to the prospective tenants, the better the chance of closing a sale.

Visit with your prospects before the tour to determine why they are inquiring with you and establish rapport or friendship. Take the time to demonstrate that you are primarily interested in finding a fulfillment of the prospects' needs rather than making a sale. Point out how your amenities relate to them personally.

Toward the end of you tour, you will want to close in. Ask your prospects if there is anything about the community that they may be uncomfortable with. Selling is a matter of identifying objections and then overcoming them. Try to ascertain exactly what they may be uncomfortable with and then solve it. For example, "Mrs. Cameron, I sense that you seem uncomfortable with our reservation agreement. If it weren't for your feeling that you may be permanently obligating yourself before you sell your house, do you think this type of lifestyle might make sense for you? If I could make arrangements to reserve an apartment in your name, risk-free, while you sell your home, do you think you might take us up on our offer?"

During the tour, the sales counselor should constantly focus on potential objections, selectively and patiently resolving them. Prospects' objections can chart your course toward getting a deposit check. To this end, here are some sample objections and responses you may wish to incorporate into your sales presentation.

TYPICAL OBJECTIONS AND SOME SAMPLE RESPONSES

Why does your prospect say, "I'm not ready yet"?

- It is a convenient way for an uninformed prospect to terminate a conversation with a salesperson.

■ Most prospects will feel the decision is premature—they desire to remain where they are more than they desire to move into your retirement community.

1. *Objection:* "I'm not ready yet."
   Response:
   • "Good, then it's just a matter of working on the timing, isn't it?"
   • "I understand how you feel. But tell me, just what do you think would have to happen to you before you felt that you were ready? Wouldn't it be comforting to you and your family that should such an event ever happen you would already be in an environment where you could receive that cushion of care right when you really needed it?"

2. *Objection:* "We would have to sell the house."
   Response:
   • "That's right. Most of our residents have sold their homes to come here and they will tell you it's the best decision they ever made. We can arrange a meeting for you with a very competent realtor who will do a comparative market analysis on your home for no obligation. Many people are surprised at how much equity they have tied up in their homes that could be earning interest for them if they sold." Barbara Kleger, president of Senior Living Associates, suggests, "Be patient; it takes a long time to grow old and a long time to make such a drastic decision as moving out of one's cherished home."

3. *Objection:* "We have too much furniture."
   Response:
   • "I know how you feel. Most of us spend half of our lives accumulating things and the other half giving them away. Most people find that when they start the paring down process it's not as painful as it seems. In fact, your new spacious apartment can accommodate many of your favorite possessions you find you want to keep. Our move-in coordinator will be happy to assist you in determining where some of you favorite furniture can be placed in the apartment. We assist you in every step of your move-in from measuring space and furniture to helping coordinate the actual moving-in process."
   • "There are a lot of things to consider, aren't there? Our residents have all faced this issue and as you can see, they've gained so much with all of our amenities, they really don't miss their excess furniture. . . . They decided they didn't want their possessions to stand in the way of getting what they knew was right for them. . . . Sort of makes sense, doesn't it?"

4. *Objection:* "I'm too old to move now."
   Response:
   • "That's interesting. We have many people here who are older than you. . . . I'll bet you're not too old to get more out of life, right? This lifestyle provides you the opportunity of a secure, enjoyable, carefree retirement, and it could be the best years of your life. Statistics prove that people live on the average two to three years longer in a retirement community than in an apartment. There are several good reasons for this. One of them is companionship. One of the saddest things about growing older is that our friends pass away. We meet new friends, of course, but if we are not in a community setting we don't have the ability to continually expand our friendships. Therefore, they are continually shrinking. If we stop driving in the years ahead, or our friends don't drive, or the weather is bad, we tend to spend a lot of time within our private residence. Many meals are eaten with our only companion being Vanna White. It's easy to see how one can slowly become a recluse over a period of time. At a retirement community, companionship is always available."

5. *Objection:* "I'm too young for this."
   Response:
   • "I see. Well, interestingly we have several people who are younger than you and they will tell you they don't know why they waited so long. . . . When do you think it is easier to make a change—when you're younger and have several options, or when you're older and possibly forced to make a decision under the pressure of time?"
   • "I understand how you must feel. Retirees who have joined us here at the Community support the philosophy that you *should not wait* until you need services such as health care to move to a full-service retirement community. Instead of being in the position of using the health care services and options provided for you among friends and neighbors, *waiting* may mean that you could find yourself in a strange nursing home several miles away from familiar surroundings. Or you may find yourself having to depend on your children or friends to take care of you, placing an undue hardship on them and taking away your independent way of life. Doesn't that make sense?"

6. *Objection:* "I've got too much energy for this." "I'm still very active."
   Response:
   • "Tell you what, take a look here at our activities calendar and let's assume you'll do everything that is listed. I'll bet halfway through the month

you'll call time out! And just because you change your address doesn't mean you'll be less active . . . . so you'll just keep on with your fast-paced schedule without the worries of keeping up with your household."

7. *Objection:* "I'm still able to take care of things around the house."
   Response:
   - "You have done all the things to maintain your household up to this point. Although you can still do them, they are probably becoming a little more difficult with each passing year. The heavier jobs such as vacuuming, laundry, and the cleaning of floors and bathrooms are the kinds of things that no one likes doing. And they will become less pleasant as time goes on."

8. *Objection:* "I'm just not sure."
   Response:
   - "There's some risk involved, isn't there? And you want to be certain you do the right thing. What information would you need to be more comfortable with your decision?"
   - "I sense that there may be something that you are uncertain about. It is the (fee, moving, apartment, etc., until you zero in). Well, if it weren't for (the objection) do you think this lifestyle here might make sense for you? If I could (fix the objection) could you take us up on our offer?"

9. *Objection:* "I'm going to look around."
   Response:
   - "Excellent. What will you be looking for?"
   - "Good idea. We encourage all our prospects to compare what we offer and our reputation with others in the business. We can show you on our comparison chart, which details how the other communities stack up. I'm sure you will recognize how much more value you get here for your dollar."
   - "I understand how you feel. It's important to make the right decision about your new home. Wouldn't it be nice to be able to reserve an option for yourself while you're looking so that if you need one, you already have one picked out to fall back on? If I could show you a way to tie up a choice apartment today, risk free, don't you think that might make good sense for you?"

10. *Objection:* "It's too much work."
    Response:
    - "Could be. Anything worthwhile is worth working for, isn't it? But we can make it easier for you by doing most of the legwork of getting you situated with us. We have some excellent resources we can work with to help you with the sale of your house and your moving

arrangements. By the way, will it be any less work in the future, or any easier for you at some time down the road?"

11. *Objection:* "I'm going to stay in my home until something happens that will make me need this."
    Response:
    - "And then what will you do? Would you rather have a choice now or leave things to chance later? I think we all like to feel that we have control of our lives."

12. *Objection:* "I don't think I can afford this."
    "I'm not used to spending this much on my housing."
    Response:
    - "At first it seems high, doesn't it? I can certainly understand how you *feel*; a number of our residents once felt the same way you do; but when they considered everything we include in our monthly fee compared to similar expenses in their own home, they found they weren't paying any more to live here . . . and in some cases, less than they were before. Here, let me show you the value on this comparison chart and you can see for yourself."

13. *Objection:* "I want to think about it."
    Response:
    - "That's fine. Obviously, you wouldn't take your time thinking this over unless you were really interested, would you?"
    - "So, may I assume that you will give it very careful consideration?"
    - "Just to clarify my thinking, what part of this decision is it that you are concerned about? Is it. . . . ?"
    - "Is it anything I may have said that I didn't make clear?"
    - "Is it anything about the community you are unsure about?"
    - "Is it the monthly fee?"
    - "Is it the moving problems?"

14. *Objection:* "I want to see it built first."
    Response:
    - "If your were simply buying an apartment that would be understandable. But we are not selling just bricks and mortar. We are selling a lifestyle along with a whole host of services that is designed to bring you peace of mind and continued independence as your every day challenges become increasingly complex. Our program is only built around the physical amenities. Your enjoyment of the community will come from the many services and intangibles it has to

offer such as, activities programming, delicious meals, housekeeping, transportation services, and other things like companionship, security, and access to health care. You see, the building is really only the location where all these things come together. It is secondary to the real benefits of living there."

In the end, overcoming objections is a process of developing a comfort level with the decision. Be patient with prospects. Listen for hidden meanings in their objections; they may be using the opportunity for a completely different motivation than just to throw out obstacles. Repeat the objection to clarify your understanding. Sometimes when people hear their objection repeated back to them it sounds worse than they really intended it to be. Confirm the objection by agreeing with the prospect. Do not try to argue or pretend to know better. Prospects like to have their objections acknowledged and affirmed. Question their real intent behind the objection and look for common ground. Answer their concerns as best you can without being smart or glib. Confirm the answer by relating the experience of others in their situation who may have had the same objection but ultimately found that it may have been overstated. Finally, close on neutral ground and leave the prospect with something that you both agree on about the situation. Overcoming objections can be a bit like handling complaints. You are seeking a positive resolution to a negative response or drawback in your program. It may also be helpful to review the checklist for handling complaints that can be found in Chapter 5.

Final Objection Formula
1. Hear It Out
2. Repeat the Objection
3. Confirm the Objection
4. Question It
5. Answer It
6. Confirm the Answers
7. Close

Follow-Through

It is not uncommon for the sales counselor to spend two hours or more with the prospect, particularly if lunch or dinner is involved. It is crucial that the sales counselor be prepared to do this. A great deal of information must be covered, and if any particular aspect

of the community is not addressed by the sales counselor (or other person who may have handled the inquiry) that cannot be found in the printed material, the prospect may wrongly assume that the service or amenity does not exist. Even if the sales counselor clearly sees that the community could meet the need very well, she still must convince the prospect of that fact.

At the conclusion of the tour and presentation, the sales counselor should attempt some trial closes. This is the most difficult part of any sales presentation. Asking for the deposit risks rejection, and most of us prefer to avoid rejection at all costs. But if the prospect has been read well and his needs have been clearly established in relation to all of the benefits offered by the community, then the sales counselor has prepared the prospect to enter the decision-making mode. At this point the prospect must have a clear feeling that she is not being sold something, but is being offered some options. Throughout the presentation, the sales counselor should be looking for common ground and making small closes on points of agreement. When the small closes have been successfully executed (the apartment selected, parking place chosen, furniture placement visualized), the decision to move ahead with the paperwork is only the next natural step. This way, the sales counselor is assuring the prospect that this lifestyle is right for her, rather than trying to convince her to sign on the dotted line.

The "feel, felt, found" answer to final obstacles is an excellent and positive way to reassure the prospect. For example, when the prospect indicates that he is hesitant to make the commitment, the sales counselor can say "Mr. Joseph, I understand how you feel. Many of our current residents have felt the same way as you do, but what they found once they made the decision and joined the community was that they should have made the decision much earlier. Would it help with your comfort level to talk to one of our residents?" This way the sales counselor has acknowledged the prospect's fears, assured him that they are not unique but common to many others who have already moved into the community, and assuaged the fears with the knowledge that others have overcome them and are glad they made the move. When the prospect decides to move, he chooses the community that more closely meets his individual needs and presents the fewest barriers.

Whenever possible, when the residency agreement is signed, the prospective resident should be passed on to operations for move-in coordination. This process should be handled delicately, inasmuch as the prospect will have already established a relationship with the salesperson and you do not want to appear to be terminating that relationship, but instead that you are expanding it to others in the community. Many communities employ a move-in coordinator in order to facilitate each transition into the community from the sales department. In such cases, the move-in coordinator will normally be introduced early in the sales process, and again later after the residency agreement has been finalized to pave the way for transition.[4] It is important to note that the move-in coordinator will need to continue to confirm the prospect's decision until well after the agreement has been signed. Seniors typically experience feelings of regret or uncertainty after they have reached a decision. This is commonly known as "buyer's remorse," and the move-in coordinator needs to learn to recognize the symptoms and continually reconfirm the decision even after the prospect moves into her apartment. Some communities will structure the move-in coordinator's compensation package to provide incentive for accelerating the move-in date. In one community, the move-in time frames were accelerated by the move-in coordinator to produce a total of 1,000 more revenue days for her community, resulting in an additional $65,000 in revenue that would otherwise have been lost. As soon as possible, salespersons need to return to the selling process.

As a courtesy, a letter should be sent to the prospect within twenty-four hours following the initial inquiry visit. This letter serves several purposes: first, to thank the prospect for her interest in the community and for the time taken for the tour; second, to prompt the prospect to recall her visit to the community (the letter should also encourage the prospect to revisit the community or contact the sales counselor regarding any questions or concerns that were not addressed during her visit); third, to show the prospect that the sales counselor is interested in his becoming a resident of the community; and fourth, and most importantly, to confirm the prospect's most recent impression of the community as a positive, professionally operated place that will perform needed services with excellence. If

for some reason the prospect chooses not to move in, the follow-up letter will leave the prospect with a favorable impression. Word-of-mouth references and referrals are also very important to the community's reputation.

Some communities send a "day after" questionnaire to the prospect in a self-addressed, stamped envelope designed to determine how well the marketing effort was executed. These are returned to the attention of the executive director, who will discuss outcomes and give feedback to the marketing director. The questionnaires are designed to be anonymous to solicit honest and objective answers. These can be especially helpful to new sales staff to fine-tune the presentation to be smooth and professional.

Approximately one week following the initial prospect visit, a follow-up phone call may be appropriate. During the conversation the sales counselor should inquire about something personal that may have been shared during the visit, and ask if the prospect has any questions or concerns. The prospect should be asked where he is in the decision-making process. If the prospect has decided to move into the community, schedule an appointment for move-in coordination. If he has chosen another community, tactfully ask the reasons for choosing the other community over yours. These responses can be very helpful in determining the community's strong or weak characteristics. If the prospect indicates that he will be moving to another community, the sales counselor should plan to make another follow-up phone call in approximately two weeks. The purpose of the call is to once again let the prospect know that the sales counselor cares enough to keep in touch. Many prospects may indicate alternate plans to delay the decision or avoid any further commitments. The sales counselor will want to be sure that the prospect is satisfied with her decision.

A "thank you for choosing" letter should be sent out by the executive director the day of the sale. It lets the prospect know that the entire community is aware that she will soon be coming to live here, and it stresses an anxiousness to serve. Little extras such as these letters are often the deciding factor that a prospect uses in selecting one community over another.

The sales/leasing office should be open at least six and a half days per week. It is important to remain open on weekends and holidays, inasmuch as these are times when families are together and in a position to influence the prospect's decision during a visit. It is a good idea to schedule all sales staff for weekend duty on a rotational basis so that the office will always be covered.

Wait Lists

Wait lists are useful to establish a commitment on the part of the prospect to your community. These can include prospects who are waiting for a specific unit type to become available, or prospects who do plan to move to the community but may not be ready yet. The prospect normally submits a fully refundable deposit that can range from several hundred to a thousand dollars or a percentage of the entrance fee (payment of interest on this deposit may be subject to local regulations). This deposit places the prospect's name on a priority list for a specific apartment type. When the desired unit becomes available, prospects are notified in chronological order and asked to sign a residency agreement within a set period (normally seven days). If the prospect does not wish to take the apartment when it is available, she will normally be kept in the same order on the list and be notified when another apartment becomes available.

The wait list prospect who is classified as "not ready yet" and does not wish to be called each time an apartment becomes available is treated as an inactive member. Inactive wait list prospects are contacted on a quarterly basis to assess their status and to encourage an upgrade to active status.

It is important to remind prospects that they are subject to normal market increases in the apartment of their choice during their wait on the list. It could cause real problems with other new residents if they find out that new residents off the wait list were locked in to a much lower rent than a new tenant.

Many communities offer additional benefits to their wait list prospects in order to demonstrate value to membership and facilitate frequent contact. Such benefits might include newsletter and event mailings, lunch or dinner at resident rates (space available), participation in selected resident programs and educational classes, or even discounts on guest apartment stays (annually limited). All these benefits are designed to keep the wait list prospect in frequent contact with the community and in touch with the value associated with living in the community.

Wait lists can be very useful to convert a reluctant prospect. The act of making a deposit on a specific apartment type is a small close. Some prospects will need to be sold in stages, and the wait list can be their first real commitment. Wait lists are generally more effective as the community becomes more fully occupied and the availability of specific apartment types becomes limited. The urgency to act becomes more real because once all the available units are sold, roles reverse: the prospect waits for the community to respond, instead of the community waiting for the prospect to get ready. In other words, during the fill-up stage, the community waits; on stabilization, the prospect waits.

Occasionally, when a specific apartment type is unavailable, the prospect may elect to move into another apartment temporarily. Normally the prospect will move into a larger apartment waiting for a smaller one. A rent reduction can be offered on the larger apartment until the smaller one becomes available. This option is normally limited in time frame depending on the occupancy status of the building. The resident is normally asked to move into the smaller apartment within 30 days of availability or to start paying the full monthly fee on the larger apartment.

Relocation within the building can be done either with community maintenance staff or by professional movers. Some communities charge the resident to relocate within the building to recover their costs. However, if time is of the essence or if someone else is waiting for the current apartment to be vacated, management can accelerate the transfer by offering to pick up the tab. As a rule, if the building is empty, the resident pays for the relocation; if it is full, management does.

Some companies pay commissions to sales counselors when wait list deposits are collected, but normally payment is structured as an advance against the commission on the eventual sale. See the compensation section later in this chapter for more detail.

Information Requests

If an interested party or prospect requests information by phone regarding the community, he or she should receive an information packet along with a cover letter. Requests for information should always be handled by a sales counselor to gauge how much information to give out and to attempt to qualify the caller. Most communities send out only a brochure in response to information requests. Sending a formal letter thanking a prospect for his interest in the community and issuing an invitation to visit will set the stage for a successful inquiry and sales process. The prospect will appreciate the time and effort put into the letter and information packet. If the prospect has any questions concerning retirement living, he will most likely look to your community for help.

Many people will call local retirement communities to gather basic information such as rates, apartment availability, and so on before deciding which communities to visit and tour in person. Therefore, it is critical to make a good impression so that your phone conversation will stand out among the rest and prompt a visit, giving the sales counselor the opportunity to complete the sales presentation. Sales counselors should resist the temptation to give their entire presentation over the phone. Most people can only remember a very small amount of information, and it is a stab in the dark for the sales counselor to guess the information that will be best received by the caller without the advantage of a personal interview. Statements should be made to give callers critical information while trying gently to persuade them to visit the community personally. After all, it is a lifestyle that they will be buying into, and it is very difficult to communicate that complex concept in a short telephone conversation. Offer to put together an information packet and set aside some time to give the caller a tour. If not, the sales counselor should try to get a caller's address and phone number and then check to see if the caller has received the packet. The sales counselor should make some suggestions on what the caller can do next and offer assurance that the counselor is there to help find solutions, not just to make a sale. If the counselor does not have anything appropriate for the caller's needs at his community, then he can assist the caller in finding the most appropriate setting. This way the sales counselor offers to perform a service rather than pitch a sales presentation.

Many inquiries will come from interested parties. These individuals are normally the children of the prospect who have already recognized a need. They will either be motivated by feelings of guilt stemming from a geographical or professional isolation from their parents or from serious concerns over their living alone safely. Many family members will visit one or several retirement communities and choose one they would like to see their parents move into. The next step is to approach them with the idea of considering such a move.

For many, this is a difficult step because of the role reversal that occurs. It is not easy to be the caregiver, offering advice and being "in charge." No one wants to push, and doing so would likely meet resistance anyway. The family member will need to recognize the importance of the decision and the fact that moving to a retirement community does not mean a loss of independence. The interested party should be encouraged to visit the community with the parent and have lunch. Many communities have guest apartments and can arrange for a trial visit or weekend stay, which will give the prospect the opportunity to experience the lifestyle and talk to a few people who live there. Many times, residents living in a community have a way of selling the place themselves.

SALES ANALYSIS

Sales analysis is the detailed study of performance-related sales statistics to evaluate strengths and weakness so that management can respond. Through sales analysis, management seeks information on the success of individual and overall marketing efforts and sales performance. Information collected and analyzed can equip management to adjust marketing tactics and allocate sales efforts effectively. As sales directors become aware of the weak areas in their sales department by analyzing the statistical results, short- or long-term contests and incentives can also be developed to focus the sales counselor's attention appropriately. Many times the symptoms of a failing community can be traced back to a lack of evaluation of the results of the marketing strategies or to productivity issues within the sales department.

Marketing departments can collect data in a variety of ways, using traffic reports, summarization of prospect lead cards, computer activity reports, and personal logs of the sales counselors. This information can be summarized by a marketing assistant or secretary, the marketing or sales director, the executive director, or even the night concierge personnel. Clearly, the most efficient way to summarize statistics and manipulate data is with the personal computer. As discussed earlier, it may be advisable to have one employee personally responsible for maintaining the computerized lead bank, marketing responses, and sales statistics. This way the sales director can ensure consistency in inputting the information and have someone who is trained to customize reports.

The evaluation of sales performance statistics is an absolute necessity of the sales management process. Although it is important to recognize that some communities will have more urgent needs than others and that each community or market is unique, evaluation of the results against industry standards can enable the sales director to quantify the relative strengths and areas of vulnerability of each sales counselor.

Phone-outs

The telephone is the single most effective method to reach the lead bank. It can be used to build relationships, initiate the sales process, coordinate appointments, prompt action, and solve problems. The average sales counselor should be able to successfully complete approximately 20 phone-outs per day. To be counted, a phone-out must reach the intended lead with at least a minimal exchange of information—either the caller or the recipient must gain some new information as a result of the call. The number of calls to each lead is established by the tickler system and urgency classification. This can be overridden by the sales counselor as is appropriate—the client may be out of town, sick, or awaiting news from a physician, for instance. If the sales counselor is not averaging at least 10 personal contacts per day, then one has to question how the counselor is spending her time. In any event, something is wrong, and that something will need to be addressed by the sales director. An excellent book on how to "reach out and touch someone," *The Phone Book,* by Richard Zarro and Peter Blum, is a good resource for improving telephone communication effectiveness.[5]

In addition to reaching the leads by phone, expectations should be established for the minimum conversion of the phone calls to appointments. The call conversion rate is the percentage of appointments set from calls to the lead bank and from phone-ins combined. For calls to new leads, this conversion ratio is a good measure of the quality of new leads responding from each individual marketing strategy. The call conversion rate for new quality leads should approximate 20 percent. This means that one in five calls to new leads should result in an appointment. For follow-up leads, the call conversion should be around 5 to 10 percent. This means that the *average* sales counselor should be able to set a minimum of one appointment per day from calls from their own lead cards.

The objective of personally contacting the lead bank is, of course, to set appointments and build relationships. The appointments must first be set, but then also kept. Occasionally, a prospect will agree to an appointment to get the caller off the phone, only to end up as a no-show. The appointments-kept statistic is a measure of lead quality and motivation as well as sales skill at booking appointments. It is often a great deal of trouble for the prospect to arrange transportation to the project, so the more difficult the arrangement, the more serious the client. Experienced salespeople will generally run a much higher appointments-kept percentage, often averaging close to 100 percent. They know the value of their time and will not be inclined to waste it on reluctant prospects and "tire kickers." Because it is relatively rare to make a sale on the first appointment (except for skilled nursing or assisted living) the appointment conversion rate to new leads is somewhat meaningless. However, the appointment conversion percentage rate for follow-up or be-back appointments is a good measure of prospect motivation and sales ability. The number of sales obtained from a single follow-up appointment should approach 25 percent. At the very least, the sales counselor should close on a wait list deposit. Some sales counselors consider a wait list deposit better than no sale at all, but caution should be exercised because this vehicle can at times provide a welcome haven for "not ready yet clients."

When the sales-activity production expectations come together, some general conclusions can be drawn to make sales forecasts. For example, if a sales counselor is making 20 phone-outs per day with an average call:appointment conversion ratio of 10 percent, she should be scheduling approximately 2 appointments each day or 10 per week (1 appointment per day should be the minimum expectation). With an appointment:sale conversion rate of 10 percent on 10 appointments per week, an average sales counselor should be able to close approximately 1 sale each week, or 4 per month (site-specific results will vary).

As the number of follow-up appointments increases for a single prospect, the sales counselor's productivity decreases. In fact, after five or six appointments without a sale, the sales director should become involved with the prospect to help determine the continued sales strategy necessary to convert the client. Some people simply like to come to the events or enjoy the free lunch. The appointment conversion rate will generally increase with the level of care. Health-care prospects are generally more need-driven and have a higher urgency level than do congregate prospects or those interested in continuing-care retirement communities. Finally, it can also be helpful to keep track of appointment conversion rates to the waiting list. This is particularly true if wait list deposits qualify for commission rewards.

Mail-outs

In contrast to phone calls, which are often considered annoying interruptions in one's day, most of us look forward to opening the day's mail. As soon as the mail is collected from the mailbox, we normally scan the contents looking for personal notes and letters and open them first. And, rather than being an interruption, the daily mail is opened and read at the person's convenience; often seniors will respond with a phone call thanking you for the personal touch.

Top sales counselors send out hundreds of personal letters and mailings each month. Most sales directors will target a minimum of 20 mail-outs for each sales counselor daily. These can include "tried to reach you" letters to unclassified mail-in leads, "day after the tour" letter, sympathy cards, "sorry to hear that you are not feeling well," "information request letters," phone call follow-ups, letters with industry news or press releases, and the like. Event flyers, newsletters, and seminar and other announcements direct mailed to the lead bank should be excluded from this count. Personal notes and cards that are handwritten have a much bigger impact than computer generated letters; so always write the letter and address the envelope by hand. Some communities even go so far as to mail small gifts and cookies to their active prospects to remind them gently of the caring atmosphere that the community offers.

Seniors are often inundated by telemarketers because many of them are home all day. It is therefore difficult to differentiate your call from the innumerable pesky calls that the average person receives. To them you become just another pushy salesperson trying to trick them into buying something that they may not need. Telemarketers rarely, however, take the time to send out a personal note; those who do can quickly cut through the barrage of advertising rubbish and get their message across. There is nothing like a personal note to communicate, "I care about you, and I'm not just in this for the sale."

The conversion rate expectations from the various contact types are discussed in the method-of-inquiry section of the Lead Sources heading earlier.

Number of Contacts

The average ratio of contacts to sale is also a good measure of lead quality and sales closing skill. The lower the number of contacts to sale, the higher the personal productivity of the sales counselor. Selling senior living, as we have seen, involves the development of trust and rapport between the sales counselor and the prospect. The more quickly trust is established, the sooner the prospect will be converted to a resident. Training sales counselors in methods of advanced communications and relationship building can serve to accelerate the rapport-building process and decrease the average number of contacts to sale and days to sale. In fact, these two statistics can be used quite effectively to evaluate the before and after effects of the training investment.

Another measure of the quality and motivation of the lead bank is the percent of sales that are generated within the first 30 days. These are essentially hot leads at first contact. Many health-care prospects interested in assisted living or skilled nursing often fall into this category. Congregate communities that are priced competitively and have good reputations in the community should expect to generate at least 30 percent of their sales within 30 days. This number should climb toward 50 percent for the more need-driven assisted-living prospect.

Table 14.4 details some typical sales performance targets for three types of communities. It should be stressed that these are only guidelines for an average community in a fill-up stage. Actual targets and relative performance will vary according to local conditions and the owners' expectations.

COMPENSATION

Designing an effective compensation package for the sales counselors will enable management to energize

Table 14.4   Sales Analysis Performance Targets

Performance category	Congregate	CCRC	Assisted living
Lead:lease conversion rate	7%	4%	10%
Average phone-outs per day per person	15–20	15–20	15–20
Call:appointment conversion rate (new leads)	20%	15%	30%
Call:appointment conversion rate (follow-up leads)	5–10%	5–10%	10–15%
Appointment:sale conversion rate (follow-up leads)	10%	5–10%	10–15%
Percent of appointments kept	95%	95%	95%
Appointment:wait list deposit conversion rate	10%	10%	5%
Average mail-outs per day per person	20	20	20
Percent of sales with interested party as initial contact	25–50%	5–10%	80–95%
Percent of sales from referral sources	10%	5%	20%
Walk-in:sale conversion rate	10%	7%	15%
Phone-in:sale conversion rate	8%	5%	12%
Phone-out:sale conversion rate	5%	5%	7%
Mail-in:sale conversion rate	3%	2.5–5%	5%
Referral:sale conversion rate	12%	7–10%	15%
Average no. contacts to sale	10	10	3–5
Average no. days to sale	100	120	60
Average no. days from sale to move-in	60	90	45
Percent sales generated within 30 days	30%	20%	50%

the sales effort and target weaknesses in the program. The single biggest factor contributing to the preponderance of failed projects has been their inability to meet occupancy projections. Operators have now reached a better understanding of the marketplace through more sophisticated feasibility studies. The remaining factor to meeting occupancy projections is in the hands of the sales staff. If the retirement community is priced right and has a good location, adequate demand, and service package that demonstrates value, then the only missing element is sales. Although these factors certainly contribute to an accelerated absorption and can help to make the sales counselor's job easier, even the best offering will take motivated and savvy people to communicate it.

Many times, management will scrutinize a $500 commission check payable to a successful sales counselor only to sign off on a $1,500 advertising invoice that produced only five leads with barely a second glance. Management may be better able to maximize the return on its considerable marketing investment by investing in its salespeople rather than the local newspaper. It is a much more productive strategy to offer additional cash incentive to sales staff to work *current* leads, many of whom may have already visited the community, than to spend additional advertising dollars and attract additional leads that may not even be qualified.

It is always better to work the existing lead bank that you have already bought and paid for. The trick is then to convince the sales counselors that the old leads have a chance to close and to put your money where your mouth is.

A good compensation plan should be designed to reward and motivate. To do this it must meet several important requirements:

■ It must provide a living wage in the form of a secure income. Sales counselors who are worried about money matters do not concentrate on doing their jobs well. Relationship-building takes time, and to be successful at building rapport with the prospect, you cannot give the impression that your sales staff is financially pressured to make sales.

■ The plan must not disrupt the harmony of the department. It is important to have a good mix of both individual rewards and team incentives so that the sales counselors will work well together. For example, the individuals can earn commissions on their personal sales, and the team can earn incentives based on total sales or total appointments scheduled, phone-outs, or conversion rates for the whole department.

■ The plan must be fair and not penalize sales counselors for factors beyond their control. It must be well balanced and provide *real* motivation for the sales counselors to seek higher levels of performance. In other words, the incentives for improving performance must be within reach and correspond to a reward amount that truly motivates. Management should not expect peak performance if the community is not competitively priced. Sales counselors who continuously lose sales to their competition due to price may be difficult to motivate with any plan. The community should be priced so that sales can be made and the sales counselors' expectations can be met if they apply themselves.

- It is critical that the compensation is easy for the sales counselors to understand, and that they be able to calculate their own earnings. Complex compensation formulas can be used as long as the sales director explains them thoroughly with several examples. The ability to calculate potential earnings in advance can allow sales counselors the opportunity to set their own performance targets and work toward them.

- The plan should include a provision that increases compensation with incremental improvements in performance. This way, there is always incentive to do more, even if the sales counselors are already having a good month.

- Finally, the compensation plan should be designed around the objectives of the sales and marketing department. It should line up with the expectations of each sales counselor, the sales director, and the executive director and the community budgeted occupancy forecasts.

The typical compensation plan will have several components: a fixed salary to provide income stability; variable elements such as commissions, bonus, incentives; and a fringe element such as vacation and sick benefits, insurance, or disability coverage. Straight salary plans, while providing management considerable control over the sales staff, also have their weaknesses. Without financial incentive, the sales counselor is motivated only to do an average job rather than maximize her earning potential. Straight commission plans pay based on performance but afford the sales director very little control over the sales staff. Most companies use a combination of the two. The proportion of each element to each other will vary,

but the minimum split between salary and commissions often works out to be about 50:50 or less for inexperienced salespeople. Clearly, the split will depend on the productivity of each individual sales counselor. Generally, inexperienced sales counselors will start with a relatively high split, but as their performance improves, so then does the level of commissions relative to their base salary. Many top sales counselors consistently producing six or seven sales per month will typically have a 20:80 split between salary and commissions.

Often the structure of the sales compensation plan is all that is required to jump-start a sales department. For example, a community with a team commission structure that split each sales commission equally among the sales staff regardless of who made the sale was consistently producing about three to four sales per month and about a 50:50 split between salary and commission income for the counselors. When the commission structure was redesigned to provide individual commissions with team incentives, the sales counselors were quick to calculate how much more they could earn if they increased their productivity. Within three months, the sales department tripled their monthly average sales to 12 per month, and due to the increase in productivity, the average cost per sale was cut in half! Although the team approach was simple to administer, there was no real reward associated with the counselor who made the sale. In fact, many productive sales counselors were very reluctant to share their hard-earned commissions with other sales counselors who may have been satisfied with only selling one or two units per month. In effect, the team approach was carrying nonproductive sales counselors. The sales compensation plan should be designed to motivate and reward top producers, not subsidize poor performance.

The base salary level should be determined through a wage survey of the local competitors. The base salary needs to be competitive if you want to attract new recruits. If the applicant realizes that the base is low and the sale price of the units (even if well commissioned) is too high, the earning potential may be limited. Management must weigh the experience of the applicants with the value of the potential productivity and make adjustments to their base-salary market rate. Some companies base their sales compensation plans on a formal evaluation process of their entire company. The danger in this is that the universal plan may not be competitive across all regions of the country and may not be suitable to address the specific performance requirements of each community. It is much better to design a compensation plan that has a basic salary and commission shell with local site specific customization of the incentive programs within budgetary guidelines.

A comprehensive sales compensation survey was conducted by Classic Residence by Hyatt; it included eighteen top retirement-housing providers representing 190 senior living communities with more than 30,000 units.[6] The objectives of the survey were three-fold: To "collect industry data on various sales compensation programs; identify sales compensation structures for stabilized communities; and identify bonus programs that maximize staff challenge and motivation and yield results in excess of projections." The companies were predominately for-profit and reported an average occupancy of 90+ percent.

Starting base salary ranges varied considerably, which is understandable inasmuch as it represents only a component of the compensation package. Sales directors' starting salaries ranged from a low of $18,000 per year to a high of $40,000. Sales counselors' salaries ranged from $12,000 to $25,000, as did move-in coordinators where applicable. Marketing assistants who are normally clerical and nonselling earned from $14,400 to $25,000 per year.

Of the eighteen companies reporting, 83 percent varied their salary structure by market or region, while 17 percent employed a universal compensation plan. Commissions were paid to marketing or sales directors, sales counselors, marketing assistants, and move-in coordinators ranging from a low of $25 to a high of $1,750 per sale.

Most companies in the industry use a sliding scale for commissions. The sliding scale is designed so that each incremental sale is worth more in commissions. The weakness of this system surfaces when sales counselors may cluster their sales together from one month to the next. This way they have a "good" month every other month to maximize their commission payment per sale.

Payment time frames for these commissions also varied by company. Forty-four percent of the companies surveyed paid the commissions upon the move-in of the resident, while 33 percent paid them to the sales staff half at the point of sale and half at move-in. Other variations, such as 40 percent payment at point of sale and 60 percent at move-in, were used by 12 percent of the companies to emphasize to the sales counselors the importance of follow-through to ensure a prompt move-in. This is understandable insofar as the revenue generated from the sale must come from the resident after she has moved into the community. Only 6 percent (1 of 18) of the companies withheld the commission check until 30 days after move-in.

As expected, types of commission plans varied greatly between the companies surveyed. Fifty percent paid commissions on the basis of the number of move-ins per month versus 33 percent on the basis of number of sales per month. Again, the emphasis is clearly placed upon move-ins, where the revenue to offset the commissions paid is collected. Other commission variations which may or may not be in addition to the above included move-in time frame (17%), occupancy level (11%), type of unit sold (6%), and monthly fee amount (6%). What this means is that some companies will use the commission motivator to focus the attention of the sales staff on critical issues of the communities. Companies willing to be flexible and creative with their commission structures can effectively respond to changing market needs and redirect the emphasis as needed.

Companies that employ a move-in coordinator were evenly split on paying commissions; half did, and half did not. The fact that 44 percent of the companies surveyed had no such position could be reflective of the overall 90 percent occupancy status. Generally move-in coordinators are employed during the fill-up stage to facilitate a smooth transition into the community after sale and free the sales counselor's valuable time up for selling.

In companies or communities where assisted living was also marketed, 56 percent utilized the same commission structure as for independent and 28 percent had a commission structure that paid less than the commission on independent living. Only 17 percent (3 of 18) of the companies do not pay assisted-living commissions.

The majority of companies (61%) do not pay wait list commissions. However, of the 39 percent of the companies that do pay commissions on wait list deposits, most paid it out as an advance only on the full commission. Wait list commission levels ranged from a low of $50 to a high of $750. Communities that experience a high level of turnover are well advised to place an appropriate emphasis on the development of a solid back-up of residents on the wait list. Although this practice can be an effective offensive maneuver to counter anticipated turnover in stabilized communities, it can also give the "not ready yet" prospect a comfortable haven in communities experiencing fill-up difficulties.

In some circumstances, a sale may cancel or a new resident may move back out voluntarily after a short period of time (less than 90 days). Companies will charge back-paid commissions to the account of the sales counselor. This is understandable because the commission should be funded from the resident's monthly fee, and if the sale is not completed in the case of a cancellation or the resident moves out quickly, possibly indicating an inappropriate placement, management should not consider this a sale. In the survey, 67 percent of the companies had charge-back policies before move-in (17%), before and after move-in (50%), and after move-in (33%). Of the 33 percent that do not have a commission charge-back policy, one-third did not pay the commission until after move-in.

The majority of companies surveyed (56%) pay their marketing or sales directors overrides on the sales generated by their staff. These payments are in addition to their own commissions received on sales that they personally make and range from a low of $25 per sale to a high of $350 per sale. Some companies (28%) even pay overrides to the marketing assistant on each sale to ensure that they are customer-driven in their job function. Of the 28 percent that pay them, these overrides range from a low of $25 to a high of $200 per sale.

In addition to the commission plan, may companies use incentives to manage their sales emphasis. The majority (72%) pay additional incentives tied to occupancy goals. Incentives tied to move-in goals were used in 56 percent of the companies as were incentives to sales goals at 50 percent of the companies surveyed. Other bonuses tied to revenue goals, phone-outs, appointments, and other performance thresholds were less common but still used by 22 percent of the more creative sales directors. Only one company surveyed did not use incentives or bonuses outside the commission structure.

The total levels of compensation achieved varied considerably. For marketing or sales directors, the low range was $37,000 and the high was $114,000 per year in total compensation from salary, commissions, and other incentives, not including the value of fringe benefits. For sales counselors, the range was also dramatic, from a low of $23,000 to a high of $83,000. This demonstrates the wide variety in compensation plans commonly used in the industry factored by the performance capabilities of the sales staff themselves.

Many companies also understand the importance of recognition in the motivation of their sales staff. In addition to their compensation plan, many organize team-oriented monthly sales contests using a theme and progressive gifts. For example, a $15 gift certificate for a new compact disk can be up for grabs when the fourth sale of the month is made, $50 at a department store to the counselor making the sixth sale, $100 theater tickets for the tenth sale, and a $300 cash bonus for a dozen sales in one month. The point here is to provide progressive incentives to improve performance incrementally, and help reduce apathy among sales counselors. Recognition dinners, additional training, motivational books and tapes, weekends away, and pats on the back are all effective at motivating employees. Savvy sales directors who identify a weakness in the sales program can creatively develop rather inexpensive and fun contests to refocus their staff. Sales staff are by nature very competitive, and many will invest *extra* hours selling to reach designated award levels.

Many companies also have a top-producers' club. These are common to most real estate offices as well. Most programs define specific performance levels with associated progressive awards. For example, a sales counselor who averages four sales per month could qualify for the minimum package to include $50 retroactive commission payments, a crystal trophy, and an award package with a letter from the president and perhaps some gift bearing the company logo. As the average sales increase to five or six, for example, the award package and trophy can be progressively more impressive. It is amazing how effective these programs can be. Salespeople crave recognition, and programs like these enable them to receive a high profile in the company while keeping them constantly aware of their production statistics. Some sales staff will work six days per week toward the end of an award period to qualify for these recognition levels.

■■■■ TRAINING

Sales training that is designed to accelerate the rapport-building process can decrease the number of contacts required before close. This can have a dramatic effect on productivity. For example, if the average number of contacts prior to close is 20 and through training and skills practice this number can be reduced to 10, you have effectively doubled the productivity of each sales counselor.

Considerable opportunity exists for improving sales through training. In many senior-living communities the training of new and experienced salespeople beyond the basics of the service package, financial options, and office paper flow receive little budget attention. Those communities will generally associate only marginal improvement in sales with their training investment. It has long been established in this relationship-oriented business that improved performance generated by training existing employees will generally exceed performance improvements resulting from employee recruitment or replacement. Then why don't we do more of it?

Perhaps the answer to this question is that people generally tend to gravitate toward activities that they do best. Activities that require them to step outside their comfort zone are usually assigned the lowest priority. Most marketing directors generally arrive at their position by demonstrating success in the selling process. This process typically involves selling in one-on-one situations. Training is also a selling exercise; the trainer is selling a thought process and ideas or techniques, the difference being that the training arena generally involves speaking before groups or leading a discussion. This is a very different environment requiring the one-on-one person to graduate to one-on-many situations. This can expose the trainer's vulnerabilities and efforts to potential criticism. Training is a whole new ball game for the marketing director; if it is not well organized and delivered, it can subject the marketing director to unnecessary stress and even hurt his credibility as a supervisor. Conversely, marketing directors who are successful at defining training needs and building effective training programs can inspire confidence, lift morale, break the monotony of the daily routine, and experience professional growth.

The typical employee-development model begins with setting expectations, then determining needs,

training to fill needs, giving feedback on performance, and coaching for career growth. The design of the specific training program should consider these elements. It can be broken down into four major components: the needs assessment, the training method, how the training should be conducted, and evaluation of results.[7] Let us explore each briefly.

■■■■ Needs Assessment

The specific training needs of the department must first be defined. The marketing director must evaluate the overall basic needs of the program and the vulnerabilities of the department. Then each individual's needs should be identified by conducting a needs assessment. The needs assessment tool should itemize the major components of the sales function. The content of the training needs should be separated into two main components: initial training and continuous training. *Initial* sales training programs typically have a very broad scope and are generally intended to orient new employees or transferred employees to the community. Categories for initial training could include:

1. Understanding the Market
2. Basic Gerontology
3. Competitive Analysis and Market Share
4. Departmental Policies and Procedures
5. Lead Management
6. Community Image
7. Service Package
8. How to Show the Community
9. Inventory and Pricing
10. Limits of Authority
11. Record Keeping
12. Orientation to Other Departments and their Services

Continuous sales training programs will concentrate on more specific aspects of the job where experienced sales counselors may have deficiencies or when new concepts are introduced. Categories for continuous training could include:

1. Relationship Building
2. Closing Techniques
3. Improving Telephone Productivity
4. Advanced Communication Skills
5. Neurolinguistic Programming
6. Personality and Temperament Testing

7. Information Gathering and Probing
8. Affirmation and Imprinting
9. Overcoming Objections
10. Handling Difficult People
11. Dealing with Conflict
12. Time Management
13. Marketing Planning
14. Community Outreach
15. Public Relations
16. Motivation and Self-Esteem

The objective of the training plan is to target weak areas that relate directly to performance, and create learning environments to influence behavior. It's a good idea to have each sales counselor rate her own skill level in each area first to determine if any patterns develop within the group. The trainer can then prioritize each subject and begin to develop a plan.

It may be appropriate to invite experienced salespeople to assist in training new recruits. This way new employees can gain an appreciation for the relative skill levels of their coworkers, which can facilitate the development of a team environment within the department.

Training Methods

The marketing director will have several training methods at her disposal. These can include group lectures, personal conferences, demonstrations, role-playing or skills practice, case studies, impromptu discussions, gaming, on-the-job training, and programmed training. Selecting the appropriate training method will be determined by the content. Some content will be applicable to the entire group, such as new policies, company direction, and skill development. Other content such as improving phone to appointment conversion rates may be of a more personal nature.

LECTURES

Lectures are generally considered by professional trainers to be the least effective training method. The lecture environment establishes a passive rather than active format of trainee participation. The emphasis of a lecture is on teaching, not learning. Studies have shown that the average retention of material disseminated at a lecture can be less than 10 percent. So even with the advent of visual aides, trainee absorption can be disappointingly low. People learn best when they are active participants and have a role to play in the

process. Brief lectures can be useful, however, to introduce new material, summarize major topics, communicate company philosophy, and provide orientation regarding the industry, the market, and the residents.

PERSONAL CONFERENCES

The personal conference is often the most effective training method. Personal meetings demand the participants' complete attention. Information communicated at these private meetings can be customized to the needs of the trainee and delivered in a manner that is not offensive or subjects the individual to the scrutiny of the group. Constructive advice and specific suggestions can be offered by the marketing director privately, which avoids potential embarrassment. Whether structured or unstructured, formal or informal, the content will determine the delivery.

DEMONSTRATIONS

Demonstrations are another method of training that are absolutely necessary to communicate how properly to conduct a tour. When training new sales counselors, the marketing director will need to demonstrate the best methods of showing the community. For example, incorporating knowledge about prospect "hot buttons" and interests gained during the initial interview during the tour can be a very effective method of assimilating the presentation into the mind of the prospect. Assimilation is a technique of incorporating an idea or thought into the subconscious; moving something external into one's cognitive process. Demonstrating how special interests of the prospects can be realized by the community amenities or service package during the tour can enhance its appeal. Demonstrating to the trainee how to steer a prospect's attention is the best method for getting your point across. Demonstration is also a very useful technique when training employees to use the computer system. Not all salespersons are computer literate, and demonstrating how to scroll through the menus can be a good way to get them started. Also, it is wise to demonstrate to staff how to operate apartment appliances, HVAC equipment, and door locks.

ROLE PLAYING

Role playing involves having trainees act out parts in contrived situations. These situations can either be problematic or structured to create awareness. Generally speaking, role playing is a very effective method used by marketing directors to problem solve challenging situations where the trainees can learn from more experienced sales personnel. This can be a great confidence builder for new employees by providing them some practice at handling difficult situations or learning closing techniques. In addition, role playing provides experienced sales personnel the opportunity to test responses out on management and to clarify company policy. Role playing, sometimes referred to as skills practice, can be fun and stimulating even for experienced salespeople who may welcome the opportunity to display their sales talents to the group. At the same time, each participant learns to accept criticism openly from others as the group realizes that sound suggestions benefit everyone.

CASE STUDIES

Case studies can be a very efficient training method when sales staff time is at a premium. Using this method, the marketing director, executive director, or senior sales counselor will write up a problematic selling situation that may be somewhat complex. Complex issues such as wheelchairs in the dining room, smoking, medical screening, family conflicts, or the application of the Fair Housing Amendments Act can be detailed for clarification using a group discussion. The case description should be concise and include all relevant facts and information to fully describe the situation. The group should then discuss the problem, clarify the facts, suggest possible solutions, and choose an alternative. The point of the discussion is not so much to reach a decision as it is for the group to gain insight into the scope of the complexity and to understand the process for resolution. Case studies can also explore problems and outcomes experienced by other operators in the business so as to learn from their mistakes.

IMPROMPTU DISCUSSIONS

Impromptu discussions can be conducted during weekly sales meetings to explore specific problems or learn new techniques. For example, the sales department should have a weekly "hots" meeting to enable each sales counselor to discuss the current status of their best leads. During these meetings, each sales counselor will describe the top 10–15 clients whom they are currently working on in terms of their personal situation,

motivation, obstacles, timing, and likelihood to close. This way the sales staff can offer suggestions on how to bring the clients to closure and discuss any conflicts they may have with move-in dates. The "hots" meeting is an excellent opportunity for sales staff to feed off of each other's excitement about pending closes and estimate the likelihood of reaching month-end targets. As the marketing director becomes aware of any problematic trends in her analysis of sales activity, she can introduce potential solutions or give direction on how the group can overcome weak areas of performance. Impromptu discussions can also be facilitated by the executive director or other department head with the intention of educating the sales people about other departments and job functions. In addition, sales staff can be kept informed about move-outs or potential problems with operations within the community so that they can steer prospects around them or be prepared to overcome potential objections. Impromptu discussions are an excellent forum in which to disseminate information about inventory availability and pricing structure or policy changes. This way management can benefit from immediate feedback from sales counselors who are in constant contact with prospects and market trends.

GAMING

Gaming is another method of training that can be fun and productive in large groups. Games such as *Jeopardy* or *Wheel of Fortune* can be adapted to highlight critical information about the community and its services. Employees from one or several departments can be brought together to participate formally or informally. Generally, the larger the group, the less structure and formality. These situations can be used effectively to break down natural barriers between sales and operations while celebrating the accomplishments of each. Gaming can also be used to familiarize employees with management's problem-solving process. The American Association of Homes for the Aged (AAHA) has developed the *Game of Aging Concerns*. This is a board game that is designed around real-life retirement housing problems, and it is intended to stimulate discussions on strategies to resolve them. Contestants quickly realize that many everyday problems are considerably more complex than they first appear. Created by Dr. Vicki Schmall, a gerontological specialist at Oregon State University, the *Game of Aging Concerns* "enables you to acquaint new managers with the kinds of problems that they can expect to encounter, develop problem solving skills, promote teamwork and sensitize staff at all levels to the perspectives of residents and their families and management."[8]

ON-THE-JOB TRAINING

On-the-job training is a cyclical process of tell, show, do, and review. Most marketing directors employ some translation of this method to train new sales employees. The supervisor will normally work together with the new employee to instruct him on the organizational structure of the department and the finer points of selling the community and its service package. Shadowing new employees on mock tours or in presentations (subsequent to orientation) provides a good opportunity to rehearse methods of overcoming prospect objections and to discuss possible responses to the vulnerabilities of the community, its service package, pricing structure, amenities, or location. Even experienced salespeople will need occasionally to practice and hone their skills when selling an unfamiliar community. On-the-job training provides supervised practice. There is simply no more effective method to learn a job or communicate expectations.

On-the-job training should ideally be conducted by the marketing director as well as other senior sales counselors, each with their own organized agenda. Many experienced sales counselors who are paid on a commission basis may be reluctant to assist with this training, as it will pull them away from money-making sales activities. This can easily be remedied by paying bonuses or overrides on the pupil's sales. There is no better role model than someone who is already successful and producing results.

Each of the training methods discussed so far represents relatively inexpensive training that will minimally impact the marketing budget. If all the training you ever did incorporated these methods in an organized and deliberate manner, the majority of your training needs could be addressed. Not all effective training has to cost money. In fact we have just explored eight methods that are considered by professional trainers to be the most effective empowerment tools available to the sales manager. The only resources they require are research, planning, creativity, organization skills, and time management.

PROGRAMMED LEARNING

Programmed learning is a training method that involves the delivery of structured instructional material in seminar format or broken down into lesson plans or units. Programmed learning or training by consultants is generally the most expensive and least targeted of all training methods at the marketing director's disposal. Still, they have some advantages. These programs are normally developed by professional trainers or consultants and are marketed as a package or in individual components. The major advantages to these programs are that they can introduce fresh ideas into the training curriculum and leave employees with the impression that they are receiving something of value. Many employees believe that these "professional" programs have inherent value and are a demonstration of the company's commitment to investing in its employees. The real translation of these invested dollars into incrementally higher productivity is difficult to measure. However, improvements in employee morale and employer loyalty can be very real outcomes. Some packaged training programs can run as high as $5,000, but I have not been able to see a discernible difference in those offered at a fraction of that price. Many good packages are available for a minimal investment.

Conducting Training

Training can be conducted with a variety of resources depending upon the material content. *Initial* training and orientation is normally conducted by the marketing director or direct supervisor. *Continuous* sales training can draw upon the resources of other successful sales persons, marketing directors and top sales producers from other company properties (that are at stabilized occupancy), executive level management, or outside consultants.

The effectiveness of the training program, however well conceived, rests in the hands of the people conducting it. The starting point for a successful training program is to train the trainers. Conducting effective training requires more refined and sophisticated influencing skills than those needed to sell the community. With training you are selling intangible techniques and ideas rather than products and services. Not all experienced and successful salespeople can become good trainers. In fact, most sales counselors tend to be very results-oriented and can become frustrated with the payback period for gratification. Training is developmental in nature and may bear fruit only after the individual has reached a level of maturity in her technique. The mechanics of teaching and learning alone do not guarantee the success of train-the-trainer programs. It also helps to have a well-planned and well-organized curriculum to assist the trainer in his delivery.

The timing of the *initial* sales training should be arranged at the time of hiring. *Continuous* sales training should be conducted informally daily and weekly as needed and formally at least monthly. If you do not do it at least monthly, then it is not *continuous!* The marketing director can develop a training series based on her original needs assessment. It can then be designed for delivery during monthly meetings with weekly follow-up modules to keep concepts fresh. The incorporation of regular skills-practice exercises will help to improve retention.

Training manuals, workbooks, and video and audio tapes can be developed or purchased for a minimal investment per employee. They can be designed with as much or as little structure as the group requires. The best programs include summaries or outlines of the main concepts, related reading materials, statements of objectives, orienting questions, and case studies.

Training Evaluation

Sales training programs can represent the investment of considerable time, effort, and expense. Although management hopes to improve morale and gain a sense of goodwill in the process, it will primarily be interested in seeing a return on its investment through improved performance. The direct relationship between training and results can take some time to take become established. It is a developmental process that may require many months to mature. Management can devise many methods for analyzing productivity, such as phone-out-to-appointment or appointment-to-sale conversion ratios, but relating results back to training is rarely conclusive.

The best method for the evaluation of any training program is to compare track records of personnel before they received their training to their current performance. It is also useful to mystery shop your sales counselors in comparison with those of your competitors. Although some sales counselors are "naturally born," for a relatively small investment, training can serve to keep your people fresh, sharpen their skills, and clarify your expectations.

As reflected throughout this entire text, managers who deliberately create a clear vision for their department, define a clear set of expectations and standards that support that vision, gain consensus among their staff, and create a sense of urgency in a positively charged environment will position their community for success. There are no shortcuts.

NOTES

1. See Chapter 13 for a discussion on reach and frequency.
2. See Chapter 4 for guidelines on running the front desk.
3. A. Robbins, *The Magic of Rapport* (La Jolla, Calif.: Robbins International, 1986) (cassette tape).
4. See Chapter 15 for more on move-in coordination.
5. R. A. Zarro and P. Blum. *The Phone Book: Breakthrough Phone Skills for Fun, Profit, and Enlightenment* (Barrytown, N.Y.: Station Hill Press, 1989).
6. M. Leary. "1993 Sales Compensation Survey," presentation to National Association for Senior Living Industries, December 1993.
7. R. R. Still, E. W. Cundiff, and N. Govoni, *Sales Management: Decisions, Strategies, and Cases* (Englewood Cliffs, N.J.: Prentice Hall, 1991), 341.
8. *The Game of Aging Concerns* and other publications can be ordered from the American Association of Homes for the Aged (AAHA) at 1129 20th Street NW, Suite 400, Washington, DC 20036-3489. Phone (202) 296-5960, fax (202) 223-5920.

Move-in Coordination

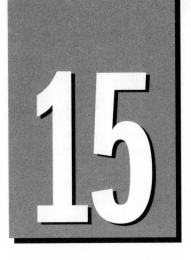

Moving can be an overwhelming experience for people of any age. For seniors it is an especially emotional process, for in many cases they are moving from homes in which they have lived for many years, raised their families, and created many memories. Because they have accumulated decades' worth of possessions, the thought of having to downsize can lead them to postpone a move to a retirement community, even though their lives will most likely be enriched by the move!

For these reasons, the move-in coordination services offered by the community are an invaluable part of the sales process. (See Exhibit 15.2 at the end of the chapter for a complete checklist to coordinate a smooth move-in experience.) Knowing that a capable professional will be there to help coordinate the move every step of the way helps erase doubts and fears in the minds of our prospects and helps to shorten the time between lease-signing and move-in.

Communities that experience an average of eight move-ins per month or more should consider hiring a move-in coordinator, especially during the fill-up stage. Even larger mature communities with 300 units and 20 percent turnover annually will need to coordinate approximately five move-ins and five move-outs each month. Managing these moves can involve a serious time commitment. Communities that use sales staff to perform this function may be wasting valuable sales time that can otherwise be committed to keeping the apart-

ments fully occupied. The volume of monthly turnover at the community will determine the allocation of staffing hours to the move-in/move-out function. Move-in coordinators can also be used to assist with activities, resident orientation, driving, concierge backup, and even night management during slow periods.

As the community reaches full occupancy, the marketing assistant can be trained to perform the essential functions of the move-in coordinator position. The ability to perform these additional duties will of course depend on the size of the community and the amount of turnover that it routinely experiences.

The move-in coordinator should introduce himself to as many prospects as possible at community tours, marketing functions, or resident programs. Depending on a prospect's needs and concerns, a marketing representative may choose to involve the move-in coordinator in the sales process even before a lease or residency agreement has been signed. At this stage, the move-in coordinator's role is to calm the prospect's fears by explaining the level of assistance that can be offered during each stage of the move.

SCHEDULING A HOME VISIT

Once a prospect signs a lease and has been officially "turned over" for move-in coordination by a marketing representative, it is important to call the prospect within three days and schedule a home visit. Because in most cases the move-in coordinator will not be able to schedule a home visit with out-of-state prospects, the initial phone call to the prospect takes on even greater importance. During the telephone conversation, it is important to do the following with each and every prospect:

- Understand and reemphasize the features of the community that led the prospect to sign a lease.
- Understand and minimize obstacles (any concerns the prospect has about moving).
- Listen for any subtle changes in attitude (is the prospect getting cold feet?).
- Look for opportunities to speed up move-in time.

Preparation is paramount to a successful home visit. It is important to schedule a briefing with the closing marketing representative to learn as much as possible about the prospect before the visit. The home visit is the best opportunity to establish credibility with the prospect and earn her trust. Keep in mind that because a prospect is likely to be more comfortable and in control at home, questions about all aspects of the community—not just the move itself—are likely to surface during the home visit. The prospect will constantly be evaluating the move-in coordinator's confidence about, and knowledge of, the community.

PRESENTING THE WELCOME PACKAGE. It is especially effective to present information during the home visit that has been personalized for the prospect. All of the following items should be included in a welcome package, although it may overwhelm the prospect to discuss more than just the most important information. *Remove barriers to getting things done.* Say, "I can take care of that for you" or "This is what we need to do now," rather than, "This is what you will need to do."

- A welcome letter personalized with the prospect's new address, including a list of the items with which you can assist during the move
- Several blank floor plans for only the apartment style the prospect has selected
- Pictures of the view from the prospect's apartment (for long-distance moves)
- A list of goods and services available in the prospect's new neighborhood (e.g., banks, dry cleaners, 24-hour pharmacies, markets, florists, places of worship)
- Local utility companies' phone numbers so that service can be canceled or transferred

- Local newspapers' phone numbers so that subscriptions can be transferred
- Change-of-address cards to send to the prospect's current post office branch and contacts
- A list of reputable realtors and moving-and-storage companies—a minimum of four each
- A list of local charitable organizations that will accept donations of furniture and household items
- A list of antique appraisers, estate sales people, decorators, resale shops, upholsterers, drapers, and so on
- Several community postcards so that the prospect can spread the good news about the move to friends and acquaintances
- A current resident newsletter and event calendar

The last item, a resident newsletter, can serve as an icebreaker during a home visit. Because it highlights exciting aspects of the community, it can help you determine which programs the prospect will find most interesting. Come equipped, too, with a scaled floor plan of the apartment the prospect has reserved, a floor plan of the common areas, a tape measure, and some imagination! Gently walk the prospect through the downsizing process. Ask questions about furniture, wall hangings, and personal possessions. Start with the items the prospect absolutely will not move without and work around the rest. Sometimes it will be necessary to ease the prospect's mind about the downsizing with comments such as, "It seems as though we spend the first half of our lives accumulating possessions and the last half giving them away. Once you start the paring down process it won't seem as big an obstacle."

WHAT TO LOOK FOR. It is during the home visit that the prospect first begins mentally to adjust to community living; observations can be made about the prospect's concerns will aid the operations staff in easing the transition into the community after move-in. It won't take long to get a feel for the prospect's temperament (e.g., is the prospect a worrier, detail oriented, indecisive, very attached to possessions?). It is important to try to gauge the level of assistance the prospect will require and then provide it without being asked. *Anticipating a prospect's needs is as crucial as being able to fulfill them.*

Take note of the prospect's surroundings during a home visit. Does the house have stairs that have become an obstacle. Is yard maintenance a problem?

Are there medical appliances in the house? Ask questions about the difficulties of home ownership and subtly reinforce those negatives: "It must be tiring to climb those stairs all the time," or "How do you manage to take care of that big yard?" Be careful not to talk about how desirable the home is other than to say that it should sell easily.

REINFORCING THE SALE. It is especially important to reinforce the sale during the home visit. Pay special attention to the way the prospect frames questions and be sure to accentuate the positive in your answers. For example, if the prospect asks, "How will I ever fit all of my dishes in that kitchen?" emphasize the dining services offered at the community, including the use of the private dining room for special family gatherings. Take inventory of the kitchen and make suggestions for downsizing pots and pans (chances are the prospect won't be cooking as much at the community). Perhaps half of the family heirloom china could be available for use/display and the rest could be stored or passed on to family members. Be sure to use an upbeat tone when making suggestions!

WRAPPING UP THE VISIT. Always close with a date for follow-up, whether it is with a phone call or an additional home visit. It is important to follow up the initial home visit with a phone call the next day to thank the prospect for his time and to reconfirm your availability to assist.

REPORTING BACK TO THE MARKETING DEPARTMENT. After the visit it is important to brief completely the appropriate sales representative who will assist the marketing department in expediting move-ins. Then set up a calendar plan that brings the prospect up to move-in day with goals along the way.

SHARING HOME-VISIT OBSERVATIONS WITH CABINET STAFF. Sharing home visit observations with cabinet staff will help them to get to know the prospect before the move-in. Perhaps a new resident is hard of hearing; if employees speak directly to her in a clear, distinct manner, she may be able to read their lips. If a new resident is visually impaired, the dining room wait staff might try describing the menu items to him in a noncondescending way. It also helps the staff to know if a new resident is recently widowed and still grieving. If employees know that a new resident loves volunteer work, they can suggest projects in which she could get involved. Being informed that a new resident is on medication that could cause mood swings can help the staff anticipate such behavior and avoid embarrassing situations. Any insight that can be offered from the home visit will help the entire staff to make the new resident's transition into the community a smooth one.

■■■ PREPARING A WELCOME PACKAGE AND COMPILING A LIST OF AREA RESOURCES

Anything a prospect has accumulated will require some type of action, whether it is to be packed up to move, updated or altered in some way, donated, given to family, or sold. It is very important to limit the involvement in this process to offering only advice and resources. Do not run the risk of offending a family member by actually becoming involved in the giveaway process personally. It is too easy to mistakenly sell or donate something that a family member may have wanted. Be careful to stay completely neutral as family possessions are distributed. *Do not offer to accept any of the prospect's belongings under any pretenses without the full approval of all family members.* To do so may constitute a conflict and could expose the community to legal liability.

It is easy to keep resources organized. Many people find that cross-referencing index cards is a good system. Developing cards under both name and type of service—for instance, Jones, Frank; Art Dealer—Consignment (Will Pick Up), *and* Art Dealer, Frank Jones—Consignment (Will Pick Up)—keeps you from having to remember the vendor's name. It also keeps like services together as they're added and removed from the list.

■ *Area Services*   The most efficient way to compile this information is through referrals. You'll probably find that existing residents from the local area will be happy to share their consumer experiences, good and bad. Next, turn to the telephone directory or a local senior services directory and look under subjects such as tailors, banks, pharmacies, and places of worship. Some services will be targeted specifically to seniors, such as hearing aid replacement and service.

Verify business hours and charges. Are senior citizen discounts available? Is the store open 24 hours a day? Is it located within walking distance? Is it accessible to wheelchairs? Will the merchant deliver goods to the community? Will the owner offer a special discount to our residents in exchange for a listing in our resident newsletter?

▪ *Realtors* Gather the names of the largest, most reputable real estate firms in town. Larger firms have more resources at their disposal and offer the broadest possible exposure to the marketplace in terms of a multiple listing service, newspaper and television ads, open houses, and office tours. Provide at least three names. If the marketing department has a realtor referral program, be sure to get the names of realtors who have referred prospects in the past or who work well with seniors. The local multiple listing service normally keeps statistics by real estate office or broker of sales volume, and on average home sales prices. With a little digging, the most productive realtors in the community can be uncovered. The faster they sell the prospects' homes, the shorter the move-in time.

▪ *Estate Auctioneers* The auction has been the traditional method for disposing of an estate. Professionals who specialize in these sales—which can be called tag sales, estate sales, garage sales, house sales, patio sales, or yard sales—can arrange for the complete or partial liquidation of residents' belongings. They will perform a valuation of the belongings to establish fair market value, then coordinate, advertise, and conduct the sale. Average proceeds from a typical sale can range from $8,000 to $15,000 and can reach a high of $75,000. The liquidator normally collects 30 percent or less depending on the valuation amount. Call around to gather the names of local auction houses that offer estate sales. When contacting them, be sure to inquire about their charges, which are usually a percentage of the total sale. Also inquire about their preference regarding the location of the auction. Should they prefer to hold the auction in the prospect's home, the prospect may have to move out by a certain date. Here are some suggested questions to ask the professional:

1. Will I receive a clear financial agreement specifying the percentage commission charged?
2. When and where will the sale be advertised?
3. How will you handle the traffic flow inside the residence to minimize theft and breakage?
4. Will I receive an inventory of the property prior to sale? (This is essential.)
5. When will the final accounting be due to the estate or owner? (The interval is usually between 15 and 30 days.)

Remember, prices in a well-run tag sale are established by the knowledgeable professional, whereas prices in an auction are established by the audience.

▪ *Antique Dealers* Valuable or unusual items that are not appropriate to liquidate at a tag sale can be sold more economically through antique dealers. Call around and secure the name of one person at each business on whom you can rely when a prospect wants to have something appraised. Get the names of at least three antique dealers so that the prospect can compare offers.

▪ *Refurbishers* Some personal treasures are in better shape than others. It is helpful to compile a list of businesses that can breathe new life into sentimental items so that prospects can still have familiar things around them. Find a local draper who can turn draperies into valances or other styles of window treatments that are currently popular; a carpenter who can fix or restore an old table; an electrician nearby who can rewire an old lamp; a frame shop that can update the look of family photos or artwork.

▪ *Charitable Organizations* Once again, the telephone directory can be a valuable source of charitable organizations for donations of household items and clothing. If your community has an affiliation with a local hospital or nursing home, either group may be able to pass along some names to you. Some churches and synagogues have resale shops for which they gratefully accept donations. The key is to work with two or three reputable organizations that will pick up the merchandise (either from the prospect's current residence or from the community) and provide receipts for tax deductions to the donors. Prospects can then select an organization from the list that you have compiled. Be sure to find out if there is anything that these organizations will not accept, so that the prospect can make other arrangements to dispose of such items.

▪ *Library* The local public library will be happy to accept used books from prospects. Call to find how to make such donations. Senior centers, nursing homes, and some university libraries also look for donations of used books. Most used bookstores will pay cash or give the prospect credit toward future purchases at the store.

- *Garage Sales* Garage sales represent big business for your local newspaper's classified section. Call the paper and inquire about any special rates it may have for garage sale advertisers; some papers even give out garage sale kits consisting of signs, price stickers, and inventory sheets. Also ask for several ad copy forms so that you can assist the prospect in preparing an ad.

- *Storage Units* The best way to research local storage-unit companies is to visit them personally. That way you can see exactly what each company has to offer and get rate schedules. Viewing the units in person will help you help prospects to decide what would best fit their storage needs.

- *Vintage Clothing and Consignment Shops* Many prospects will have vintage clothing, and shops specializing in such goods have increased in popularity over the past few years. If there are any in the area, call them and find out which types of items they will accept, and whether they will pay for them. Consignment shops will offer to sell the items for the prospect in exchange for a percentage of the sale price. A third option for prospects is to place a classified ad in the local paper under the clothing section.

- *Post Office* Ask the local post office branch for several change-of-address forms and stamps-by-mail order forms and distribute them to prospects.

It is crucial that all potential resources be thoroughly screened before they are referred to prospects. And, because all businesses do not conduct their affairs in the same fashion, it is crucial to evaluate resident satisfaction with the services that were recommended. When a resident uses a service or purchases goods based on the community's referral, find out if he would recommend the service to someone else and if he was satisfied with the level of service provided and with the price charged.

■ DEVELOPING A LIST OF REPUTABLE MOVERS

The primary goal when contacting movers should be to find several that understand senior-living communities and their prospects' special needs. The first step is to set up screening interviews with reputable, long-

standing companies that are able to provide references and that hire only full-time workers, as opposed to seasonal part-timers. Offering prospects three local and two long-distance movers from which to choose is sufficient. Emphasizing up front the expectation of good service will help to establish a positive working relationship with the movers from the start.

When interviewing these companies, inquiries should be made about employee professionalism. Do they wear uniforms? Are they friendly and patient enough to deal with seniors? Perhaps a crew can be assigned to work exclusively at your community during fill-up months so that a strong rapport can be developed.

UNDERSTANDING RATES. How are rates established? Are the mover's rates competitive? Why do some movers charge more than others? Will the mover provide a guaranteed estimate, meaning the final charge cannot exceed the estimate? Some companies will "lowball" a bid, meaning they will offer a low estimate in order to get the job then charge more on delivery. Sometimes an extra charge is assessed because the items being moved actually weigh more than the estimator thought they would. Finally, ask if the mover will drop off goods at a local charity free of charge if the resident has items to donate.

GETTING COMPETITIVE BIDS. Explain to each moving company that a minimum of two competitive bids will be solicited on all moves.

SECURING INSURANCE. All movers must be insured, bonded by the state, and able to provide you with documentation of such. Inquire about insurance for moving specialty items—pianos, works of art, and the like—and request that the insurance coverage be thoroughly explained to the prospect by a representative of the moving company. Keep copies of the moving companies' documentation on file.

SHARING INFORMATION. Each company should be evaluated according to the type of move for which it is best suited. For example, Mrs. Jones will not be able to do any prepacking or unpacking; recommending the company with the most efficient packers/unpackers will save her time, money, and stress. If everything is left in boxes on the day of her move she will be overwhelmed with the clutter, and it will take longer for her to get settled. If Mr. Smith prefers to prepack his belongings, perhaps the less costly, "bare-bones" moving company is sufficient for his needs.

UNDERSTANDING SPECIAL CHARACTERISTICS OF LONG-DISTANCE MOVES. Because of the distances involved, residents who move to the community from out of state most likely will not have received a home visit before their moves. This dictates that the welcome package be sent by mail the same day after first making contact with the prospect.

One of the most important things to remember when dealing with long-distance movers is to get them to *guarantee* a delivery date. Keep in mind that the new resident will need to stay in a guest apartment or hotel until her belongings arrive. The sooner delivery can be arranged, the sooner the new resident can get settled in and make your community her home.

Long-distance movers frequently give a two- to three-day window for delivery. Many are reluctant to guarantee a delivery date, but this point is negotiable. Insist on it. If the company wants the business, its representatives will be flexible.

Several factors determine the date of delivery: the size of the load, the route it will take, and the maximum possible shipment per truck. For example, if a resident has a large load that will fill a truck, the delivery date will be based on the time it takes to travel straight to the community. If it is a relatively small load, as is normally the case, other loads will also be collected to fill up the truck. The delivery date in that case will be based upon where the load is in line for removal from the truck.

Long-distance will typically arrive first thing in the morning. The driver will undoubtedly want to unload as soon as possible, so plan to be available and have the loading dock clear by 7:00 A.M. Be sure to coordinate the delivery schedule with the new resident. If he is not an early riser, you may want to suggest a wake-up call.

Long-distance moves require extra time and attention. Residents will not only be new to the community, but to the surrounding area as well. If possible, arrange to have a resident/volunteer with similar marital status and interests show the new resident around the neighborhood. A driver could be assigned to spend a few minutes driving the new resident around the local area and pointing out things of interest. Your welcome package will go a long way toward making new residents who have moved from a distance feel more at home.

SCHEDULING MOVE-INS

Because most long-distance movers will arrive in the morning for delivery and unpacking, it will be necessary for high-rise communities to schedule the freight elevator to avoid conflicts with other deliveries or move-outs. Schedule no more than two move-ins or move-outs per day. Meet with the movers to inform them that their company will be held responsible for any damage they may do to facility walls, corners, or carpeting. Movers can make a building look shabby after only a few move-ins if they think they do not have to be careful. It is usually advisable to ensure that a maintenance employee is on site during all move-ins to hook everything up and see that everything runs smoothly after the resident moves in.

COMMUNICATING WITH OTHER DEPARTMENTS

Once a move-in date has been confirmed, it is important to inform other departments about the upcoming move-in. A smooth move-in can happen only when all departments are involved and committed to doing their parts to see that all bases are covered. The move-in coordinator is the point person and is responsible for coordinating this process.

ENGINEERING. Completing a maintenance request update on a weekly basis will keep the engineering department informed as to who is moving into which apartment, when the new resident is moving in, and what type of assistance will be required from the engineering department (for instance, grab bars installed or fixtures hung). Apartments should be added to the list as soon as a lease is signed regardless of the move-in date (within reason). This gives maintenance a chance to schedule apartment work conveniently, avoiding a "crunch" should the resident move up her move-in date. This list should be distributed to the housekeeping supervisor as well. Engineering staff should clean up their own maintenance messes.

HOUSEKEEPING. Residents often bring a few personal items to the apartment before their actual move-in date;

therefore, the apartment should be cleaned and presentable a few days prior to the scheduled move-in date. If a new resident is moving in on a Tuesday, the apartment should be ready no later than the Friday before so that the new resident can use the weekend to set up kitchen items, have a sofa delivered, or bring over some clothes. If this is the case, a notation must be made on the maintenance request update so that both maintenance and housekeeping will know when they need to have their work completed.

Incorporate into the maintenance request list any deliveries, decorating, or customizing that is to be done to the apartment. Avoid double work: request that housekeeping clean the apartment after painting is complete, or that additional closet organizers be installed after any wallpapering is done but before closet doors are rehung.

DINING ROOM. Be sure to let the dining room manager know which dinner seating the new resident has selected. Inform the manager that dining certificates will be needed for the new resident to use for lunch and dinner on moving day. Tell the dining room manager whether other residents or family will be dining with the new resident on move-in day. Any special dietary concerns should be discussed as well.

Finally, on a weekly basis, prepare a list of who will be arriving during the upcoming week and distribute it to all staff. This will help the staff become familiar with names and apartment numbers. Residents also take an interest in knowing when the next move-in will be—it's easy to get them excited about the new kid on the block.

CONDUCTING ORIENTATION

Because moving can be an unsettling experience, it is important to be sensitive to the fact that new residents will need some assistance in becoming acclimated to the community. New residents will usually have toured the community several times before move-in and will be relatively familiar with it. Nonetheless, they will appreciate having important information reiterated to them. There is a big difference between going on an escorted tour of the building during the sales process and having to find their way around the building once they have moved in. In the case of long-distance moves, orientation may be a resident's first introduction to the community. Either way, orien-

tation for every resident should include all of the items on an orientation checklist. (An example of an orientation checklist can be found at the end of this chapter.)

EMERGENCY INFORMATION

A multiple-copy emergency medical card (Exhibit 15.1) should be completed before move-in. The information can be obtained at the time the lease is signed or during the move-in coordination process. The card should be kept in an emergency card box at the concierge desk and/or in the personal care/assisted living center. In the event of an emergency, the card will be readily available so that the concierge or other responding staff can relay pertinent information to emergency medical personnel via telephone. A copy of the emergency medical card should go into the resident's file. For quick reference, attach the emergency medical card to the front inside cover of the resident's file. The emergency medical card can also be packaged in a clear plastic bag and attached to the front of the resident's refrigerator where the paramedics can have quick access to it. A piece of red paper in the bag will help draw attention to it.

UPDATES. The emergency medical card should be updated on an as-needed basis. Staff should make themselves aware of changes in residents' doctors, medications, allergies, family phone numbers, and so on. Memos requesting that residents update their cards should be distributed twice a year.

NOTIFICATION. Only the executive director or cabinet staff should notify family members of a resident emergency or illness. All consideration must be given to the residents' privacy.

UNDERSTANDING THE HOME SALE MARKET

The principal goal of the move-in coordinator is to *accelerate* the move-in time frame and to facilitate a *smooth* transition into the community while releasing the sales staff to pursue other prospects. Many residents will need to sell their homes before moving into their new apartments. It is helpful for the move-in coordinator to be familiar with some basics about the home-sales marketing strategy and the subsequent escrow closing. Understanding the home-sales market and methodology will equip move-in coordinators to

---

Exhibit 15.1   Emergency Medical Card

Name: _____   Apt. no.: _____ Phone: _____

Date of birth: _____   Marital status: _____

Living will? ☐ Yes ☐ No

Known medical conditions (stroke, heart attack, diabetes, etc.):

_____

Known allergies or reactions to medications:

_____

_____

Pacemaker? ☐ Yes ☐ No

Diet restrictions? (list)

_____

_____

- -

In case of emergency, please notify:

Name	Name
Address	Address
City, State, Zip	City, State, Zip
Phone number	Phone number
Physician	Office phone
Address	After-hours phone

Hospital preference: _____

Copy of supplemental insurance cards   *Copy of Medicare card*

---

advise prospects on the marketability of a prospect's home and provide counsel to prospects whose homes may be slow to sell.

Many prospects have owned their homes for years and have watched their values increase dramatically, and for most their home equity represents their single biggest investment. To offset fears of outliving their equity, and as an excuse to delay their decision to move, they will sometimes list their homes for sale considerably above market value. Realtors will accept these listings because they will receive a commission if *anyone* sells the home.

THE LISTING. Normally, when prospects sell their homes they utilize the services of a residential realtor. Although they may charge the resident up to 8 percent of the sales price as a commission (less as the price of the home increases), the realtor they select will have the ability to market the home professionally through the multiple listing service. The multiple listing service is an organization that publishes a monthly listing and description of every home on the market for sale by professional realtors. This advertisement gives the home much more exposure than could be achieved through a "for sale by owner" strategy. The home will be listed according to price and area. This list is distributed to every real estate agent in the area. The primary source of marketing the home is to other real estate agents in the market area. Several top realtors should be asked to prepare a listing presentation, which normally includes a *comparative market analysis,* a detailed analysis of value based on comparative home sales in the area. It includes the essential elements of a home appraisal and recommends a listing price and a sales strategy. If the homeowner is unsatisfied with the suggested sales price, then it may be advisable to have the home appraised by a certified Member Appraisal Institute appraiser. The listing agent should also create an information guide to the home, complete with an attractive photo, to serve as a handout for people who visit. The homeowner should evaluate the presentation not only on the recommended price but also on the realtor's track record and projected length of time to sell. A listing agreement is usually signed to establish the parameters for selling the home and the fees charged. These agreements are usually made for a minimum of six months. Shorter agreements usually will command more attention by the real estate agent. Normally, the listing agreement may be terminated before its expiry date, without obligation, by the seller if she is dissatisfied with the listing agent's progress in selling the home.

PRICE. The single biggest factor affecting the length of sale of the property is the list price. When the home is priced above its market value, the number of prospective buyers who want to see the home is reduced. When it is priced below market value, the amount of interest increases. The key is to match the list price with the selling goal. If the seller wants a quick sale, then the home should be priced competitively. For example, in any given market, a home priced at fair market value will attract about 60 percent of the prospective buyers looking to purchase. At 5 percent *below* market the home will attract 80 percent, and at 10 percent *below* it will attract 90 percent of the prospective buyers. Conversely, if the home is priced at 5 percent *above* market value it will attract only 30 percent of the prospective buyers, and at 10 percent *above* it will attract virtually no one. A high price on the home can make other homes more attractive; fewer salespeople will show the home, fewer prospects will respond to ads, and the seller may run the risk of losing buyers who

may be willing to negotiate. The maximum attention that a home will receive will be from the second to the fifth week. After the fifth week, if the home has not had an offer, the activity level will decline sharply. Therefore, it is critical that the home is priced accurately during the first five weeks. If the home has not had any offers during this period, something is wrong and the price should be reevaluated.

THE SALES PROCESS. Upon listing the home, the listing office will erect at its expense a "for sale" sign on the property and announce the new listing to its office realtors during their weekly meetings. All agents of the listing office preview new listings of the office each week. The listing realtor will hold a broker's open house where the other real estate companies are invited to view the home before the general public. Food is usually served at this function to entice other agents to view the home, and it is held midweek (usually on Thursday). Normally, other agents will come to see the home if they have a current client in that price range— or if the food is good! The agent who sells the home generally receives a 3 percent commission. The listing agent will receive twice the commission (6%) if he sells a listing, but this rarely happens; obviously, the more the exposure the quicker the sale. Each time a home is visited, or "shown," the law requires the visiting agent to leave her business card. The listing agent should follow up with salespeople who have showed the property and communicate their responses to the seller. Therefore, the more cards and the more showings, the more likely an offer will follow. Too few cards may indicate that a listing is too expensive, poorly marketed, or undesirable for some other reason. Agents who already have more than 10 listings will have little time to pay proper attention to each. If the listings are not worked aggressively they quickly become stale, and clients may be well advised to terminate the listing agreement and hire another realtor.

In addition to brokers' open houses, the agent should also hold twice monthly public open houses on Sunday to expose the home to passersby and neighbors. A desirable home with good curb appeal in a good location should attract between 50 and 100 prospects on a sunny day. The public open houses should be advertised in the Sunday paper, along with a photo. Some larger real estate firms even advertise Sunday open homes on television.

An *earnest money agreement* is normally used to establish intent by a buyer to purchase the home and provides a nominal deposit (1–5%) to the seller. This agreement outlines in general terms the proposed price and method of payment. After negotiation, the agreement is followed by a *purchase and sale agreement* for cash sales or a *real estate contract* if the seller is offering terms to carry back a note on all or a portion of the sales price. Once the purchase agreement or contract has been signed, the deposit is normally increased to 10 percent of the purchase price. The real estate agent should continue to market the home and solicit backup offers in the event the sale falls through. This can happen quite often owing to the buyer's inability to consummate the deal or failure to perform on a contingency. A contingency is a clause in a contract that protects the buyer against unforeseen difficulties in closing. For example, the sale may be contingent on the sale of the buyer's existing home, on the buyer's ability to secure acceptable financing, or on an engineer's inspection and approval. If any of these should fail, the deal is normally off; all deposits are returned and the seller and the buyer have no further obligations to each other. Depending on the nature of the contingency, some sales may be tenuous at best. After contingencies have been cleared, the transaction is turned over to an attorney or escrow agent for closing.

ESCROW AND CLOSING. Deals can be killed in escrow as well. During this time, the buyer will have selected a title insurance company and applied for a loan to finance the purchase. The mortgage broker will conduct research on the buyer to determine creditworthiness and submit the loan application to the company's underwriting committee for approval. This committee will assess the risk and recommend approval or rejection. If the loan is rejected or some problem is discovered during the title search, or if the engineer discovers some irreconcilable problem that cannot be negotiated to resolution, the deal can dissolve.

The point of this description of the pitfalls of real estate sales is to emphasize the importance of continuing to market the home. The move-in coordinator needs to be in constant contact with the prospect to ensure that the sale of the home moves quickly toward its logical conclusion so that the subsequent move into the community can be made without delay. If the home is not showed on a regular basis, then the problem needs to be uncovered. That problem is usually its price. The seller may need further counseling or advice on the opportunity costs associated with holding a home on the market too long. In fact, lengthy delays caused by unrealistic price expectations could work against the marketability of the home altogether. Realtors look for a good deal for their clients and will avoid overpriced homes in favor of those to which they can steer their clients toward a quick sale. Conversely, a sales price resulting in lower than expected net after tax proceeds may effect the prospect's ability to qualify financially for the senior living community.

During the fill-up stage of a community, sales counselors are typically very flexible on scheduling the move-in date. The longer the delay, the less likely the sale will result in a move-in. Move-in time frames allowing longer than 60 days do not create any sense of urgency in the prospect to move in, and actual dates become meaningless. The prospect should be encouraged to pick out a particular unit and be prepared to pay rent on that unit if someone else becomes interested in it, or else run the risk of losing his *choice* unit. During the home sales process the move-in coordinator should periodically ask the prospect about the frequency of showings and other sales activity of the home. If the home does not have activity at least weekly, then there could be a problem that could ultimately further delay the eventual move-in. On receipt of a bona fide offer, it may be helpful to advise the prospect of the importance of backup offers, especially if there are any contingencies.

■ MANAGING MOVE-OUTS

Moving a resident out of the community should be given as much care as moving a new resident in. The move-out is likely to be more traumatic than the move-in, so considerable attention should be paid to the resident or family to help organize the move.

Residents are responsible for removing all furniture, food, and personal belongings from the apartment. The apartment should be left in "broom clean" condition. Small picture holes and marks on the wall should be repaired when the apartment is being repainted; these constitute normal wear and tear.

Residents should be held responsible for removing all garbage to the outside bins, inasmuch as other residents may not be able to get to the garbage rooms when they are cluttered with large amounts of move-out debris. The housekeeping department should be on call to provide assistance if the resident wishes to have the garbage removed for a small fee. In addition, the maintenance department should be notified in advance to assist with any furniture breakdown that the movers will not provide.

There should be no prorates allowed on move-out. Most states will allow more than a 30-day move-out time, but some states require that the apartment be vacated five days before the lease expires to allow the landlord to return the apartment to rentable condition. This means that the lessee may need to move out on the 26th for the apartment to be available on the 1st. If the community maintains a waiting list, the new lessee should pay rent starting when the apartment is in move-in condition, if possible. If the lessee is not willing to take the apartment it may go to the next in line. In other words, move-ins should not be prorated to minimize the possible loss of revenue on the unit.

The security deposit should not be considered the last month's rent. Upon move-out, the resident services director or maintenance personnel should inspect the apartment for any damages. Normal wear and tear is not considered a damage to the premises. Chargeable damages normally include damage to carpeting less than five years old, damage to window coverings that belong to the building, and damage to wallpaper. Any room that has been painted a color other than white should be returned to its original color. Any structural changes to the apartment must be undone to return it to original condition unless the change has been approved by the executive director in writing. The resident can arrange to have the damages repaired if the executive director approves this in advance. The security deposit should be returned within 30 days of the *actual* move-out, unless otherwise specified by state law.

All turnover apartments should be given priority above all except emergency work orders to return the unit to move-in condition within 48 hours of move-out. Any painting and repair work should be scheduled in advance of the lease ending date. Be sure to obtain the resident or responsible party's permission to enter the apartment for this purpose prior to the lease expiration date. The vacant apartment should be thoroughly cleaned immediately after maintenance is finished and should be left in "showable" condition. Maintenance should anticipate the need to order parts or fixtures for the unit. With the resident's or family's permission, apartments should be made available to the marketing department so that they can be shown before the residents have vacated them. Maintenance should clean up their messes so that the apartment is always in "showable" condition.

As the community nears full occupancy, the ability to manage the final few units proactively can make a big difference to the bottom line. For example, the difference in cash value of 95 percent occupancy of a 200-unit project and 100 percent occupancy at an average rate of $2,100 per month is $252,000 per year. At an 11 percent capitalization rate, this can add $2,291,000 value to the property. The incremental expenses associated with these additional units are minimal at this occupancy level. In addition, marketing should evaluate the current market rate for each vacated apartment as they become available and at least semiannually for all units in the community. All re-leased reduced-rent apartments should be moved up to the current market rate, regardless of the budgeted percent rate increase or average revenue per unit projections. The vacated unit should be repriced at *market rate,* not the rate the previous tenant was paying.

A follow-up call to the family should be made by the resident services coordinator or the executive director to confirm receipt of the security deposit, to offer the community's best wishes, and to ask for an evaluation of their experience at the community. Upon the death of a resident, the family should be asked if they would like to have the move-out coordinated and the apartment cleaned.

Exhibit 15.2 **Checklists**

MASTER CHECKLIST

Name _____

Apartment number _____

_____ Review client's special needs with marketing representative.

_____ Make initial contact with client.

_____ Make sure the medical form and application for residency are complete and that file has been approved by the executive director.

_____ Confirm that a realtor has been contacted (or that notice has been given if the client lives in an apartment).

_____ Schedule home visit to measure furniture and develop floor plan.

_____ Confirm that mover has been selected.

_____ Plan garage sale, estate sale, or other method of disposing of property.

_____ Locate storage facility, if needed.

_____ Contact telephone company to transfer service.

_____ Complete change-of-address card; contact post office.

_____ Transfer newspaper subscription.

_____ Call utility company to cancel existing service (done by client).

_____ *Important!* Make sure that the family has marked all clothing, glasses, and assistive devices with the resident's name before move-in.

_____ Conduct apartment walk-through.

_____ Confirm mover.

_____ Deliver amenity basket to apartment (toiletries).

_____ Check phone jack to be sure service is connected.

_____ Contact welcome committee.

_____ Be sure orientation package is complete.

_____ Visit new resident and schedule an orientation date.

MOVE-IN CHECKLIST

Resident _____

Apartment number _____

30 days before move-in

_____ 1. Sit in on lease-signing to meet with and establish a personal relationship with the lessee. Deliver and discuss resident handbook policies.

_____ 2. Schedule a home visit to counsel the lessee and discuss the move-in process. Establish a move-in time frame. Provide moving company referrals.

_____ 3. Be present in the lessee's home when moving company estimates are given.

_____ 4. Arrange with several real estate companies (if appropriate) to do a free comparative market analysis of the lessee's home and make listing presentations.

_____ 5. Make personal phone contact weekly to answer questions or concerns. Keep lessee updated on any maintenance requested on apartment—e.g., painting, wallpapering, etc.

_____ 6. Be sure all forms required for residency (e.g., application for residency, medical form) are submitted on a timely basis and that the resident's file is approved by the executive director prior to move-in.

(continued)

Exhibit 15.2 Checklists *(continued)*

Two weeks (minimum) before move-in

_____ 1. Inspect the apartment. Notify in writing appropriate departments (housekeeping, maintenance, dining room) of arrival.

_____ 2. Notify the resident relations staff so that they can be ready with welcome information/orientation for new resident.

_____ 3. Confirm that telephone service (and any other utilities) will be transferred on the date of the move.

_____ 4. Notify the community's postal carrier for the community of the new resident's name and apartment number.

_____ 5. Mail change-of-address cards to the local postmaster.

_____ 6. Call and confirm the mover.

_____ 7. Include the new resident in the community resident directory.

_____ 8. Order a name tag for the new resident. This will help existing residents get to know the new resident and will also help the new resident begin to feel like part of the community.

Two days before move-in

_____ 1. Conduct apartment walk-through: check all light fixtures, activate appliances, set clock on stove, etc.

_____ 2. Assemble a move-in package and attractively display the contents in the kitchen of the apartment: collateral and basket of amenities, resident newsletter and activities calendar, complimentary meal tickets, resident directory, telephone directory, Chamber of Commerce information (for out-of-state moves), cable television information, a welcome card signed by the staff. Post transportation schedule and dining room hours on refrigerator.

_____ 3. Involve welcome committee or arrange for a resident with similar interests or hobbies, to escort the new resident to dinner on move-in day.

_____ 4. Write maintenance ticket for television connection.

Moving day

_____ 1. Provide two folding chairs for the apartment.

_____ 2. Check to see that a welcome snack/fruit basket and beverages have been placed in refrigerator by the housekeeping staff. Provide coffee for the resident and family.

_____ 3. Place a welcome plant on a shelf outside the resident's door, or have a member of the welcome committee deliver it personally.

_____ 4. Turn on heat/air when appropriate.

_____ 5. Notify concierge staff of resident's name, estimated time of arrival, apartment number, and telephone number.

_____ 6. Check the resident's mailbox to see that a previous resident's mail is not in it.

_____ 7. Greet the new resident, escort her to the apartment, issue keys, have her sign the new-resident form, and get her situated.

_____ 8. Be sure to have lunch certificates available for the resident and family or friends who are helping with the move.

_____ 9. Greet movers, show them to the apartment, and restate any appropriate policies (damage, elevator availability and lock-off, refuse disposal, any time constraints).

_____ 10. Reconfirm the new resident's dinner escort.

_____ 11. Install telephones and confirm active telephone service.

_____ 12. Stay with the new resident until after the bed is made up, bath linens have been unpacked, apartment has sufficient lighting in place, traffic paths have been cleared, alarm clock and telephone are placed by bed, necessary medications and toiletries have been unpacked, the television has been connected, the emergency response system has been tested, and the new resident feels secure.

_____ 13. If the new resident seems overwhelmed, offer room service on the first night at the community.

(continued)

Exhibit 15.2 Checklists *(continued)*

Upon move-in

_____ 1. Review the resident handbook with the new resident, including policies and procedures, a map of the community areas, and the community's organizational chart.

_____ 2. Schedule appointments for all cabinet members to personally visit the new resident and discuss the services available through their respective departments. (These meetings should ideally take place within one week of move-in.)

Department	Contact	Date
Resident relations		
Dining room		
Kitchen/chef		
Maintenance		
Housekeeping		
Programming		

_____ 3. Send a notice to all residents with some general information about the new resident (where from, hobbies, etc.). Be sure to get the new resident's permission first!

_____ 4. Post a photo (a Polaroid is fine) of the new resident near resident mailboxes along with a "welcome" sign. (Again, get the new resident's permission first.)

_____ 5. Post a photo of the new resident in the employee cafeteria so that employees will begin to associate the new resident's face with his name.

_____ 6. Schedule two hours to help the new resident get acclimated to her apartment, unpack, hang pictures, and so forth. Some general comforting will be in order.

_____ 7. Schedule resident orientation.

If a new resident must stay in a guest room while waiting for furnishings to be delivered, no charge should be assessed. Rent and meal allowances, however, should begin at this time.

RESIDENT ORIENTATION CHECKLIST

Resident _____

Apartment number _____

Community areas

Tour of all common areas and refer to the types of activities that occur in each.

_____ Concierge desk and the services coordinated there (transportation, parcel deliveries, maintenance requests, program sign-up, etc.)

_____ Administrative offices and functions performed there (billing, etc.)

_____ Cabinet members' offices (reiterate who handles what)

_____ Dining areas (select seating time)

_____ Mail area (explain use of in-house mailboxes)

_____ Commissary (hours, information on volunteering)

_____ Beauty shop (hours, services provided)

_____ Library (policies for use)

_____ Art Studio (describe classes, activities)

_____ Health Club (hours, classes, use of equipment)

Also discuss the following:

_____ How to sign up for events

_____ How to sign up for and use transportation

_____ How to make lunch/dinner reservations for guests

_____ How to arrange for room service

(continued)

Exhibit 15.2 Checklists *(continued)*

Orientation: Resident's Apartment

Many aspects of a resident's own apartment will take some getting used to before he or she can feel settled. *Apartment orientation* should take place just before the move or on moving day itself and should cover the following:

_____ How to lock and unlock the door properly
_____ How to open mailbox
_____ Location of light switches and corresponding sockets
_____ How to set and reset electrical outlets
_____ In-depth demonstration of climate control system
_____ Explanation of circuit breaker box
_____ Explanation of emergency generator

_____ How to work kitchen range, timer, overhead hood (fan and light)
_____ Refrigerator setting and icemaker operation
_____ Garbage disposal operation
_____ Bathtub stopper
_____ How to open, close, and lock windows
_____ How to operate window blinds
_____ Emergency assistance pull cords
_____ Garbage collection procedures
_____ Use of laundry facilities

MOVE-IN COORDINATION SERVICES

- Organizing the details of your move
- Providing information about moving, packing, storage, and furniture rental companies
- Coordinating the logistics of your move with the moving company
- Assisting with the planning and organizing of garage sales and/or estate sales
- Assisting with furniture measurement and placement
- Helping with the selection and placement of household items
- Transferring telephone service or ordering new service
- Handling details at the U.S. Post Office, such as change-of-address forms
- Transferring newspaper and magazine subscriptions
- Conducting apartment and community orientation

CHANGE-OF-ADDRESS FORMS

Enclosed in this packet you will find a change-of-address form to be sent to your local post office branch. The form has been filled out and needs only your signature in order to start the change.

If you like, you can request that your mail be sent to the community beginning a few days prior to move-in. Please send this form to the post office as soon as your move-in date has been confirmed.

Once you send in your change-of-address form, you will receive a moving kit from the post office. It will contain change-of-address notification cards to be used to inform all sources of correspondence of your new address.

Your mail will be forwarded to the community by the post office for six months, beginning on the start date provided on your change-of-address card; therefore, it is very important to send out the notification cards on a timely basis. If you would like assistance filling out the cards, please bring them by on your next visit, or I will come to your home and help you fill them out.

It is recommended that you inform Social Security in writing of your new address.

Your new address will be: *Your address including apartment number:*

_____   _____

_____   _____

_____   _____

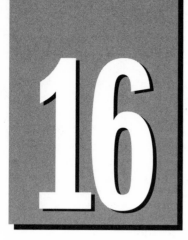

16 Aging in Place

Operating and Marketing Stabilized Communities

The issue of aging in place and its resulting effect on lowering facility census is a constant battle affecting retirement communities. Understanding the problem from the conception of the project, evaluating potential risks, and being prepared with specific operational solutions can substantially improve your financial results.

As many Americans age, their ability to perform the normal activities of their daily lives becomes restricted. The daily routine of caring for themselves and their living environment can become difficult. As seniors become less able to meet these challenges, they turn to their families for help and support, and chores such as home maintenance, cleaning, grocery shopping, and transportation can therefore become a burden on seniors and their families alike. This can lead to stress in the relationship and feelings of guilt because seniors do not want to impose on their families' already busy schedules. In the end, their quality of life usually suffers. The fact is, the Handling of Everyday Life Problems can spell HELP for many of America's seniors.

It is not hard to understand why an ever increasing number of seniors and their families have turned to retirement centers for answers. It can be argued that when seniors inquire at independent-living retirement centers, they are in fact taking a major step for the first time in their lives toward declaring their own dependence.

■ ANALYSIS

All too many retirement housing projects were developed in the 1980s by uninformed analysts whose idea of the typical resident was someone over the age of 65 with an annual income in excess of $25,000 per year. Demographic studies were carried out to support a tremendous demand for alternative lifestyle choices among this population, and new projects popped up in major cities across the country. Those seniors who were already aware and in need of a supportive lifestyle were quickly absorbed. Consequently, operators who were slow to fill their projects progressively lowered their selection criteria to admit more frail residents, in efforts to fill their buildings as projected.

Newly developed retirement communities market to primarily active, healthy seniors through stringent admission standards with the proviso that lease agreements will be terminated if impairment develops. These communities encourage independent behavior through management and programming. Where strong markets exist, this scenario will lengthen the average stay and consequently reduce unit turnover. In competitive markets, however, admission standards tend to become more relaxed, and additional services are offered to cater to a more independent population. The active residents who moved in when the project opened will eventually age in place and be joined or replaced by new residents who fit the current, more frail profile in the project. Continuing-care retirement communities have been successful at creating a balanced community that accommodates all levels of care while maintaining an environment for active, independent seniors. As the average age and acuity of residents increases, attracting and marketing to younger retirees can be a considerable challenge. Over time, if left unchecked, as the project struggles to reach cash flow, the average stay for each resident shortens, resulting in an ever-increasing percentage of the resident population turning over annually. This problem is further compounded by the construction of new and modern retirement centers in the same service areas that initially attracted the active market, leaving the older facilities to absorb the frail and limited-income constituents of the market population.

DESTINATIONS

All discharges from retirement housing facilities can be categorized as either involuntary or voluntary.

Involuntary discharges are normally those residents who expire or need higher levels of care than can be provided in retirement communities. Involuntary discharges account for about 78 percent of all discharges from facilities nationwide. Studies have shown that disability increases dramatically as people approach the age of 85 and older; 65 percent of this age group has some disability, compared to only about 15 percent disability in the 65–75 age group. A report on retirement housing published by Laventhol and Horwath indicates that residents with an average age of 81 live in retirement centers. This number increases to 85 for facilities built before 1970. As a project ages, you can expect an increase in the proportion of involuntary discharges.[1]

Voluntary discharges account for the remaining 22 percent and can be broken down by family, cost, unhappiness, and miscellaneous reasons. Family discharges include those residents who move to be closer to their families or actually move in with them. Follow-up surveys have revealed that the primary motivation for this type of discharge may be financial. In depressed areas of the country, we have seen the children of the residents discharging them to their own care, often depending on their parents' Social Security check to help make ends meet. Or the retirees exhaust their savings and are unable to live in a retirement community on Social Security, even if supplemented by their families. Many residents are discharged to a long-term care facility that accepts Medicaid residents simply because they can no longer afford to live independently in a retirement community. Family discharges account for 70 percent of all voluntary turnover. The remaining 30 percent may leave because of cost considerations, resident dissatisfaction, or other reasons (Figure 16.1).

Discharges for cost considerations are the result of rent increases and can be significant in price-sensitive markets. When pricing the service package, it is prudent to tailor the facility's amenities to the image and affordability of the local target market. Any change to the pricing structure should reflect quality while demonstrating value. Residents who are living on 80–90 percent of their monthly income can be significantly impacted by rent increases. The introduction of optional programs such as long-term care insurance may also restrict the facility's ability to increase rents, inasmuch as the monthly premiums could absorb any remaining disposable income the resident may have.

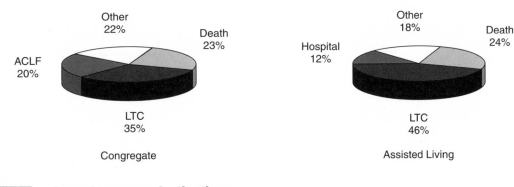

Figure 16.1   Annual turnover destinations

Source: Data from the Assisted Living Marketplace: A Report to Ciba-Geigy Corporation, *Marketing Solutions,* March 22, 1995.

Resident satisfaction is the best retention and marketing tool. Although you may not be able to please all of your residents all the time, this turnover rate should be less than 1 percent.

Other reasons for voluntary discharge may involve transportation issues, problems with a sense of belonging or assimilation into the community, recuperation, moving back into a home or to an apartment, or even marriage.

GEOGRAPHIC DIFFERENCES

It is important to understand how geographical differences and their corresponding motivations can affect facility turnover. The southern regions of the country are usually retirement destinations. More than half of the elderly persons who migrate to other states move to Arizona, Florida, and California. Seniors who move to these areas to retire are generally more active, affluent, and motivated by desire. Discharges to assisted-living facilities from independent retirement communities can represent up to 30 percent of the total annual turnover in the southern regions, versus 13 percent in the northern and midwestern states. This can be explained by the affordability of this option to the more affluent transplants. Conversely, in the northern regions, we find significantly more discharges to long-term care facilities or back to the care of the family. Seniors will remain living in their homes until forced to seek alternate living arrangements for health reasons. The typical resident admitted to the local retirement community is generally need-driven and is influenced to a large degree by his family or personal physician. Northern-region facilities will experience a considerably higher voluntary discharge rate primarily due to the depletion of residents' personal assets.

As seniors' physical dependency increases, their financial burden will rise concurrently. Inflation is the greatest enemy of a fixed income. The purchasing power of each dollar of a 65-year-old's income will be reduced 50 percent by the time she turns 80, just about the time she starts looking to retirement centers for answers to health and lifestyle concerns.

COSTS OF TURNOVERS

The effect of turnover is manageable in a full facility, but the longer it takes to fill a facility, the greater the risk aging in place can have on census-building efforts. Projects that cannot achieve full occupancy in 18–24 months will experience the combined effect of marketing empty apartments plus replacing apartments vacated by discharged residents admitted when the facility first opened. For example, a 200-unit project with a 25 percent turnover will need to rent 4.17 units per month just to break even with its turnover (Figure 16.2). At an average marketing cost per unit of $2,000, a $100,000 budget in advertising and marketing will be required without increasing your net census by one unit (Figure 16.3). The accumulation of working capital on the balance sheet under this scenario has tipped the scales between success and failure on many well-conceived projects that were slow to fill. In facilities that are one to nine years old, overall averages for turnover per 100 ranged from 1.7 units in newer projects to 35.2 units in the oldest projects, with a national average of 16 units. Northern states' facilities generally have higher involuntary turnover when compared to Sunbelt states due to a higher acuity level.[2]

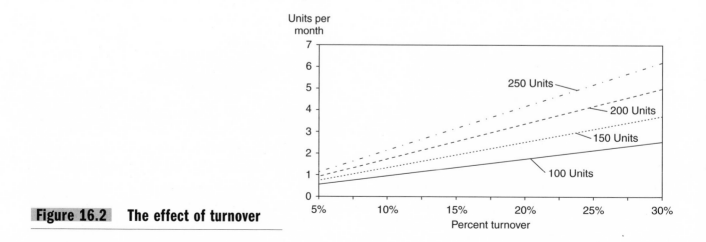

Figure 16.2   The effect of turnover

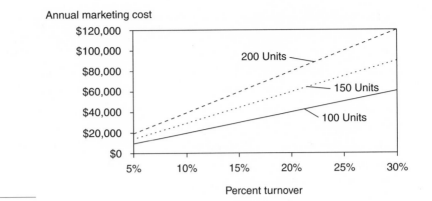

Figure 16.3   Costs of turnover

SOLUTIONS

Before Admission

The best way to minimize the effect of resident turnover is through proper marketing planning and prequalification. Focus groups, independent surveys, and thorough research of the community in which the project will be constructed are essential. Such studies will enable the developer to focus accurately on the needs and perceptions of the existing residents without second guessing 10-year-old census data. Armed with this feedback, the developer will be better able to match the facility unit mix and amenities to target the local market. Appropriate market positioning and image development that emphasize value and cater to the local resident profile can significantly shorten the project fill-up period.

Upon opening the facility, establish specific selection criteria for whom you can accept and how this kind of person fits into your service package. It is helpful to establish an admission evaluation committee to review each applicant to ensure appropriate placement. Medical profiles or doctor references can be useful to determine the applicant's condition of health and his ability to live with relative independence. Some facilities have financing that may require compliance with certain income-eligibility requirements. Routine financial information provided by the residents can alert marketing staff to the eventual need for financial counseling and allow management to calculate turnover as various rent increases are imposed.

Guest apartments can also be useful in providing respite care or admissions on a trial basis for questionable applicants. Gift certificates for respite care or beauty-shop appointments offered to the family will not only allow you to evaluate potential applicants, but also help dispel "buyer's remorse" on the part of those on deposit by quickly assimilating them into your community lifestyle. It is much easier to convince a reluctant prospect to "try it for a few weeks and keep your home. If you like it [60–70% of short-stay visitors convert to permanent residents], then you can execute a lease." This approach provides the family with a welcome opportunity to solve their crisis through a series of gradual steps rather than trying to convince a parent to leave her home, sell the house, dispose of her belongings, and assimilate into a community environment all at once.

After Admission

For many seniors, the adjustment after years of living alone to living in a community environment can be difficult. A thorough orientation to the facility by each department head and a resident hospitality committee can help assimilate new residents to the retirement-community lifestyle and generate a sense of belonging. The process should last a minimum of three months, and, if handled well, can result in additional referrals as new residents communicate their experiences to family and friends. Teach your staff to recognize these first few critical months and reward them with a resident-retention bonus, if appropriate.

One of the biggest challenges management faces is dealing with preconceived attitudes about aging among residents and staff. It is commonly perceived by both that upon admission to a retirement community, the resident's health will deteriorate over time. Proper orientation to an active, healthy lifestyle by the staff can cut turnover significantly. If residents think they are happy and healthy, they generally are.

Conversely, if they are focused on their personal limitations, their health usually suffers. In addition, negative feedback of management's performance can occur as the health of a resident or the resident's spouse declines. Enrichment programs designed to slow the aging process and encourage independence can be a significant retention tool. Leisure-interest surveys taken on admission can be used to develop activity programs of interest to the residents and can generate a sense of purpose.

Personal-care and concierge programs that provide assistance with dressing, bathing, medication reminders, and the like are usually welcomed options that can provide a cushion of care to your residents should it occasionally be needed. The balance between frail and active residents is a delicate one. Management must be able to provide services to those who require them while keeping the community image intact. Recuperation from a fall or illness can be handled discreetly within your facility for short periods of time. However, if the problems become chronic, it is advisable to discharge the resident. The emphasis on admitting appropriate residents should also apply to discharging those to whom you can no longer give the needed level of care. Resist the temptation to hold on to your marginal residents, inasmuch as this attachment may hurt your overall resident profile and may expose you to legal or ethical liability.

Wellness programs designed to promote health awareness can alert management to potential problems and position the facility with a rehabilitation focus. During the flu season, the risk of sickness that can trigger a permanent discharge can escalate. Annual flu inoculations for all residents should be scheduled in the fall to minimize this risk. It is advisable to obtain a written physician's order before the injection. A registered nurse consultant visiting weekly to monitor blood pressures, body weights, and exercise programs can also be warmly received by the residents and their families.

Issues of transportation to families, doctors' appointments, shopping, and church meetings may become restrictive in larger buildings and may also trigger a discharge. Many communities have well-developed transportation resources sponsored by the metro bus service, church groups, senior advocacy groups, and volunteers. A well-organized referral directory to these options should be able to accommodate just about everyone.

Many facilities convert all or a portion of their physical plant to assisted living to help slow their "back door" traffic. Two very important considerations must be addressed before such a conversion is made. First, in most states assisted living is regulated under the jurisdiction of state health departments. These regulations are usually specific regarding the physical plant, and consequences for noncompliance or non-licensure can be severe. Second, it may be inappropriate to mix independent residents with those in assisted living, particularly at meal times. A separate dining room and activities area must be provided to run a successful program. Retrofits can provide a profitable vehicle to drive up facility census, and developers would be well advised to consider assisted living specifications when designing independent retirement communities for maximum flexibility. Remember to step up marketing efforts after converting to assisted living, inasmuch as the higher acuity level in those units will surely accelerate unit turnover.

Before Discharge

Problems that could lead to discharge must be dealt with swiftly. Quarterly review conferences should be held with the families and key facility staff to discuss potential problems and concerns, if appropriate. Many issues can be quickly resolved with early intervention. These conferences can be a valuable source of information about resident satisfaction and health, dietary, and affordability issues. Many creative solutions can be found to ease certain financial restraints. These options range from cash subsidies to reverse mortgages, sale-leaseback agreements, and other strategies that may even offer tax breaks for the family. Facilities that have researched the community for legal resources specializing in these areas can substantially control affordability-related discharges.

Resident endorsements are the best advertisement. Residents define quality as simply the difference between what they expect and what they get. If management consistently delivers more than they expect, residents will perceive the community as a quality operation. Frequent resident meetings and annual satisfaction surveys can help keep lines of communication open and allow management to tailor services and programs to meet and exceed residents' expectations. The more management can find out about what residents want from the community, the better job it can do at delivering it. As a rule, never overpromise and underdeliver. Teach your staff to represent the facility competently. The facility should not lose any residents as a result of satisfaction issues if all residents are treated fairly and consistently.

Senior advocacy groups can be found in most communities that specialize in providing support services to the elderly. Facilities that organize a directory of information on these sources not only have a database to draw on for their own residents' needs, but also position themselves as a source of referrals and information on senior issues in their community.

Where appropriate, shared living or semiprivate occupancy in larger units can be a solution for financially or emotionally unstable residents. Simultaneously, this concept can add substantially to the average revenue per unit while reducing turnover.

A monthly visit by a physician advisor is an invaluable source for handling sensitive issues. The physician can check in on health problems and evaluate medication compatibility. We have found that many discharges can be caused by illness resulting from overmedication or incompatible medication. Residents or their families will purchase prescriptions from different pharmacies that check history only on medications they have dispensed. In a recent case, one resident who was feeling very ill was found to be taking 44 different medications from three pharmacies! Routine medical evaluations and medication monitoring will enable facilities to retain these residents and keep them healthier.

Home-health agencies have been useful in providing assistance with rehabilitation and activities of daily living where the facility is marketing to a frail population. The introduction of a home-health agency will have the effect of increasing the acuity of your average resident profile and over time develop a dependent population at the facility. The advantage to the residents is that they can receive Medicare-reimbursable care while remaining in their apartments. Be sure to check state licensure requirements before contracting this service on behalf of the residents.

After Discharge

Many residents or their families will be unclear about the reasons for their having been discharged. Proper counseling at the first sign of a problem will help uncover the best solution for all concerned. Additionally,

should issues be resolved that can lead to readmittance, the transition can be dealt with smoothly.

Facilities that have developed reciprocal arrangements with local nursing homes and acute-care hospitals have found these relationships beneficial to their existing residents. Short-duration admission to higher levels of care when health problems are first identified can make the difference between a temporary or permanent discharge. Allowing residents to keep their belongings intact in their apartments can facilitate an easy readmission during periods of reduced demand for resale of their unit.

Facilities that maintain contact with discharged residents on birthdays and other holidays, and through newsletter mailings, not only build good will in senior circles but also generate a family atmosphere that can draw voluntarily discharged residents back to the facility. Combine this with random follow-up exit interviews of residents or their families to give management the proper feedback to determine if discharge counseling was handled appropriately.

Retirement communities rely heavily on community support and endorsement for their livelihoods. Residents who are appropriately admitted, treated fairly, and discharged professionally and consistently will positively represent their experience to the community. The needs and wants of each resident must be held in balance with the objectives of the retirement community. Resident turnover is an integral element in this balance, and if planned for, evaluated, and understood, it can be a stabilizing factor necessary to keep your population thriving.

Along with aging in place come increased costs of operations and difficulty in recovering these costs from long-term residents. Clearly, as residents age and become more frail, they also experience a heightened sense of vulnerability and fear. This usually translates into more requests for additional staffing, night management coverage, and additional security. Normally these are the residents who have lived at the property the longest and are the least equipped to finance these increased operating costs through rent increases. Operators who can effectively manage the level of care at their property can avoid some of these potential pitfalls.

To meet the challenges resulting from the aging process successfully, facilities must create a clear vision of exactly where it is they want to take the business and define their critical operating assumptions.

Operators who understand the basic human problems associated with aging and are prepared with specific solutions can significantly manage their operations to reduce the impact that resident turnover can have on their performance.

In some circumstances, some turnover is actually healthy for the congregate operation. This is particularly true in operations marketing themselves to a younger, more independent clientele. Residents who have access to supportive services and home health care in their "independent" apartments are certainly entitled to do so under the protection of the Americans with Disabilities Act. The number of residents who will actually do so is in reality very low indeed. Operators who have limited physical options to provide a continuum of care on site and choose to deal with the aging in place phenomenon in-house need to understand that they may be changing the entire market position and image of their property over time. This is a very dangerous strategy, for not only does the operator expose herself to criticism from existing residents who will complain that "the place is starting to turn into a nursing home," or "this is not the type of lifestyle that I was sold on when I moved in two years ago," she also runs the risk of having to compete with some developer with a bright, shiny new facility for the independent, active, and affluent prospects in the marketplace. Many independent retirement communities have been run into the ground financially after defensively marketing to manage their turnover rather than offensively building a waiting list to manage their level of care and revenue.

OFFENSIVE VERSUS DEFENSIVE MARKETING: The Stabilized Community

Traditional approaches have employed "defensive" marketing tactics to sustain occupancy upon community stabilization. "Defensive" marketing is a *reactive* marketing strategy for managing ongoing turnover and is widely employed in the industry. Defensive marketing assumes significant cuts to the marketing budget, minimal staffing, and minimal sales compensation levels once the community finally fills. Although in most circumstances it may be advisable to scale back somewhat on marketing budgets, the potential disadvantages of assuming a defensive posture can outweigh the obvious cost-saving advantages. As with everything else, a

long-term winning strategy will seek to achieve a financial balance in the marketing program.[3]

As the marketing and advertising expenditures are scaled back, fewer leads are generated for a community. If the leads and subsequent closing ratios on each lead type are insufficient to cover turnover, several serious problems can result:

- Insufficient leads may result in longer time frames to obtain sales and move-ins, thus reducing anticipated apartment revenue. Difficulty in obtaining leases breeds potential for price concessions, which can result in further revenue shortfalls. More important, vacancies restrict the community's ability to command premium rate increases due to high supply.

- Communities may try to retain failing residents longer than is appropriate, raising ethical and regulatory concern regarding the provision of care in the most appropriate setting. As noted earlier, frailer residents may also erode the active image of the community, jeopardizing resident referrals and attracting frailer new prospects.

- Smaller marketing budgets often force sales staff to work harder with fewer resources and lower compensation levels. Staff members are then easily attracted to competitor communities, resulting in the loss of the invested time, energy, and money invested in training the top salespersons, who are the best human resources in the area at selling your community. This is also complicated by the need to retrain their replacement(s) and orienting them to the community's assets and character.

Offensive Management and Marketing

An alternative to succumbing to the pitfalls of defensive marketing is "offensive" marketing. Whereas defensive marketing manages turnover, "offensive" marketing is designed to manage proactively the profitability of a community. Offensive marketing tactics seek to minimize marketing expenditures without compromising a community's ability to maintain stabilized occupancy and maximize revenue. Offensive marketing provides the following assurances:

1. Sufficient leads are generated to keep pace with turnover. Sale and move-in time frames are minimized, thus achieving or exceeding apartment-revenue projections.

2. Resident acuity levels are optimized, such that failing residents are placed in the most appropriate care settings. By retaining the integrity of the community's "active" image, a community is better positioned to compete against new communities. This is particularly important for congregate rental communities that do not have the internal transfer option that continuing care retirement communities have for maintaining a more active profile, that is the ability to transfer from independent living to assisted living or nursing care as the resident's needs for additional support are realized.

3. Monthly fee increases on turnover units are maximized. Monthly fee increases on lease renewals can also be aggressively managed because turnovers can be filled quickly.

4. Price concessions are minimized because lead generation efforts generate sufficient demand to build a strong waiting list.

5. Top sales producers are retained because they have the resources to generate sufficient new leads to fill turnover, have the necessary sales staff to facilitate the sales process, and receive compensation that is competitive. Staff recruitment, training, and orientation costs are avoided.

The offensive marketing approach to the aging-in-place issue reduces a community's financial exposure by proactively managing turnover and its impact on revenue. Specific offensive strategies include maintaining a marginally higher staffing complement to work existing leads adequately and minimize staff burnout. Each lead represents the community's current assets, and, other than resident referrals, each lead represents money spent in advertising or other media that may result in future move-ins. Some communities have spent literally millions of dollars to build this lead bank and their presence in the marketplace. By reducing staffing levels too aggressively at stabilization, operators may be compromising the investments they have already made. All leads must be worked monthly in order to keep them fresh; operators should pare down staffing levels slowly as the size of the lead bank diminishes over time. At stabilized occupancy, lead banks are usually at their all-time high. Keeping a "baseline" presence in the media to avoid starting from scratch to rebuild awareness also protects the community's market position.

Operators should guard against the possibility of losing their top talent (and potentially many of their hot prospects) by maintaining a competitive and compelling compensation program that rewards staff for reaching goals in excess of budget. In addition, conducting ongoing sales training to reduce sale and move-in time frames and to keep staff motivated and challenged will also help to maintain the productivity momentum.

Offensive marketing reduces a community's financial exposure by proactively managing turnover and its corresponding impacts on gross revenue. An example of *not* following an offensive marketing approach is found in Table 16.1.

Offensive marketing offers the opportunity to add significant value to a senior-living investment. Through offensive marketing, these defensive-marketing pitfalls can be avoided—and $317,200 more in net annual operating income could result from our example. At a 12 percent capitalization rate,[4] approximately $2,643,000 in increase property value could be realized. Conservative reductions in the marketing budget at stabilization would clearly be justified.

An alternate way of examining this issue is to analyze the opportunity cost related to marketing defensively. Vacant units will result in lost cash flow and ultimately lost investment value for a community. For example, if 75 percent of the monthly fee is typically needed to cover fixed operating expenses and debt service, then each vacant unit reduces the contribution to those costs. A 200-unit community that stabilizes at 94 percent versus 99 percent represents an opportunity cost of $180,000 in lost revenue or $1,500,000 in lost value for the investment at a 12 percent capitalization rate (200 units × 99 percent = 198 units) − (200 units × 94 percent = 188 units) = 10 units × $2,000 per month × 12 months = $240,000 × 75 percent contribution to fixed operating expenses and debt service = $180,000/0.12 = $1,500,000.

A karate expert will tell you that the way to put your hand through a board is to focus beyond the board.[5] The only way to achieve 100 percent occupancy is first to convince the staff that it is possible, then look for opportunities to reach that visualization. The clearer the vision, the closer the goal.

Communities have traditionally focused on reducing operating and marketing expenses as buildings mature. However, only so much value can be added to

Table 16.1 **Defensive Marketing Pitfalls**

	Annual Loss
2 fewer units occupied in a month (e.g., $2,000 lost revenue × 2 units × 12 months)	($48,000)
2 slower move-ins (e.g., $2,000 lost revenue × 2 units × 12 months)	($48,000)
2 leases lost because existing residents look "too old" (e.g., $2,000 lost revenue × 2 units × 12 months)	($48,000)
No increase in unit turnover versus 5% increase (e.g., $2,000 × 5% = $100 per month × 12 months × 36 turnover units per year)	($43,200)
1% less on lease renewal rents because building not full (e.g., $2,000 × 1% = $20 per month × 12 months × 200 units)	($48,000)
Lease concessions equivalent to one month's rent (e.g., $2,000 × 36 units per year)	($72,000)
Cost of recruiting/training new marketing staff (e.g., $10,000 recruitment/training cost)	($10,000)
TOTAL	**($317,200)**

the investment by cutting expenses. The more aggressive the cuts, the less transparent the effect these cuts will have on the residents. They may soon notice that the service package is being reduced while their rents continue to go up, and they will react negatively, which will at least have an effect on referrals. In other words, at some point efforts to incorporate "operational efficiency" into the expense management could have diminishing returns as the residents are affected. A balance may be the best option. Communities that focus on a defensive expense-management strategy combined with an offensive revenue-enhancement strategy will better be able to provide additional value to the investment in the long run. The leveraged benefits of either revenue enhancement or expense reduction can be transparent to the residents while greatly enhancing the investment value. Even a modest combination of $50 per unit per month in increased revenue/or decreased expenses yields $10,000 per month, or $120,000 per year for a 200-unit project. The enhanced product value is over $1 million using

an 11 percent capitalization rate. This type of expense management can be made in most communities with minimal impact on residents or the marketing budget.

In summary, offensive marketing is a revenue-enhancement strategy, whereas defensive marketing is an expense-management strategy. Although both are important, potential revenue-generation opportunities clearly outweigh aggressive marketing-budget cutbacks for a stabilized community.

NOTES

1. B. W. Pearce, "How to Slow the Revolving Door," *Contemporary Long Term Care* 15(5) (Sept. 1992): 36.
2. B. W. Pearce, "Resident Turnover," *Retirement Community Business* 1(2) (Summer 1992): 12.
3. M. G. Leary and B. W. Pearce, "Offensive versus Defensive Marketing," *Retirement Community Business* 3(3) (May 1994): 10.
4. See Chapter 2 for a detailed analysis of capitalization rates.
5. D. Smith, "On Senior Housing," *Selling to Seniors,* January 1995, 5.

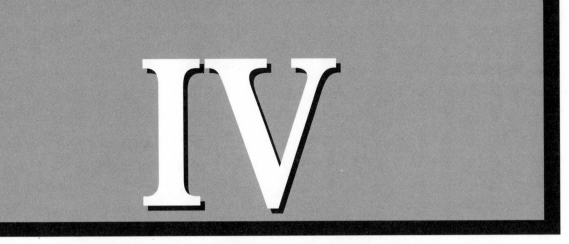

IV

Other Services

Personal Care

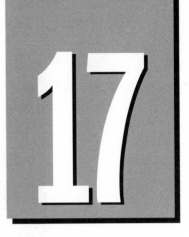

The introduction of personal care to the retirement community or the development of a freestanding assisted living community can be very attractive to seniors looking for cost-effective alternatives to home health care or institutionalization in a nursing home. As a rule, the cost of assisted living is only about two-thirds of equivalent care in a skilled nursing facility. The cost of delivering personal care in a multifamily residential environment such as an assisted-living community, as compared to purchasing home-health services that are individually delivered to each resident's home, is also driving the current boom in assisted living.

The typical resident of an assisted-living community is an 83-year-old female with 3.06 activity of daily living (ADL) deficiencies and some cognitive impairment. Residents stay an average of 2.38 years (28.5 months). Most (46%) are discharged to a nursing home or to a hospital (12%), which could involve a readmission.[1] A smaller number of discharges (24%) are due to death.

As people live longer, their personal care needs increase. Figure 17.1 illustrates the average personal-care needs for seniors 85 years of age and older from the general population. Fifty-seven percent of the population will require some assistance with the activities of daily living. Thirty-five percent need assistance with one or more ADL.

Acuity levels for residents in assisted living communities are considerably higher than those in the general population. Figure 17.2 illustrates actual residents living in assisted living communities in 1995. According to the figures, the highest assistance need is in bathing and medication reminders, followed by dressing and escort services.

The most common disease states encountered in the assisted living setting are arthritis (42.6%), dementia/emotional illness (33%), hypertension (28.1%), asthma/pulmonary disease (11.5%), and diabetes (10.6%).[2] The assisted living residents in the study averaged 2.9 diagnoses per resident. The percentage of residents suffering from incontinence has doubled from 15 percent in 1993 to 30.2 percent in 1996, indicating the effects of aging and increased acuity.[3] The most common are listed in Table 17.1. These residents are most often given cardiac drugs / diuretics (48.6%), CNS medications (46.3%), and laxatives/cathartics (17.2%). Thirty-five percent of residents had four to seven prescription records, and 19 percent had eight or more. These residents have clearly identified the need for assisted living and will have higher personal-care needs than those who may be living at home with family or other support.

The methods of delivery of the personal care component of assisted living vary greatly among providers, as does the staffing assignment. Typically, the equivalent monthly service package, which includes 24-hour supervision and 45 minutes per day in personal-care services, will only purchase about 6 hours per day of

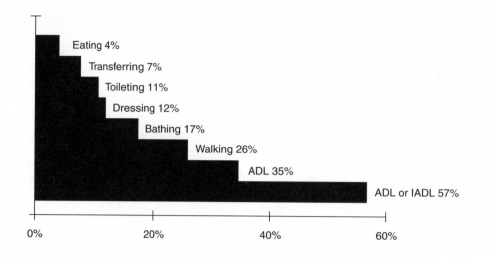

Figure 17.1 The need for assistance in the population 85 and older

Source: Data from U.S. Department of Health and Human Services, Agency for Health Care Policy and Research, "Functional Status of the Noninstitutionalized Elderly: Estimates of ADL and IADL Difficulties." Publication No. PDS-90-3462 (June 1990).

home health services delivered to the home. Clearly, for those seniors who have extensive needs and can afford it, assisted living can be very cost effective while providing the added benefit of companionship and 24-hour emergency service.

The decision to move into an assisted-living community is generally made by adult children seeking a more affordable alternative to nursing home placement. The advantages of a private residential unit and the non-institutional, homelike environment can help to ease feelings of guilt often common to families considering institutionalization.

ALTERNATIVE SERVICE DELIVERY METHODS

As the assisted-living business has grown and matured, the complexity of service delivery and billing methods also has evolved. Assisted living originally developed as a concept in response to congregate or independent-living communities that were looking for ways to maintain their occupancy and manage the aging in place of their existing residents. As their lifestyle challenges become increasingly complex, those residents required additional services. Some communities met this challenge through the introduction of home-

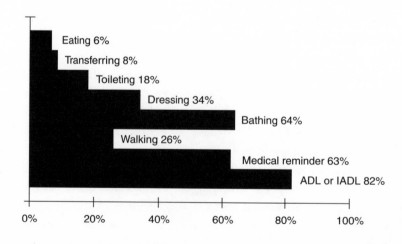

Figure 17.2 The need for assistance among residents of assisted living communities

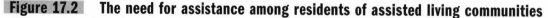

Source: Data from Coopers and Lybrand, ALFAA, acuity study within assisted living communities

Table 17.1 **Common Diagnoses among Assisted Living Residents**

Cardiac, circulatory	44%
Arthritis, osteoporosis	42%
CVA, stroke	28%
Dementia	26%
Depression	16%
Diabetes	11%
Chronic obstructive lung disease	<10%
Thyroid irregularities	<10%
Cataracts and other eye disorders	<10%
Anemia	<10%
Hearing impairments	<10%

health agencies; others discharged these residents to a "more appropriate level of care," while still others segregated their independent community by designating a separate floor or section of the property to personal care or assisted living. In the continuing-care retirement community the progression was planned, and a full continuum of care, including assisted living and skilled nursing, was offered. Subsequently, developers recognized that prospects were becoming more aware of the limitations of traditional congregate communities and began developing properties with both independent-living apartments and a separate assisted-living component. This, of course, was more popular to many seniors who were interested in gaining access to services if they needed them but who did not want to live in an environment with other elderly people who had become infirm over time. Ultimately, freestanding assisted-living communities grew in popularity, primarily designed for those seniors who had the financial resources to gain access to health-care services in a residential setting while avoiding nursing home placement.

Although there is a wide variety of service-delivery methods employed by assisted-living communities to deliver the care residents require, most are a derivative of one of four basic methods. The following discussion will describe each and itemize the advantages and disadvantages.[4]

Home-Health Option

The home-health option segregates the basic service package from the personal-care component. The developer or manager will provide the basic service package, such as meal service, housekeeping, maintenance, laundry, activities, and transportation, and subcontract out the personal-care component through a Medicare-certified home health agency. This way, residents of the community can have access to personal care services using their collective purchasing power. This option is attractive to home health agencies because they can deliver a wide array of services, many of which are Medicare reimbursable, to a captive audience without the expense and inconvenience of travel time.

The home-health option enables the community to deliver a much higher level of care than would be possible under assisted-living regulations in most states. This care is not delivered by the management of the community directly as a component of the package included in the monthly service fee. The involvement of a Medicare-certified home health agency can provide benefits for both residents and ownership. Residents can use Medicare benefits that they would perhaps otherwise pay for separately. This arrangement can provide relief to those residents who may be experiencing financial pressure as their health-care needs accelerate. The community can benefit from reduced turnover, stabilization of the assisted living population, avoidance of nursing care transfers, control of the continuity of care, and differential billing structures.

This concept is very attractive to owners looking to defray expensive nursing costs, particularly during the ramp-up period until stabilized occupancy is reached. During the start-up phase of the operation occupancy is continually changing, which makes it difficult for management to optimize staffing at the most efficient level. By contracting with a single Medicare-certified home health agency, ownership and management can also have some influence and control over personal care-service delivery. Without this arrangement, an assisted-living community will be subject to the risks of a wide array of different home health agencies delivering Medicare services to its residents with little or no control over the quality of these services or the qualifications of their personnel. Should a medication error or resident abuse occur at the hands of a home-health staff person, the community may be exposed to the resulting liability and bad reputation that invariably accompany such an incident. In one assisted-living community no fewer than fifteen home-health agencies were delivering services to its residents, making the community vulnerable in terms of control and quality assurance.

Careful steps must be taken to avoid being viewed by Medicare as an abusive practice. Medicare and Medicaid anti-kickback provisions contained in U.S.C. 1320 a–7b(b), Section 1128B of the Social Security Act are enforced by the Office of the Inspector General. Because of the broad scope of the federal anti-kickback laws, the secretary of Health and Human Services issued regulations on July 29, 1991, commonly known as the "Safe Harbor regulations" (Federal Register 56 F. 2d Reg. 35951), which provide clarification as to the applicability of the federal regulations specifically. It is critical to document the arrangement with the independent contractor through the use of a "safe harbor" agreement to protect against any possible infringement of the Social Security Act.

The home-health arrangement must be kept totally separate from ownership and management of the business. First, there can be no duplication of services that the facility is obligated to provide under the existing contract. The contract can, however, be modified to exclude those services so long as the home-health agency provides for those residents who may not qualify for Medicare. Medicare also does not allow any inducement to residents for the provision of Medicare-reimbursable services. Therefore, it is absolutely necessary for the community not to gain financially or receive any services in exchange for or as a condition of this subcontract. An arrangement where the community is delivering personal-care services with its own staff in conjunction with a preferred home-health agency that manages the program through nursing staff provided to the community at no cost may be in violation of federal regulations by receiving services in exchange for access. Providers cannot legally deny any Medicare beneficiary the freedom to choose among health care providers. The agreement must be a nonexclusive arrangement in which the certified agency may engage other contractors to provide similar services or provide access to other certified home-health agencies to provide its services. The provider must at all times refrain from recommending or referring patients (residents) to any single agency, but because the owner or manager is not providing personal care services, the residents are free to choose whomever they wish, and most if not all will choose the main contracted agency out of convenience and because they may already be familiar with the home health agency staff. Finally, the ownership or management of the community cannot receive any payments from the agency, a stipulation that takes into account the volume or value of any referrals or business generated between the parties for which the payment may be made in whole or in part by Medicare or a state-funded health program. Ownership and management should also avoid creating a supplemental staffing company and billing the home-health agency for the nurse and home-health aide who provide the Medicare services. This is also viewed by Medicare as an abuse of the system and considered an inducement for referrals. However, the occasional use of specific subcontracting services can be allowable. The community can provide office space for a Medicare home-health agency as long as it charges the agency a reasonable and customary rent.

By contracting out the personal-care component of the service package, the community relinquishes any operating margins that could be reasonably expected through the delivery of these services with its own staff. Under most circumstances, the delivery of personal-care services by a community's own employees is more efficient than if accomplished through a home-health agency. Efficiently operated, a personal-care delivery component offered by the assisted-living community with its own staffing should produce a 70–80 percent margin in loaded costs. Another disadvantage of this home-health option is realized after the community has been opened and the resident acuity profile increases. It then becomes difficult for the community to attract residents other than those who are nursing home candidates, thereby limiting its marketability.

Service Levels Option

Most assisted-living communities include some level of personal care in their basic monthly service package. The amount of this service can range from 30 to 90 minutes per day of assistance with activities of daily living (ADLs) with the overall average for most communities about 45 minutes. For most residents this amount of service works well, and for those who need extra personal care, the community can provide it more economically than can an outside agency. Be aware that some home-health agencies will seek to provide private services that are not reimbursed by Medicare and will bill the resident separately.

Personal-care services normally include bathing, dressing, escort or tray delivery, medication reminders, additional housekeeping, personal laundry, dementia support, orientation and cueing, grooming, scheduled toileting, and safety checks. Upon admission, residents are assessed on their personal-care needs, and a personal-care service plan is created to deliver those services. Under the service level program residents are reevaluated periodically as their needs change and are assigned to a service level—called level 1, 2, 3, etc.; or basic, intermediate, enhanced, comprehensive; or some other such ascending scale. Premiums for each higher level of service are usually based on additional personal care time required per day by the resident, translated to a monthly rate. For example, for an assisted-living community that includes 45 minutes per day of personal care in the basic monthly service package may charge an additional $120 per month for an intermediate level that provides up to 60 minutes per day ($16.00 per hour aide cost ÷ 4 = $4.00 per 15-minute increment × 30 days per month = $120.00). This can continue for each 15-minute increment to $240 additional per month for 60 minutes, $360 additional for 75 minutes, and so forth. Any significant change in a resident's status that requires an increase in care on a long-term basis, or a significant increase in care on a short-term basis, triggers a service plan review with the resident and family.

Although this system works fine for residents who normally use 45 minutes or less per day of personal care, some providers have found that it can be difficult to convince families and residents that those residents need to move up to the next service level and incur the additional expense. Residents will often argue that they need additional services because they are suffering from a temporary setback and that there is no need to adjust the rate. Many residents will also request escort service or demand to be catered to personally, attention that should trigger a service-plan review. In addition, because the monthly service fee is adjusted with increasing levels of service, a service-plan review that comes at the same time as a lease renewal and normal rent increase can be a tough sell to the resident and family.

Staffing the service level option can also bring challenges insofar as it is difficult to quantify exactly the number of service hours per shift actually delivered to the residents. Personal care aides are con-stantly being pulled in many different directions to service residents on demand. Management will find that some basic-level residents require more care on an intermittent basis, while higher service-level residents are always demanding special attention because they pay more.

Point System Option (ADL Acuity Guide)

The point system is normally determined by a baseline assessment tool used to classify each resident's needs. A numerical score is determined based on progressively higher levels of staff intervention, each assigned a point value, usually 1–5. The higher the point value, the higher the acuity level. The final score is derived by adding the acuity points from each service category, then dividing by the number of categories, usually 10. For example,

Category: Bathing and Dressing

1 Point: Independent in bathing and dressing.
2 Points: Requires assistance only in transferring into and out of bath, and can bathe self.
3 Points: Requires assistance in bathing and dressing but does most of the work.
4 Points: Requires considerable assistance with bathing and dressing.
5 Points: Completely dependent on staff for bathing and dressing.

Resident acuity scores for all categories are added together and averaged. Each acuity level is generally assigned an additional monthly fee of, say, $200 or $300. Acuity levels of 4 or 5 can demonstrate a need for nursing home care and trigger discharge planning. Assessments are conducted upon admission and periodically thereafter on a scheduled basis. If the personal care director waits until an obvious reassessment is needed, chances are that the personal care aides are already providing higher levels of service without recovering the additional costs associated with delivering the service to the resident. Consequently significant amounts of care are given away and the staffing of the unit is always short.

Like the service level option, the point system leaves significant room for interpretation. Residents and family may contend that the point system is based on conjecture and can vary widely from one week to the next depending on how the resident may be feeling. Management needs constantly to stay on top of regularly scheduled assessments for every resident and resell the increase in fee structure many times throughout the lease term. In addition, the time to perform activities of daily living can vary widely between residents. One resident may require 20 minutes to bathe and get dressed for breakfast, while another may need 45 minutes to accomplish the same task with assistance. There is simply no way to directly correlate nursing time expended to each resident and fully recover the cost to deliver that care.

Actual-Care Option

Under the actual-care option, residents are allocated a daily time limit of, say, 45 minutes included in their monthly service fee. Any additional care is billed in arrears for the actual care delivered. Upon admission, residents are assessed and a personal service-care plan is developed. The service plan measures the amount of personal care the resident needs in a seven-day period, normally Sunday through Saturday. The plan itemizes each daily assignment such as bathing, dressing, daily housekeeping, personal laundry, dementia support, daily orientation and cueing, grooming, and other recurrent activities such as scheduled toileting, breakfast, lunch, or dinner escort or tray, and morning, noon, or night medication reminders.

An initial seven-day time study, performed by the personal care aides assigned to the resident, serves as the foundation of the service plan. The total number of minutes is added up for the week; if the total exceeds 315 minutes per week (45 minutes per day for seven days), the excess is billed to the resident's account. The time study is repeated for this resident only if one or more of the following exist: (1) the resident returns from the hospital after a short stay, (2) the resident's physician alters the resident's major medication or treatment regime, (3) the resident's overall personal care needs either increase or decrease, or (4) the resident experiences a cognitive decline. If any of these conditions exists, a care conference is called between the personal care director, personal care aides, family, and physician to update the personal service plan. Normally, personal care assistants account for every minute of their day during the time study (and the tool can also be used to monitor performance). This way all possible interactions between personal care assistants and their residents are documented.

Another time study is completed on the revised service plan as the services are delivered the first week.

The total time that exceeds the allotment in the monthly service fee is then billed separately, for example, at 35 cents per minute ($21.00 per hour). This system is very beneficial to the resident and families because it allows for the fact that on certain days a resident may need more than 45 minutes of service (such as days when assistance in bathing is required) and on other days the service needed is considerably less. This way, the resident is charged only for the care that exceeds 315 minutes per week even if he or she needs one hour or more on any given day.

Delivery times for the same service will vary widely between residents. This system allows management to recover the cost for actual time of service delivered rather than impose a flat fee, as in the service-levels option discussed above. Upon completion of all time studies, management also has a very accurate tally of the total staff hours actually required to deliver services to the resident so that the most efficient level of staffing can be scheduled or budgeted. An accurate tally of the total service time by category can be an effective method to quantify the overall acuity of the resident population.

Each personal-care assistant is assigned specific residents and has a daily schedule transposed from the weekly service plan. The daily schedule will include the time of delivery, apartment number, resident name, assignment detail with check-off boxes, and minutes allocated to perform the service. The personal-care assistant's entire day is fully scheduled, and he is expected to complete his assignments before clocking out. Under this system, it is not unusual to reach 90 percent efficiency in service delivery. Schedules do have some flexibility to allow for unscheduled service and personal attention. Some companies use computers to develop the personal service plan, schedule each resident, assign a staff person to the residents, and generate a billing statement, personal information sheet, medication record, and acuity report. Programs such as these can also be used to optimize staffing and manage the overall profitability of the ancillary-care delivery system.

Upon completion of the time study, a daily schedule is completed for the week that documents the actual time needed to deliver each service to the resident. The actual service times and additional billing amount should be discussed with the family or resident. By reviewing the service plan and approving it in advance, management can reach consensus before the resident receives a billing statement. If the resident or family feels that the additional billing amount is objectionable, management can ask which services should be deleted from the plan and explain the implications of such actions. If family members have been involved in the care-planning process from admission to discharge, they should be prepared to understand their options and the cost of alternatives rationally.

QUALITY ASSURANCE

Quality assurance must be part of the culture of a senior-living community. It comes from management's commitment to communicate standards of excellence and painstakingly follow through on this commitment. It must be a component of everyday life at the community. The long-term success of the community absolutely depends on its reputation for problem-solving and consistent delivery of quality care and service.

In contrast to skilled nursing, where quality assurance can be managed through traditional rounds, the assisted-living environment is considerably more challenging. As the compression of acuity has resulted in a frailer clientele, communication becomes paramount in the delivery of care to residents who live in the equivalent of an apartment building where access to them is limited by the structure of individualized units.

Management should not wait until it hears of a problem from the resident's physician or family member before taking corrective measures. The offensive approach involves the development and periodic evaluation of personal-care service plans for each resident designed to ensure that the appropriate level of care is planned for and consistently delivered. In a community with individual apartments, management must take a systematic approach to the delivery of personal-care services and rely on effective communication from the nursing assistants to update the personal care director on changes in residents' conditions. This will involve continuous communication about residents' needs in which both positive and negative information is shared. Personal-care assistants must alert management to the changing health conditions of the residents they visit each day.

The use of a senior caregiver or LPN to supervise the implementation of the care plan and its scheduled personal care services can help to guarantee that the services in the care plan were in fact delivered. This individual can also be available for emergency response and to help with aides' questions regarding the need for medical intervention for their residents as they identify problems. In particular, residents who are identified as high risk can be visited regularly throughout the day.

Another good technique to ensure quality of services is to schedule care-plan reviews periodically. This will involve the reevaluation of all the care requirements of the resident. Each service will be evaluated in terms of timing, frequency, duration, and resident response. This should be done at least every six months, or sooner as changes in the resident's needs or condition are observed. From an operations perspective, residents have a habit of asking for small amounts of extra care that are routinely provided by the nursing staff. As resident health declines incrementally over time, these requests will become more frequent, contributing to higher costs. Personal-care plans that are reviewed frequently will ensure that the cost to deliver this additional care can be identified and consequently recovered from the resident.

Quality assurance is even more challenging in assisted-living communities with special-care units, such as those that cater to residents suffering from Alzheimer's disease or related disorders. In later stages of the disease, residents lose the ability to communicate health complications and pain. Common disorders such as urinary tract infections can go undiagnosed for long periods until they become quite serious in nature.

STAFFING

There are three basic ways to categorize staff assignments: universal worker, rotation, and primary care. All three systems are commonly used within assisted-living communities but are rarely mixed.

Universal Worker

In a typical assisted-living community, services from bathing and grooming to meals, housekeeping, and activity programs need to be delivered every day. The traditional operation accomplishes these tasks through departmentalization. For example, the housekeeping department cleans the community, the food and beverage department prepares and serves the meals, the activity department organizes leisure interests and events, and the nursing department delivers the personal care. Each service is generally supervised by a separate department head, who can become territorial and bureaucratic. Because staff members are trained or experienced only in one discipline, there is very little crossover from one department to the next. Consequently, the entire service package becomes compartmentalized and segregated. The more the residents' needs are passed from one department to the next, the more likely the risk of a communication breakdown that will result in a problem for the resident.

Under the universal-worker concept, which has become popular among providers, employees are hired as "care managers" and cross-trained in several departments. This way they are conditioned to accept responsibility for the total care needs of the resident and there is little "buck passing" on service requests. An employee is hired as a care aide, for instance, then cross-trained as a housekeeper or wait person in the dining areas. She can come to work and spend the first four hours of her shift bathing and dressing residents, then move to cleaning apartments or assisting in activities. In assisted living–based Alzheimer's or special care units, the care manager normally handles *all* of the care needs of the residents to whom she is assigned. Facility management or department heads can then act as facilitators and trainers, assisting the care managers in a "service rich" environment. The system is designed to build accountability to meet the residents' needs, whatever they may be, by each and every one in the operation. This effectively breaks down traditional hierarchy and bureaucracy replacing it with an attitude of customer service. Some technical skills, such as maintenance, cooking, and bookkeeping, are difficult to cross-train, but the majority of services that are delivered to the residents in a community can be performed by universal workers.

Clearly, it is easier to set up a new community under this structure than it is to break down the paradigm in an established community. The introduction of the universal-worker idea is often met with resistance from established employees who may feel that management wants them to work harder for the same pay. People are by nature resistant to change, because change itself forces them to step outside their own comfort zones. Some operators have restructured their compensation plans to overcome this objection. They hire for attitude, then train for skill; employees are hired

in one specialty and then as they learn and pass competency tests on each new discipline, their base compensation is increased. For example, a personal-care assistant may be hired at $7.00 per hour, then cross-trained in housekeeping for an additional 25 cents per hour, then as a waitperson for 25 cents more or a dishwasher for 15 cents more. This way, as the employees learn and grow in their positions, they become more flexible to management and consequently more valuable. As employees move up the learning curve, they are motivated by a sense of accomplishment and reward.

According to *The State of Seniors Housing, 1994,* the typical assisted-living community requires approximately 0.46 full-time equivalents per resident. Under the universal-worker concept, some operators suggest, this figure could drop to 0.356 FTEs providing care for residents who usually need help with the activities of daily living.[5] One operator suggests that segregating job functions can result in a productivity loss of up to 40 percent. In the competitive assisted-living environment, it is no wonder that operators are embracing this concept on a grand scale.

The difficulty in managing the universal-worker concept is in quality assurance and convincing employees to embrace the idea. Service to the residents can become inconsistent when employees skilled at performing one job are learning another skill. Staff can become frustrated, believing that they are doing a lot of different tasks, but not any one particularly well. Management must respond to this frustration with continuing skill testing and retraining until proficiency is reached. Management must play an active role, continually reinforcing the merits of the concept to residents and family members throughout the start-up or transition period.

Rotational System

The rotational system is designed to have staff assigned on a task basis. Many operators rotate their personal-care assistants from resident to resident. Aging residents may experience a heightened sense of vulnerability and be suspicious of a new personal-care assistant, but rotation does have a number of advantages. Rotating allows for variety and can break the monotony of dealing with the same residents every day. To have all care assistants trained to the personal-care needs of all the residents makes rescheduling and call-in coverage easier. In addition, if residents become attached to a personal-care assistant and the employee leaves the community, separation anxiety may result. The employee turnover rate does not become known to the residents with monthly rotation. Rotation also discourages favoritism on the part of the resident and the personal care assistant. This allows for the workload to be shared equally among the personal care assistants so that the same aides do not shoulder the burden of heavy-care residents. It also allows for the maximum scheduling flexibility.

Primary Care Assignments

Also known as modular nursing, the primary care system assigns specific personal-care assistants to specific residents. The daily personal-care needs are scheduled for several residents, then assigned to one personal care aide on each of three shifts. This way accountability for service-plan delivery can be allocated to a minimal number of employees. Residents will always prefer this system. The delivery of personal-care services is a very intimate business. It requires a considerable amount of trust and is best accomplished through the development of personal relationships between the resident and the caregiver.

People who are attracted to the personal-care business are normally very compassionate human beings. They are motivated by their ability to influence the lives of the residents they serve and often become quite attached to their residents, as the residents will be to them. Each becomes the support system of the other. The patient generally receives the best quality of care that the assistant is capable of giving.

Spending so much time with their residents, personal-care assistants become intimately aware of the resident's condition and overall health. Personal-care assistants who work with the same residents day in and day out will recognize minor changes in their resident's health, activity level, and even bathroom habits, much the same as they would at home with their own children. Spotting these changes as they occur positions personal-care assistants to alert management and families so that problem can be diagnosed and treated immediately. This is the very essence of quality care: It is not about people delivering purchased services to residents in a consistent manner, but about people caring about their residents personally and taking responsibility for their health and happiness because

they want to. Families will also feel more connected to personal-care assistants whom they know and are better able to support them when residents exhibit difficult behaviors. Families are generally suspicious of management when employees are constantly rotating or turning over.

When staff members are rotated, even the best-intentioned caregiver has no baseline to use in evaluating the present condition of their residents. They can go only on what they can see today and what their instincts, training, and experience have taught them. It is nearly impossible for them to recognize the often subtle changes that can lead to big problems. More important, it is not easy for the residents constantly to remind their ever-changing caregivers about their inability to perform specific activities for which they depend on assistance. As soon as the resident becomes accustomed to a personal-care assistant, the assistant is rotated on to a whole new set of residents. This system is really quite disturbing to the residents and their families.

CALCULATING STAFFING REQUIREMENTS

There are several ways to calculate staffing requirements in the personal-care department. Staffing can be calculated based on the amount of minutes per day included in the residents' monthly fees; on coverage in the building throughout the day; on actual care scheduled in each resident's care plan; or on ratios of caregivers to residents.

In a community that offers 45 minutes of personal care in the monthly service fee, a fully occupied 90-unit assisted-living community with four second residents requires staffing of 70.5 hours per day if every resident uses exactly 45 minutes and the night shift is completely utilized for care delivery. This works out to a ratio of about 1:23 on the day shift and 1:45 at night. The problem is, of course, that rarely does anyone ever use *exactly* any amount of care.

The best way to calculate staffing needs is to develop assignment sheets for each personal-care aide matching the needs and preferences specified in the care plan. These assignment sheets can then be translated into hours or minutes of service and scheduled accordingly. For example, one personal-care aide can during an eight-hour shift deliver approximately 400 minutes of care (480 minutes less 60 for lunch and breaks, less 20 for transferring assignment documentation to the residents' files). This 400 minutes can be delivered in 20-minute modules to each of the 20 residents to whom she is assigned. Other personal-care aides will then pick up the care needs on the other shifts to complete the care plan. With the exception of the night shift, when the residents are mostly asleep but coverage is still required, the personal-care aides should have this 400 minutes of care time fully scheduled. At night, in smaller communities, one person may be adequate provided there are no residents requiring two-person transfer. If two persons are required, one or both can be kept busy during slow periods with marketing or administrative projects such as stuffing and labeling direct mailings or assisting with other business office projects that are not of a proprietary nature. Some communities have one personal-care aide and one housekeeper on during the night shift. The housekeeper can do common-area housekeeping and the entire day's laundry and be available to assist with emergencies or transfers.

It should be understood that at times there will be distractions, refused care, or care that takes a longer or shorter time than is anticipated and is not generally predictable. This can be noted by the care aide, and the personal-care director will then adjust the overall assignments accordingly. It is critical that all of their time be accounted for, including travel time between residents. When service times become longer as the residents age in place, the personal-care director must recognize these changes and ensure that the proper staffing is scheduled. When residents are transferred to the hospital, move out, or require less care, staffing needs to be cut or aides reassigned to assist with other residents. It's a good idea to schedule some part-timers on the morning shift, when the care requirements are highest, who can have flexible hours that increase or decrease in accordance with the assignment requirements.

The management of staff cost is as important in assisted living as it is in home health care. A home-health agency would not remain in business very long supporting staff that does not have billable hours. Whether the care delivered in the assisted living community is included in the monthly service fee or is billed additionally, it all must be balanced against the total recoverable revenue from the residents. The margin of profitability can very quickly be erased with inefficient management and the use of in-house staff not delivering countable care. The personal care department

must be operated as if it were a separate home health agency so that all minutes of staff time scheduled are either billable or attributable to and covered by the monthly service fee.

Scheduling residents for personal care is also an important consideration. In the example above, 94 residents requiring 45 minutes per day will require most of their service during the morning shift. At this time of day, residents will be needing assistance with bathing and grooming before going to the dining room for breakfast. Those who are unable to accomplish this process during the breakfast hours will order room service. They will, of course blame management for not attending to them in time in an effort to have the tray-delivery charge waived. At the same time, personal-care aides can be found in the kitchen waiting for the trays that were already ordered, which creates a bottleneck in the kitchen and delays service to the residents who did manage to make it to the dining room and who are now complaining about slow service. As the personal-care aides are forced to wait, still more residents waiting for help in their room will miss breakfast. The entire cycle of poor service can be avoided or minimized by encouraging some residents to rise earlier for their bathing and dressing assistance, and by limiting the number of morning baths to a more manageable number. The expectations of the residents must be managed so that everyone can be serviced without adding staff. Many of the residents can be scheduled for their bath after dinner, before they go to bed, so that they need assistance only with dressing the next morning.

Creative scheduling can often improve service to the residents *and* reduce the cost of delivering that service. For most residents there are 14 to 16 hours available in which to schedule their care. Although some of it must be scheduled at certain times during the day, typically around mealtimes, some of the heavier care can be distributed throughout the day or evening. If the resident were purchasing the supportive care from a home health agency out of their home, it would be cost-prohibitive to have it delivered to them in small increments throughout the day. The use of part-time personal-care aides during the busy morning rush between 6:00 and 10:00 A.M. can also help to defray care-delivery costs. Some operators will run an 11:00 P.M. to 9:00 A.M. shift (10 hours per day four days per week) so that they will have two care aides on to help during the morning rush. This will add four hours to the night shift but will eliminate two four-hour morning shifts for a net savings of four hours per day.

Another important consideration should be to focus staff efforts on improving residents' self-care ability. There needs to be an acceptance of less than perfect performance from the residents who can learn to become more independent in some tasks and less dependent on their personal-care assistant as a servant. Start or complete difficult tasks for the residents and encourage them to do the parts in the middle. This builds strength and self confidence in the residents while easing the burden for staff. Residents respond well to encouragement and to recognition for small victories over the effects of aging. The resident's service plan should also integrate some family involvement so that they can contribute to their parent's well-being. Families who are willing and interested can often be encouraged to perform small services routinely. These tasks, once integrated into the service plan, can formalize the family's efforts to assist and generate some sense of teamwork between families and the staff. As problems arise or the care needs increase, the family is right there to observe the problems firsthand and can be involved in the solution or more easily accept the cost of additional care.

When confronted by employees with personal scheduling problems such as child care, transportation needs, or other such issues, the personal-care director will normally accommodate these difficulties through creative scheduling. Creative scheduling almost always results in higher cost to the operation through less than efficient utilization of staff. It is crucial in this low-margin operating environment to match the employees to the job requirements, not the job to the employee's requirements. It is simply much easier for the sympathetic personal-care director to incur additional cost in the name of better care or to keep a good employee than it is to find a creative solution to the employee's schedule conflict or need for additional hours or overtime. It is vital to make sure that the staff schedule has the same amount of hours scheduled as the assignment sheet of personal care to the residents, which should also agree with the staffing budget for the department. If the level of care increases, the staffing level can also increase provided the additional cost to deliver that care can be recovered through additional billing. The executive director should do a weekly or bimonthly audit of the time cards against the schedule, assignment sheets, and budget for the department to keep a

handle on this inevitable cost creep. Teach staff to be flexible so that the community can deliver the best care that it can with the resources that it has available. Often is simply a matter of learning to adapt an old routine to a new one. In the long run they will receive better care and be more satisfied.

There has been much study about the most efficient number of units in an assisted-living community. Too few units and the overhead in supervision cannot be fully amortized by the residents' monthly service fees; too many and the complexity of supervision to maintain quality control becomes prohibitive. As described earlier, quality is difficult to monitor in the private-apartment setting of an assisted-living environment. In sharp contrast to a skilled-nursing facility, where patients are available throughout the day, the assisted-living residents are more secluded in the privacy of their own apartments. Therefore, as the number of units increases, it becomes increasingly difficult to keep track of their individual care needs.

A nurse supervisor (RN or LPN) can reasonably cover approximately 60 residents. This includes care planning, supervision, scheduling assignments, medication monitoring, dealing with families and physicians, emergency response, and some direct care. Larger units will require additional supervision depending on the overall level of acuity and cognitive impairment. Communities with more than 100 units will also tend to develop higher acuity among the residents as they age in place and management holds on to residents longer to maintain higher occupancy. The problem then builds upon itself: as acuity increases, so does the need for additional supervision; the turnover rate increases as the average length of stay decreases, costing more marketing dollars to refill the units. (For maximum coverage, schedule the LPN to work daily from 1:00 to 9:00 P.M. daily, and from 10:00 A.M. to 6:00 P.M. weekends. Schedule the personal care director from 8:00 A.M. to 5:00 P.M. daily. This way there is nurse coverage most days from 8:00 A.M. to 9:00 P.M., when the residents are most active and during normal family visiting times.) In a competitive environment, this trend can lead to financial difficulty. A stand-alone assisted living community should not exceed 60–80 units for maximum efficiency, unless there is a special-care unit associated with it on the same site. This way, nursing supervision and other staffing can be shared for both units.

STAFF TRAINING

Training personal-care assistants never seems to receive the attention it deserves. Many companies talk a lot about training, but few ever perform much of it. Some states such as Massachusetts require six hours of training before a personal care aide can work with the residents, then six additional hours of training annually thereafter. Although this can become expensive, what management is really investing in is employee satisfaction and ultimately, longevity. It is up to management to teach employees specifically about the expectations of their jobs and to eliminate guesswork.

Several textbooks, training manuals, and videos are available on the market. Each community should develop its own training program consistent with its own management and care philosophy, a program that can be easily communicated in several short orientation sessions. The coursework should include the following topics:

1. Philosophy of Independent Living in an Assisted-Living Community
   - Choice
   - Dignity and respect
   - Right to privacy
   - Fostering independence
   - Promoting individuality
   - Resident freedom
   - Responsibility of sharing information
   - Quality expectations and service outcomes
   - The role of the personal care aide and how it looks when it is done well
   - Overview of the job's specific requirements
   - A place to call home: the residential environment
   - Resident and family involvement
   - Relationship to the wider community
   - Confidentiality

2. Resident Bill of Rights
   - Residence responsibility
   - Grievance procedures
   - Ombudsman

3. Communicable Diseases, including AIDS/HIV and Hepatitis B; Infection Control in the Community and the Principles of Universal Precautions based on OSHA guidelines.
   - Defining a communicable disease
   - Examples of communicable diseases
   - Infection control guidelines
   - Universal precautions: instruction and procedure
   - Sanitation
   - Basic personal hygiene

4. Communication Skills
   - Changes due to aging that affect communication
   - Communicating appropriately with residents
   - Communicating with families
   - Communicating without words; nonverbal tools
   - Barriers to communication
   - Talking about death and losses
   - Listening skills
   - Handling resident complaints

5. Review of the Aging Process
   - Normal versus pathological changes in aging
   - Common diseases and issues
   - Common myths and stereotypes
   - Coping with loss and the grieving process
   - Dealing with sensory loss
   - Death and dying; dying as a stage in life; the needs of the dying resident; hospice care

6. Dementia and Cognitive Impairment
   - Overview of Alzheimer's disease and related dementias
   - Effective communication techniques, verbal and nonverbal
   - Safety and environmental issues
   - Coping with difficult behaviors
   - Stress and taking care of yourself as a caregiver
   - Role of the caregiver

7. Medication Management
   - Common geriatric medications
   - Medication reminders
   - Abuses of medications
   - Liability
   - Documentation
   - Medications and the cognitively impaired

Topics such as these can provide the caregiver and other employees with the basic understanding of their position and the needs of those whom they serve. The more vivid the picture of the expectation, the more likely the desired outcome.

MEDICATION MANAGEMENT

In most assisted-living communities, an essential element of personal-care services involves the coordination of self-administered medication management. A quarter of all prescription and nonprescription drugs in this country are consumed by only 12 percent of the population—people over the age of 65. Approximately two-thirds of the residents in a typical assisted-living community will require some help with their medications. Where regulations exist, most states define medication management to include the tasks of reminding or cueing, opening containers, reading labels, observing, checking, and reassuring residents in connection with taking their medications. These activities are not generally considered to be a skilled health service.

As residents of assisted-living communities age in place, their health-care requirements will accelerate. Ultimately, communities currently not licensed to provide health-care services will begin to do so to keep up with their residents' needs. Residents become attached to the community after months or years of residency and begin to identify their assisted-living community as home. Residents become reluctant to leave the community when they become ill, and the community responds by increasing the amount of personal care or by bringing in home-care agencies to augment their services. The increase in acuity raises the complexity of their care and medication regimen. As this occurs, the exposure to and responsibility for medication errors increases for the owner and manager of the community regardless of who administers the medications.

Medication administration involves determining the appropriate medication at the appropriate time, taking it out of the container, and handing it to the resident. Medications can be administered through crushing and mixing with food, injection, topical lotions, eyedrops, gastrointestinal tubes, IVs, or other methods. These are normally administered by licensed staff and are generally contracted for by the resident. Medication administration and documentation errors arise when there is a difference between the doses dispensed and those documented as given. Such errors often involve omission and use of the wrong drug, dose, or schedule.

Normally in assisted living, the community may coordinate, supervise, and observe, but it may not dispense or administer. The more involved the assisted-living community is with its residents, the more liability it will accept. Some communities will insist that the pharmacy deal directly with each resident and deliver medications directly; others accept medications centrally and distribute them from medication carts.

Clearly, as the acuity levels in assisted-living communities have increased, so also have the complications of managing the resident's corresponding dependency upon pharmaceuticals. There are a number of options available to help minimize this dilemma. Pharmacists can now dispense medications ordered by the physician in ways that portion out the individual pill or pills custom sorted and hermetically sealed into clearly labeled medication cups with a soft foil backing; doses are to be taken as directed when prompted by the caregiver. These are often referred to as bingo cards or foil packs. Strip packs can also be set up that package one or more pills in individualized rolls like old-time penny candy. The prepackaged individual dose is simply rolled out and torn off, opened, and taken. The contents of each packet, along with the dose amount, patient, physician and patient name, frequency, and other information are printed on the outside. The disadvantage with this system is that, unlike with foil packs where the caregiver can easily see if the medication was taken, the strip packets are removed upon use so that one cannot visually determine if the medications were taken or not.

Normally, Medicare or the patient will pay the pharmacy a dispensing fee. This dispensing fee can be payable by unit dose or in a 30-day dose amount. In states where unit dose is allowed, the cost of changing the prescription can be minimized. But where 30-day dose-dispensing fees are utilized, substantial amounts of medications are wasted because 30 days of medications are dispensed and packaged together, and these may become obsolete and require disposal. With the unit dose, prescriptions can be easily changed with minimum waste. Unit doses are more expensive to dispense and so are preferred by the pharmacies. For example, the state of Massachusetts will reimburse the pharmacy $3.25 for a 30-day dose of a prescription, but Medicare pays 55 cents per day for the dispensing fee on a single prescription, or $16.50 per month.

The use of medication boxes is a great solution to medication management in assisted-living communities. A medication box is a clear or colored plastic pillbox with individual compartments for every day of the week. The medications are normally taken from their individual containers and distributed into each compartment according to the frequency of dose and time. The disadvantage to the boxes is that there is no way for the pharmacist to guarantee that the dispensed doses have not been tampered with by residents or staff. Until recently, the family or home health agency had to accept the responsibility for setting up the resident's medications, for this service is beyond the license capability of assisted living in most states. With several different resources handling medications, as discussed earlier, there is a wide margin for error. Pharmacists eager to capture the larger market share and convenience of serving assisted-living communities are now willing to dispense unit doses into these Mediset boxes or unit-dose packets such as Medicine on Time.

Pharmacists, in fact, may be so eager to tap into the captive one-stop mass market of the assisted-living community that they will offer to provide a consultant pharmacist, an additional fax machine, and a fax line at no cost to the community! The consultant pharmacist will essentially manage the entire medication program for you. Their free services can include answering questions about medications, performing a monthly drug regimen review to see that the residents are taking their medications according to prescription, and performing computerized compatibility checks to identify potential cross-reactions. In addition, consultant pharmacists are often aware before physicians of new drugs that can replace what two or more other pills were prescribed for, thus saving the resident or insurer money and possible discomfort.

Large drug companies such as Merck have money in their marketing budgets for sponsoring continuing-education seminars on a variety of current health and medical topics for local nurses, physician assistants, and other health-care professionals. These seminars, arranged and conducted by the local pharmacy, are normally held in local hotel conference rooms and are poorly attended. The pharmacy may hold its seminar in the assisted-living community if offered free meeting space. The assisted-living community can then benefit from being exposed to visiting professionals, and from a hot lunch catered by the community and paid for by the pharmacy and the drug company at a 30 percent premium. Attracting resident referral sources to your community has now become a profit center!

■ POLYPHARMACY

Most states do not have extensive regulations concerning the distribution, administration, and delivery of medications to assisted living residents. In fact, there is a wide disparity in regulatory approaches from state to state. Any true control of medical services, and especially medication flow, remains nebulous. One study found that 73 percent of staff who reported passing medications within an assisted-living setting were not licensed nurses (RNs, LPNs), and that 28 percent of the staff giving injections were not licensed nurses. The researchers also tested those who passed or administered medications to residents on correct procedures and recognition of signs and symptoms of adverse reactions. Only 14 percent of the operators and staff scored 75 percent or higher; and 39 percent of the staff provided correct answers for half of the questions or fewer.

Approximately 25 percent of all medications are inappropriately selected and dosed in the elderly,[6] resulting in an estimated 28 percent hospitalization rate due to inappropriate drug therapy in the elderly.[7] In fact, more than one in six older Americans are taking prescription drugs that are not suited for the elderly and may lead to physical or mental deterioration and even death.[8]

The assisted-living industry is highly exposed to drug-related problems involving their residents. These communities are largely unregulated and offer medication assistance or reminders that are frequently interpreted by the nurse's aides as administration. Personal-care aides eager to please residents will inadvertently overstep their authority and training to assist their residents in taking their medications. Medication errors occur at the hands of the residents as well. They can occur throughout the drug-use process and can be made by the resident, family, caregiver, prescriber, and even pharmacist. Drug-related problems are defined as any unwanted or unintended consequence of the administration or nonadministration of medications. There are two general types of drug-related problems: (1) medication errors and misuse by any person associated with drug prescribing, filling, administration, amd assessment, and (2) adverse drug reactions and interactions.

Polypharmacy is a term used to describe the use of multiple medications to treat chronic illnesses of the elderly. It is the principal drug-safety issue of the elderly, especially those with multiple disease states. Management must actively manage the risks of medication errors by educating staff and outside caregivers on the potential problems that residents can encounter. In the administration of medications by the community or outside professionals, omissions, wrong dosage, unordered medication, wrong time, outdated medication, number of drugs per resident complicated by the number of passes per day, and poor communication can all spell big problems for the resident, and liability for the community. Also drug–food interactions can result in consistent undesirable weight loss, poor appetite, chronic infection, or insufficient caloric or protein intake, with insufficient vitamins and minerals necessary to ensure nutritional balance. As residents increase in acuity they may experience adverse reactions or altered desirable therapeutic response to drug–drug interactions in their increasingly complex drug regimen. This is commonly caused by residents using drugs of similar pharmacologic action. A resident may refuse or be unable to take chronic-care medication, which can be very detrimental to the patient.[9]

As the assisted-living industry continues to expand rapidly, and competition forces providers to retain their residents longer, it is inevitable that medication-related incidents will occur. Many residents currently in assisted-living communities are reluctant to move to a more appropriate setting as their health-care needs grow beyond the scope of assisted-living providers. Both residents and their families will avoid the relocation for fears of losing independence and the financial implications of long-term care settings. Management should be proactive in dealing with these complex issues and manage resident and family expectations as the problems arise rather than waiting until their actions are dictated by crisis. Provisions of the Omnibus Budget Reconciliation Act of 1987 require that state Medicaid programs have prospective and retrospective drug-use review programs in place. These programs require pharmacists to screen prescriptions for therapeutic duplication, drug-disease contraindications, incorrect dosage or duration of treatment, drug allergies, and clinical abuse or misuse. An integral part of the law is a requirement that pharmacists offer to counsel all Medicaid patients about their prescription medications. Since the law was enacted many states have amended their pharmacy practice acts to require that pharmacists offer these same services to all patients, not just those covered by Medicaid.

Consultant pharmacy services, and especially drug-regimen review, can have a significant impact on the accuracy and suitability of medication management in the assisted-living community. In the assisted-living environment, individual independence is often stressed over patient safety. Although medication management of the residents in assisted-living communities should be monitored by a consultant pharmacist, the likelihood of these services' becoming mandated by regulation is remote. Implementing a comprehensive medication management and monitoring system can help reduce the operation's liabilities, as well as help the community retain clients by preventing unnecessary hospitalization due to adverse drug reactions.

Several excellent training programs are available to operators. The state of New Jersey has developed a medication training program/policy and procedure manual for personal care assistants that is an excellent resource and training guide to familiarize laypersons with common medications and their effects on the elderly, and Institutional Consulting Pharmacy Services has developed a medication administration training video for personal care assistants. Most institutional pharmacies also have reference libraries with videos and guides of common geriatric medications that can be checked out for the education of staff.

NOTES

1. "The Assisted Living Marketplace. A Report to Ciba-Geigy Corporation," *Marketing Solutions,* March 22, 1995.
2. E. Clemmer, "Assisted Living and Its Implications for Long Term Care," *AARP,* Dec. 1994, 1–15.
3. *Overview of the Assisted Living Industry: 1996* (Assisted Living Federation of America Publication) (Fairfax, Va.: Coopers & Lybrand L.L.P., 1996).
4. B. Pearce and T. Grape, "Checks and Balances," *Assisted Living Today* 4(2) (Winter 1997): 30.
5. *Briefings on Assisted Living. Special Report: Flexible Workers: A Solution for Assisted Living* (Marblehead, Mass., 1996), 5.
6. S. F. Clackum, "The Quest: Preventing Adverse Drug Events," *Provider* 22(8) (Aug. 1996): 58–59.
7. GAO/AIMD-96-72. *Automated Prescription Drug Review Systems* (Washington, D.C., 1996).
8. GAO/HEHS-95-152. *Prescription Drugs and the Elderly* (Washington, D.C., 1995).
9. J. W. Cooper, *Drug-Related Problems in Geriatric Nursing Home Patients* (Binghamton, N.Y.: Haworth Press, 1991).

# 18

Home Health

Over the last several years, our nation's health-care system has consistently moved toward residential and community-based health care and away from institutional inpatient care. Preliminary discussions in Washington indicate that the forces shaping health-care reform, such as reduced cost, improved accessibility, and quality care, are at work within the new Federal Health Care model designed to move dramatically toward in-home residential health-care services, an attractive and popular option. This drive is fueled by economic concerns as well as by considerations of the patient's dignity. A recent national survey by the American Association of Retired Persons found that three out of four respondents preferred home care over institutionalization.

The nation's burgeoning aging population requires government to consider every elderly person's residence to be a potential site for health-care services. The country will never be able to build and support institutional facilities in quantities sufficient to accommodate the need. The 1983 revisions in Medicare reimbursement, combined with the move by private insurers to encourage shorter hospitalization, has forced patients to seek nontraditional sources to serve their health-care needs. In-home services are by far the most universally flexible method of providing temporary, interim health care services to the growing numbers of citizens needing this type of long-term care. Other economic factors include the continued

pressure on the acute-care system to discharge patents much earlier than before; they will be in need of follow-up post–acutecare services. The creation of Diagnostic Related Groups by Medicare now dictates the length of hospital stays and has made it more profitable for institutions to discharge patients sooner. In addition, more families have become spread out geographically and are increasingly unable to care for each other.

Controlling federal spending on Medicare's home-health benefit will require major changes in how home care is reimbursed. The home-health benefit is broadly defined, permitting large discretion in its interpretation. Once approved, beneficiaries may receive an unlimited number of qualifying services so long as they are provided pursuant to the physician's plan of care. Physicians must review and re-affirm the plan of care at least every 62 days. There are no limits on the number of days of care or visits, and beneficiaries currently pay no coinsurance or deductibles. Medicare pays home health agencies the lower of their costs or a limit. The limits are established at 112 percent of the average cost per visit for free-standing agencies. Some of the initiatives that are currently being considered to control home health costs include the introduction of beneficiary copayments, a case-mix adjusted prospective payment system (episodic rather than cost-based), and monthly limitations on per visit payments. Each of these changes will, if implemented, place limits on home health utilization and encourage seniors with chronic conditions to consider assisted living for these long-term needs. In addition, the use of personal care services among the elderly tends to be intermittent in nature. Seniors require such services at irregular intervals throughout the day. These services are more efficiently delivered in an assisted-living environment where staff is available when the services are required, rather than regularly scheduled through home health care.

Caring for patients at home is the fastest growing part of the nation's health budget, representing $16.5 billion in 1993, up 30 percent over 1992 as reported by the Commerce Department.[1] The report goes on to say that medical and health services accounted for 14 percent of the country's gross domestic product. Nursing-home payments will see annual increases of 13 percent, which is in line with health-care costs overall. The American Medical Association reports that for each patient in a nursing home there are three more severely impaired patients being cared for at home. The National Center for Health Statistics recently published the *Chartbook on Health Data on Older Americans,* which analyzes data on activities of daily living, long-term care, prescription drug-use patterns, the costs of health care, and their payment sources.

Today, home care has come of age. An ever-increasing number of patients are finding that even "sophisticated" convalescent care can be had at home in familiar surroundings at a fraction of the cost of a hospital room. In addition, elderly people who may need only the services of a nurse's aide can in most cases save considerable money and dignity by avoiding nursing-home placement, in which they pay for skilled staff whether they need them or not. Use patterns suggest that some home health users have intensive health-care needs for a short period of time associated with an acute condition, while others have less intensive needs associated with more chronic conditions brought on by the aging process.

▬▬ HOME HEALTH CARE OPTIONS

Home health services are typically divided into two forms of organizations. The first are Medicare certified home-health agencies, which provide in-home skilled nursing and therapy services inclusive of intra-venous feeding and pharmacy services. Patients may qualify under Medicare Part A and B for home health services, such as part-time or intermittent skilled-nursing care, physical therapy, speech therapy, occupational therapy, medical social services, medical supplies, and some rehabilitation equipment. These services may be paid in full by Medicare when the patient meets the following four conditions:

1. It is for intermittent care, and
2. The patient is confined at home, and
3. The services have been prescribed by a doctor, and
4. The services are rendered by a certified Medicare approved provider.

Unlike skilled nursing services, the patient is not required to have a hospital stay before home-health services are covered. Medicare does not pay for the cost of 24-hour skilled nursing in the home, meal delivery, or homemaker services (except where provided under hospice and respite provisions). Certificates of Need for Medicare-certified home health agencies are becoming increasingly difficult to secure as legislators continue to identify opportunities to control the expansion of state and federally sponsored health care.

Medicare coverages are normally short-term and can run out in 60–90 days, after which the resident normally converts to a fee for service basis. This continuum of care can produce profit margins from 20 to 25 percent, while still providing reasonably priced services to the residents, less than the "street rate" of a home health agency. For example, home health visits can be billed to residents at $11 per hour, which may cost $8.60 to deliver ($7 per hour plus 23 percent benefits—less for per diem employees).

Second are noncertified agencies that can provide all of the same services as the certified facilities without the authorization to recover charges from the Medicare program. The noncertified agency's income sources are typically private pay, insurance (industrial), and contract services. The highest use of noncertified agencies is by elderly individuals needing occasional in-home companion or aide assistance. The agency acts typically as the employment agent for the client and pool employee, executing a contract by and between the agency and the contractor as an employment assistance agency and with the client as a provider of service. Quite often, those clients consistently using a specific individual for care would buy out the contract of the contractor, very similar to a true employment agency arrangement. Under greater IRS scrutiny, most agencies have gone to a pool on-call employee relationship. The employee can and often does "register" or become employed with several agencies. The agency that markets its services more effectively is able to retain individuals in its pool. There is inherently very little company loyalty with this type of employee group. Employees specifically prefer the independence and self-determination of this type of employment, as well as the typically higher wage, even without benefits.

Most residents do not relish the thought of a nursing home and will prefer to purchase their own home health care out of their apartment. This can present a myriad of challenges to management in their efforts to control the continuity of care, the quality of care, and the depletion of resident's resources by potentially unlicensed, unbonded, and unsecured contractors. The establishment of a community-based home health agency can and does lend management opportunities for considerable control.

The home health industry has continued to grow steadily over the last six decades from the hospital-based Visiting Nurse Association (VNA), which followed up with patients post-hospitalization or in rural areas where acute care facilities were unavailable, to the Public Health Nursing programs of the 1940s through the 1960s, to for-profit national home-health agencies such as Upjohn, Health Care Personnel, and "The Kelly Girl" company. Many hospitals, physician joint ventures, and other health-care organizations have, over the years, entered into the home health-care industry. Typically, the most successful organizations are those with a national organization and/or a built-in referral source, such as hospitals or physician groups.

Opportunities in the home health industry continue to develop as changes in national attitudes and governmental objectives continue. This is a fairly competitive business that has a great deal of room for creativity and quality. Customer service at its purest form is the product of the home health-care industry. There are essentially two delivery methods practiced within senior living communities: the community-based operation designed to service the existing residents' needs as they age in place, and the storefront opera-

tion set up to deliver its services to the outside community. Let us explore the advantages and disadvantages of each.

■ COMMUNITY-BASED HOME HEALTH CARE AGENCY

Many senior-living communities have chosen to introduce home health care as an alternative to improve revenues and to augment resident turnover as their tenants age in place. As interest rates climb, operators who financed their projects with float rate debt will look to add revenue-generating services to help offset their increasing interest obligations. Home health care is an attractive option that is normally well received by residents. Operators will continue to expand the scope of services to achieve these goals while improving the quality and continuity of care for their residents. Other revenue generators could include respite care, hospice, special-care wings, banquet services, community-based maid and maintenance services, and meals on wheels. The long-term financial viability of these investments will depend on the innovation of ownership to meet the revenue needs during normal interest rate cycles.

The development of community-based home health agencies has met with considerable success in both congregate and continuing care communities. In congregate and assisted living communities, home health services have allowed the residents to age in place while bringing stability to community turnover. A well-run home health agency can ensure the highest quality of nursing, provide continuity of care, and protect patients' rights.

The establishment of a noncertified home health agency that subcontracts with a certified Medicare provider can provide benefits for residents and management alike. Residents can use Medicare benefits that they may otherwise pay for separately. This arrangement can provide significant financial relief to those residents who may be experiencing financial pressure as their health-care needs accelerate. The community can benefit from reduced turnover, stabilization of the assisted living population, and avoidance of costly nursing care transfers by establishing a continuity of care and differential billing structures.

The community can set up a licensed, noncertified home health agency through the applicable state licensing agency. The subsequent survey and approval process can take up to four months depending on the current backlog of applications. Upon licensure, the certified agency would then conduct an initial assessment, set conditions of participation and frequency, develop a care plan, communicate with the physician, and provide the services through the facility's own staff to each eligible resident after the medical necessity of such care has been substantiated through documentation and physician order. The facility then bills the certified agency back for the use of its staff at fair market value. Medicare will reimburse no more than what it would cost to provide those services by a prudent operator through any other qualified contractor. Therefore, if the market rate is $41 per visit for a registered nurse and $23 per visit for a nurse's aide, then that is what the facility can expect in reimbursement from the certified agency for the use of its staff. Medicare will compare reimbursement requests in two ways: primarily to ensure that the visit rates are at fair market value, and secondarily to ensure the prudent use of government resources.

In summary, the overall process involves obtaining a license for a home health agency, hiring or contracting staff to perform home health services, negotiating a preferred provider arrangement with a Medicare-certified agency, and maintaining employee records only (the Medicare-certified agency is responsible for patient records). Essentially, the community-based, licensed, noncertified home health agency provides registered nurses, licensed practical nurses, and home health aides to perform services for the certified agency's Medicare-eligible patients residing both within the community and nearby. Residents are considered patients of the Medicare-certified agency, and as such the agency assumes all of the regulatory requirements demanded of a Medicare-certified home health agency related to the delivery of home health services such as initial assessments, care plans, and supervision. (See Tables 18.1 and 18.2 for a financial analysis.)

Several restrictions apply to this type of arrangement:

1. There can be no duplication of services that the facility is obligated to provide under the existing contract. The contract can, however be modified to exclude those services so long as the community provides for those residents who may not qualify for Medicare.

2. Medicare does not allow any inducement to residents for the provision of Medicare reimbursable ser-

vices. Therefore, it is absolutely necessary to disclose to the residents that the community participates in the delivery of home health services, and that they have the right to choose any agency of their preference for the delivery of their services. Providers cannot legally deny any Medicare beneficiary the freedom to choose among health care providers.

3. The agreement must be a nonexclusive arrangement in which the certified agency may engage other contractors to provide similar services, and the community-based nonlicensed agency may contract with other certified home health agencies to provide its services. The provider must at all times refrain from recommending or referring patients (residents) to any single agency.

4. Payments cannot be determined in any manner that takes into account the volume or value of any referrals or business generated between the parties for which the payment may be made in whole or in part by Medicare or a state-funded health program.

Careful steps must be taken to avoid the risks associated with becoming viewed by Medicare as an abusive practice. Medicare and Medicaid anti-kickback

Table 18.1   Creating a Community-Based Home Health Agency

	Scenario 1	Scenario 2	Scenario 3
Total visits	**500**	**750**	**1500**
SN visits	200	300	600
HHA visits	300	450	900
SN revenues	8,200	12,300	24,600
HHA revenues	6,900	10,350	20,700
Total revenues	**$15,100**	**$22,650**	**$45,300**
SN costs	2,133	3,200	6,400
HHA costs	2,100	3,150	6,300
Total costs	**$4,233**	**6,350**	**$12,700**
Monthly net income	$10,867	$16,300	$32,600
Annual net income	$130,400	$195,000	$391,200

NOTE:

Scenario 1: Maintain volume of 500 home health visits, and set up a community-based agency to participate in the delivery of care.

Scenario 2: Increase volume of home health visits to 750 monthly through early detection of problems and through providing temporary rehabilitative services to other residents within the community and in the local geographic vicinity, via a community-based agency.

Scenario 3: Average visits possible in a 200-unit comparable facility.

Table 18.2   Assumptions

Number of beds	90
Visits per month	500
Average monthly visits per bed	5.56
% visits that are skilled nursing (SN)	40%
% visits that are home health aides (HHA)	60%
Reimbursement rate for SN visit	$ 41.00
Reimbursement rate for HHA visit	$ 23.00
Direct cost of SN per hour*	$ 16.00
Direct cost of HHA per hour*	$ 7.00
Average SN visits per hour	1.5
Average HHA visits per hour	1.0

*Note: Costs do not include benefits or administration.

provisions contained in U.S.C. 1320 a-7b(b), Section 1128B of the Social Security Act are enforced by the Office of the Inspector General. Because of the broad scope of the federal anti-kickback laws, the secretary of Health and Human Services issued regulations commonly known as the "Safe Harbor regulations" (Federal Register 56 F.2d Reg. 35951, first published July 29, 1991) that provide clarification as to the applicability of federal regulations. It is critical to document the arrangement with the independent contractor through the use of a "safe harbor" agreement to protect against infringement of the Social Security Act. *Providers who are considering entering into such arrangements with an independent contractor to provide Medicare-reimbursable services to their residents are strongly encouraged to seek competent legal advice.* They should also be sure to check applicable state regulations, as this arrangement may not be permitted in some states.

In continuing-care communities, the introduction of a home health agency can substantially prolong or even avoid the transfer of residents to the high cost nursing home segment of the life care community. This is particularly advantageous to nonprofit communities where healthy residents are in effect subsidizing the care for those in the nursing home. As more residents are transferred to the nursing home due to the lack of supportive services in their apartment, costs to provide that care are borne by all members. In addition, overcrowding in the medical center can be virtually eliminated by the implementation of a home health agency. Also, by increasing the level of care to residents in their

independent apartments, life-care communities can keep beds available for rehabilitative care for nonresidents, creating an additional revenue source to help offset rising expenses.

■ MARKET TO CURRENT RESIDENTS

It is possible to set up a noncertified home health agency within the confines of the retirement community to provide services to community-based residents so that it will cash flow after 60 days. The community must comprise at least 200 units and be at a stabilized occupancy of at least 95 percent. It will be critical for management to understand the potential effects that a supportive-care environment such as home health care will ultimately have on the resident profile over time. Once implemented, it is not easily withdrawn. Supportive-care services, when introduced to a relatively independent population, can change the image of the community permanently and should not be employed as simply a method to boost revenues. Eventually it will be more difficult to attract and keep more active residents, and the community will make the transition over time to a more frail population. This will, of course, result in a shorter length of stay, and consequently a higher turnover percentage will result. Be sure to step up marketing efforts so as not to compromise the stabilized occupancy of the community. If occupancy slips too far, the home health services designed to enhance revenue may turn into a financial burden. A preliminary survey should be conducted among the resident population to ascertain demand and to educate the residents to the potential costs involved. Try to obtain commitments from several residents sufficient to cover the initial costs to staff the project. As more residents join the plan, the margins will improve due to the economy of scale. The introduction of supportive services to congregate communities will serve to increase turnover which will require aggressive market planning to offset this effect. In the CCRC environment, home health care may serve to delay nursing-home placement, which when funded by the resident can significantly reduce overall exposure. In models where the owners realize a return on their investment through the resale of turned-over units, the home-health model will initially lengthen the residents' occupancy. However, over years of operation, resident attrition will rarely exceed 8 percent annually.

MARKET TO HOMEBOUND ELDERLY

The community-based home health agency can also be set up to market to homebound elderly. To the host community the advantage of improved cash flow with little start-up cost can be very attractive. The major disadvantages will include competition for quality staffing, complicated by the difficulty in supervision and associated travel expenses. Home health care provided within the grounds of a host retirement community will have little nonproductive travel time, depending on the geographic proximity of the homebound client base. Travel time can represent up to 40 percent of the costs of running the operation and can be difficult to recover in a reasonable hourly rate to the client. Nevertheless, there is a tremendous demand for the services by residents who do not want to leave their homes, and by government officials looking for cost-effective alternatives to institutionalization.

THE ORGANIZATION

Management Requirements

The administrator or executive director is an individual preferably with hands-on experience with the day-to-day operations of a for-profit certified home health agency or, at a minimum, senior management experience in a home-health environment. For congregate projects, the personal care or assisted living director can serve in this function; in the absence of these positions, the executive director can fill this role. In a continuing-care retirement center, current administrative configuration of the CCRC setting would require additional supportive staff if the facility administrator is to operate several health-care entities. Freestanding community agencies normally require significant amounts of marketing efforts from the administrator.

The director of nursing must be a registered nurse with a minimum of one year of administrative and supervisory experience, and preferably experience in home-health management and supervision. The start-up agency is typically staffed by the director of nursing, who also acts as case manager. Based on obtaining certain operating levels, an additional case manager should be employed part-time.

The R.N. case manager preferably has one or more years' experience in home care or public health patient care. Additionally, one year of supervisory experience is preferable. The R.N. case manager supervises the agency staff in clients' homes and coordinates and manages the patients' care plan. The case manager also provides direct patient care services for patients requiring skilled-nursing services. Generally, one R.N. case manager can appropriately manage between 25 and 35 cases, depending on the level of care each patient requires. Therefore, it is appropriate to add case managers incrementally with part-time employees.

In general, support-services needs are variable according to the level of automation available to the organization. Certainly, the home health environment lends itself to the use of computerization. Billing, scheduling, and charting are all highly repetitive processes that are easily computerized. The staffing coordinator office assistant function is a very demanding part of the organization that requires good organizational skills and follow-through. The individual best suited for this position preferably has had some experience in the home health environment. Although not essential, a home health background will give the coordinator much needed insight into staffing flexibility. Once the agency obtains a staffing level of approximately 1,500–2,000 hours per week, the combined position of staffing coordinator and office assistant should be divided into two positions, again staging in from part-time to full-time status. The office assistant is the primary clerical support position of the agency.

Depending on the location of the agency—that is, whether it is located within the CCRC or retirement community or freestanding—such as accounts payable and receivable and payroll, the typical business office functions need to be provided. It is advisable to use the existing business-office staff and simply hire a part-time clerk as the need arises, rather than have two separate accounting functions on a property. Again, the computerization of these functions allows for significant accuracy and coordination of scheduling, billing, and payroll and can be easily incorporated into one set of books.

Depending on the agency's state regulations or lack thereof, the in-home labor force is a pool of employees available for specific assignments. The in-home labor force consists primarily of licensed practical nurses (LPN), home health assistants (HHA), companions, and homemakers.

Each state has its own unique standards, qualifications, and service limits for both the agency and the caregiver. The pool labor force is typically a non-benefited class of employees who register with a variety of different agencies at the same time. Recruitment and retention is a much more challenging prospect than the facility-based health care worker presents. Flexibility is the key enticement to the home health worker. Wages are typically as high as 25–30 percent greater than for the equivalent facility-based job descriptions. The key for management is to identify the quality individuals in the home health organization and provide them with the number of hours that they require to develop a long-term association with the agency.

Recruitment methods are also very important. A small agency can very quickly run into financial problems by utilizing the local newspapers as its primary source for applicants. The agency should be as aggressive in its outside marketing efforts for employees as it is for clients.

Operational Policies

Home health employees and the work environment present a unique management challenge. The structure of the agency's personnel policies is significantly different from all other directly supervised employment relationships. The home health environment requires specific personnel policies. The employee/employer relationship is typically very thin and requires clear, itemized policy statements to ensure the highest potential employee compliance.

As with all health-care facilities, the home health industry has its share of regulated administrative requirements. The administrative policies are those company policies that make up a regulated position statement that is a statement of business practice for the knowledge of the client. These policies typically cover the following areas:

1. Admission/retention
2. Discharge policy (voluntary and involuntary)
3. Business standards
   a. Billing
   b. Refunds
   c. Discrepancies
   d. Truth and lending
4. Civil rights policies

5. ADA and EEOC
6. Statements of liability
7. Any other regulated patent notifications

Patient Care Procedures and Standards

In general, every act of patient care requires an in-depth explanation of the agency's approved procedures and standards of performance. The typical areas of content include:

- Infection control
- Hazardous waste
- Direct patient care
- Emergency procedures
- Life safety procedures

Many of these standards are universal in the health care environment, although a specific agency may choose to intensify the standard for purposes of setting itself apart from other providers.

Licensure Requirements

Each state and governmental program has its own specific licensure or certification requirements. The individual agency will need to specifically identify those requirements and develop systems, policies, or protocols to accommodate those requirements. A copy of the administrative codes for the legal operation of home health agencies is readily available from the office of the state licensing body. Great care should be exercised during the planning stages to determine the financial impacts of the regulations on the overall operations before opening shop.

MARKET ANALYSIS AND PLANNING

The colocated agency has a very unique opportunity to develop a clientele within the retirement community. Otherwise, the general market demographics are of significance in the success of the agency. In general, the key success indicators are:

1. Per capita income or other income indicators.
2. Age distributions and diversity. Obviously, the private in-home care industry is most used by the affluent elderly, in the 70+ age group. Other minor sources of use are the over-60 post-hospitalization group, although this is typically the segment most captured by the certified agencies.

3. Geographic distribution. It is highly desirable to operate in as small a geographic area as possible. The higher concentration of the target market group provides significant management and supervisory advantages.
4. Other key market analytical indicators are available through local, state, and regional planning organizations. They provide nearly all statistical information needed to identify the target market location.

Obviously, other competitive interests may have already identified the same market location as their target. The success of the agency is solely dependent on client attraction and referral. Many community hospitals have developed their own home health agencies and provide noncompetitive advantages to their own interest. Typically, these agencies are certified and compete for the Medicare business first and the private market to a much lesser degree.

Identification of the agency's market resources is one of the major keys to success. Hospitals, physicians, and other health care providers provide great opportunity for referrals. Additional resources can include:

1. Trust departments
2. Financial advisors
3. Private case management
4. Pharmacies
5. Rehabilitation organizations
6. Nursing homes
7. Attorneys
8. Assisted-living and congregate communities

A comprehensive marketing program must be developed and planned to take optimal advantage of both resources and opportunities to promote the agency. The marketing program must be designed to encompass external client resources, external employee resources, and internal-staff marketing consciousness. The typical agency relies primarily on the administrator and director of nursing to coordinate all agency marketing activities. The more aggressive (and potentially the more successful) agency will allocate a specific position for marketing and will empower and incorporate the entire agency staff in market and client development. Incentive programs, uniforms, car-signage, employee functions participation, or anything else that can be used to include the agency staff broadens the agency's marketing force.

FINANCIAL ANALYSIS

Start-up capital requirements are relatively modest compared to other industries of equal revenue potential. Most of the capitalization requirements are simply to cover the cost of operations during the agency maturation process, which can range from 12 to 18 months.

1. Equipment needs can most appropriately be satisfied by lease rather than by capital purchases.
2. Office needs can be as modest or as elaborate as is required by the unique opportunities of the individual agency. Obviously, the colocated agency would require a relatively attractive office space due to the opportunity for walk-in traffic at the retirement community. Otherwise, typical home health operations are in storefront locations centrally located within their service area. It remains more important to be convenient for the employees than for the client.
3. Other operating capital requirements:
   a. Start-up payroll: It is anticipated that the start-up agency would require approximately 60 days of start-up time to bring the agency to opening status, then an additional 30–60 days for market awareness to develop and income potential (cash flow) to be established.
   b. Operating overhead: Utility expenses, licenses, tax, fees, and assessments. Supply cost, i.e. charting forms, charge/payroll slips, and other administrative and personnel documentation.
   c. Marketing cost: A significant percentage of the start-up capitalization would be allocated to production and development cost associated with marketing. Collateral development, advertising, sponsorships, and memberships fall into this category. Many of these costs will be ongoing throughout the agency's maturation period.

   A well-developed marketing program is essential to the eventual success of the agency. An appropriate and significant allocation of resources must be made available to the start-up agency for name recognition and market saturation. A beginning agency requires a very large spectrum of referral sources that can later be narrowed as it more soundly develops its market niche.
4. Typically, home health agencies do not have large capital assets available for attachment through liability litigation. Therefore, the primary assets

available are name, reputation, future earnings, cash reserve, and owner assets. Liability exposures are significant in the home health business and can include:

a. Negligence
   1. Owners
   2. Management
   3. Caregiver
b. Abuse and/or theft
c. Employee injury
   1. Worker's compensation
   2. Employer negligence
d. Vehicular incidents

It becomes obvious that a strong umbrella insurance and bonding package be in place for the protection of the entity. Required types of coverage would include:

a. General business liability
b. Medical malpractice
c. Employee bonding
d. Workers Compensation

Another issue involving insurance is the use of client and/or employee property for the purpose of providing service, i.e., automobiles. There are generally three approaches to this issue:

a. Agency provides umbrella coverage
b. Employee's car insurance primary
c. Client's car insurance primary with a no-fault disclaimer

Certainly, the highest protection and the most expensive for the agency would be agency-provided umbrella coverage.

NOTE

1. "Home Health Care Expenditures to Increase 30% in 1993," *Health News Daily,* January 6, 1993.

Appendixes

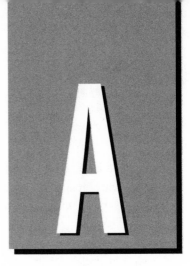

50 Questions Frequently Asked by Residents and Families

1. How many residents do you have?

We have about _____ residents signed up; however, many apartment sizes and locations are still available. We have 100 apartments and expect that 110 residents will live here when we are full.

2. Who owns this place?

The property is owned and managed by Talisman Senior Housing.

3. What kind of security do you have?

You'll find a very sophisticated emergency alert system in each apartment for an immediate response in case of need. Also, we have staff on duty 24 hours a day, 7 days a week, and cameras on all doors.

4. How many square feet are in each apartment?

We have more than 10 apartment sizes in several floor plans, depending on your needs. Of course, monthly fees are based on the location and size of each apartment.

5. How often do you raise the monthly fee?

Raising the monthly fee is a concern to all our residents. Of course we try to be very sensitive to that, but we don't want to cut costs by reducing the services or quality of food. We do require a 60-day cancellation notice. All monthly fees are guaranteed through your residency agreement against increase for 13 months; you also have the opportunity to sign a three-year agreement with capped increases.

6. Do you have an entrance (membership) fee?

Yes, the entrance fee is used to cover the costs of the initial assessment, income verification, preliminary care plan, and administration. It is not intended to be used as a security deposit and is not refundable upon move-in.

7. Are the apartments quiet?

You'll find that your apartment is especially well insulated to reduce and eliminate sounds. This is a high-quality structure. All ceilings and floors are eight-inch solid concrete, as are most of the walls between apartments. They are well insulated to ensure your privacy.

8. Are there kitchens in the apartments so that residents can cook if they choose?

A continental breakfast is included in our monthly fee along with 30 additional meals, lunches or dinners, to be eaten at your leisure. More meals can also be purchased. Each apartment has a fully appointed kitchen so that you can cook if you'd like to.

9. Is there a place to park my car?

Yes, there is parking available in our indoor garage. Special discount rates are available for our residents and their guests.

10. Do you have laundry and valet service?

Laundry and dry cleaning services are available to all residents for a small additional fee. A flat linen service is included in the monthly fee.

11. How many apartments are empty and how many are occupied?

We have 100 total units. About 90 percent of them are leased at this time.

12. Do you have storage areas for the residents?

Yes, each apartment is provided with extra closet space. We also have additional locker storage on the ground floor.

13. What about housekeeping service? If it is available, how much does it cost?

Included as a standard service at no additional cost are weekly vacuuming, dusting, cleaning of the bathroom(s) and kitchen, and a change of bed linens.

14. Do you have cable television?

Yes, cable television will be available at an additional charge. We also have a master television antenna to ensure good reception.

15. Are your deposits refundable?

No, the entrance fee is not refundable when you leave the community.

16. Do your two-bedroom apartments have two baths?

Yes, all of our two-bedroom units have two baths (one bathtub, one shower stall).

17. Are the apartments furnished?

Residents usually prefer to bring their own furniture and personal belongings; our models are furnished to give you an idea of how things might look. Rental furniture packages are available at reasonable rates.

18. Can I have guests stay in my apartment for a few days?

We welcome your guests. There is no problem with their visiting, but we do ask that you give us advance notice.

19. Do you have guest rooms?

Yes, they may be reserved at the front desk. The daily charge for a guest room is $50.00, which includes bed linens and towels. We also have respite suites, which provide our full range of services; they are available on a temporary basis.

20. Are my guests permitted to eat with me in the dining rooms? If so, what is the cost?

Yes, your guests are welcome to join you in the dining rooms. All you need to do is call ahead (a day in advance if possible) to make a reservation. The fee for guest meals can be found in the schedule of charges in the resident handbook.

21. Do you cater to special diets?

We consider your diet. We plan our menus for nutrition and health as well as for flavor and appeal. Our Heart Smart menu at each meal features low-fat, low-salt, and low-cholesterol dishes.

22. Is there assigned seating in the dining rooms?

You are free to choose any table that has been set up. Our dining room manager may also suggest the best seating to facilitate efficient service.

23. Do you have a workshop? Can I bring my own tools?

We will have an arts and crafts room where residents will be able to make minor repairs and work on their hobbies. These projects can be worked on with either your tools or ours.

24. When I'm out late how will I get in? Will I get a key?

The night staff will be able to let you in. However, for security and safety reasons we ask that you advise the concierge at the front desk if you will be late.

25. Are waterbeds permitted?

Our building is structurally sound and can accommodate waterbeds.

26. Is there an age limit?

We have no maximum but do have a minimum age requirement of 65.

27. Is smoking permitted?

You are free to smoke in your apartment, out of doors, and in designated smoking areas.

28. Can we have pets?

We accept cats if you currently have one; dogs, however, are not allowed.

29. Are there individual heating and air conditioning controls in each unit?

Yes, all apartments are equipped with individual controls. The common areas are controlled by a computerized energy-management system for your comfort.

30. Are personnel on duty at night?

We have personnel on duty 24 hours a day, seven days a week.

31. If I become ill, what happens?

Our staff is on call around the clock; each apartment is provided with emergency pulls in both the bedroom(s) and the bathroom(s). If you require additional care temporarily we will help you arrange for it through our home health agency.

32. If I'm ill, will meals be brought to my apartment?

Yes, we would be happy to accommodate your request temporarily, for a small delivery charge.

33. How are the meals served?

Meals are served by our professional, friendly wait staff in our dining rooms. Choices of a variety of entrees are available in both our cafe and our main dining room.

34. If I am away for a period of time, do I get a food credit?

Yes, if you are away you get a credit against your meal account. This credit will begin on the fourteenth day of your absence, as outlined in the resident handbook.

35. Do you furnish transportation?

There is free scheduled transportation in our community van within a five-mile radius. We also have a van to accommodate special events and weekly tours.

36. Is there public transportation nearby?

Yes, a bus stops at the corner and travels south to shopping areas and downtown.

37. Are there recreation and exercise rooms?

Yes, we have an exercise room and an art studio, multipurpose room, card room, billiard room, and library for the use and enjoyment of all our residents.

38. What kind of activities do you have?

Activities are held within our building and elsewhere. Our full-time program director will develop a full program of recreational activities, trips, special events, and seminars, which provides for a wide range of interests.

39. Do you go on tours and trips?

Yes, we have our own van which is used for a variety of purposes—shopping excursions, day trips, special events, and tours of the many tourist attractions within driving distance.

40. Do you provide medical services?

We prefer to allow our residents to continue to rely on their personal doctors. We will, however, have a wellness office on the premises staffed on a scheduled basis. There is also an examining room for regular physician visits.

41. Do you allow wheelchairs?

Twenty percent of our apartments are designed for wheelchair use. We will try in every way possible to serve your needs and to keep you as part of our family.

42. Do you have a beauty salon or barber shop?

Yes, we can accommodate the needs of both male and female residents in our salon.

43. Is there a swimming pool?

There is no swimming pool in our building; however, we do have an arrangement with the YMCA. It is within walking distance. Our courtesy car will drop you off and pick you up if you'd like.

44. Who pays for the utilities?

Electricity charges are included in the monthly fee. Your only utility expenses are your personal telephone and cable television.

45. What is done in the event of a noisy disturbance by a neighbor?

Because of the quality of construction, we do not anticipate that to be a problem in our buildings. If it ever is, you may be sure that management will follow up as a matter of courtesy and will attend to the problem.

46. Are young children allowed to visit?

This is your home. Family and friends are always welcome.

47. Is this property run by the Hospital Corporation?

The community is an affiliate of the Hospital Corporation and provides our residents with access to a host of health-care services.

48. Do any of the residents play bridge?

Bridge is very popular. We have several groups and several levels of playing ability.

49. Am I ready for this type of community yet? I don't think so.

We've heard that often from our residents when they were first considering moving here. Now they wish our building had been built years earlier. Residents find that our community offers a wonderful lifestyle with services and amenities that afford them freedom and enjoyment.

50. What is assisted living?

Assisted living is a new retirement-living alternative that offers seniors and their families the security and peace of mind they deserve. Residents are able to live independently in their own private apartments while receiving just the right level of service they need to stay independent.

Assisted-living communities offer an extensive and varied program of services tailored through a service plan to each specific individual. The services range from help with simple chores to a comprehensive program that enables each resident to have access to 24-hour-a-day personal care assistance in his or her private apartment. Other services include medication reminders and help with daily activities such as dressing, grooming, bathing, and ambulation.

In addition to living in a comfortable, secure setting, residents may join in a variety of social and recreational activities and enjoy the companionship of friends and family in their own apartment or in community areas.

There is no endowment or other large up-front fees at our communities. All services and amenities are included in the monthly rental fee.

"Our assisted living communities are a cost effective alternative to extensive home care," claims Ben Pearce, senior vice president. "For what the typical resident at one of our communities would pay for our services and amenities with 24-hour supervision, they could only purchase about six hours per day of home health care." This clear financial advantage has led seniors and their families in large numbers to inquire about these residential alternatives.

Operations Audit

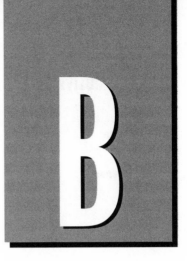

Key Result Area
Departmental Operations Audit

▪▪▪▪▪ INSTRUCTIONS

This operations survey is designed to assist executive directors and their staffs in reaching excellence in all aspects of managing a facility. It should be used as a self-evaluation tool that will assist managers of facilities and department supervisors in understanding the expectations of operational performance and help them reach the goal of providing quality services for residents.

Each line item number should be rated from 0 to 10, 10 being best and 0 being poorest. In some instances more than one question will make up the total rating. An example would be the following:

- Are staff meetings and department head meetings being held?
- Are minutes of these meetings on file?

If the answer to both questions is yes, a score of ten (10) would be appropriate provided the meetings are held *consistently*. If the answer to the second question is no, then perhaps a score of five (5) would be correct.

Each section of the survey will be scored separately and rated as follows:

92–100%	Excellent
83–91%	Good
74–82%	Fair
65–73%	Poor
0–64%	Disaster

The final page of the survey will be used to total the results and arrive at a rating in the same way as explained above.

For those areas where improvement is needed, the department head will be responsible for completing a plan of correction using the attached form. This plan should be proactive and address the standard alone, not the behavior or personality of the supervisor. People work best when expectations are clearly defined, standards are communicated, and consistency is the norm. The better the job we can do as managers to take the guesswork out of what specifically is expected of our staff, the better the job they can do of delivering.

▰▰▰ EXECUTIVE DIRECTOR

	KRA	Standard	Score
1	**Budget**	All departments consistently meet expense budget guidelines each month.	_____
2.	**Revenue**	The community maintains occupancy levels as budgeted. All rollover units are repriced at the maximum marketable value.	_____
3.	**Business plan**	The facility has a completed business plan in effect that is being followed for the current fiscal year.	_____
4.	**Hourly wage plan**	The facility has a completed hourly wage plan in effect that is being followed for the current fiscal year.	_____
5.	**Communication**	A formal system of communication is in place to ensure routine and emergency information is efficiently distributed to staff, residents, and corporate.	_____
6.	**Meetings**	Weekly department-head meetings, monthly all-staff meetings, and all resident meetings are consistently held and planned with an appropriate agenda. Minutes are kept, distributed, and maintained on file.	_____
7.	**Orientation**	All employees have a current job description and employee handbook and have been fully oriented to their positions. Supporting documentation for this orientation is in each employee file and is current.	_____
8.	**Employee files**	All employee files are current and complete. All new employees have been personally interviewed before hiring. Vacant positions are replaced on a timely basis.	_____
9.	**Sales management**	The performance of the sales department is monitored daily. Weekly sales meetings are held with the marketing/sales staff to review and strategize on the closure of all hot leads.	_____
10.	**Community relations**	The performance of a community-relations function for the facility with particular attention to the medical, legal, financial, and religious communities who have influence on the senior market is carried out in a focused and systematic manner.	_____
11.	**Regulations**	The community is fully complying with all government laws and regulations regarding the operation of the property.	_____
12.	**Analysis**	Relevant operational data is consistently analyzed and effectively presented with recommendations and conclusions in a timely manner. Reports are clear, concise, and thoroughly researched.	_____
13.	**Management control**	Monitors departmental systems, goals, and objectives designed to report on and analyze the performance of all service components and individuals under direct supervision.	_____
14.	**Motivation discipline**	All management staff are challenged and motivated in their positions using a systematized approach with regularly scheduled follow-up. All management staff are disciplined, if necessary, in a proactive and positive manner using written plans of correction and review.	_____

15. **Service delivery** — All aspects of service delivery to the residents are monitored on an ongoing basis. Changes are made to assure resident satisfaction and achieve optimal profitability. _____

16. **Competition** — Semiannual reviews and evaluations are conducted of consumer purchasing behaviors, pricing sensitivities, and differentiation of facility services from competitor services. _____

17. **Goals and objectives** — All departmental prior-period goals and objectives have been met. _____

18. **Resident survey** — How well did management score on the resident opinion survey? There is a written plan of corrective action for fair/poor responses. _____

19. **Consistency/response** — All staff are fully informed and rehearsed on the appropriate responses to the most frequently asked questions by prospects, residents, and their families relating to key facts and information about the facility and its services. _____

20. **Policies and procedures** — The facility has a full set of departmental policy and procedure manuals. The manuals are kept current and are referred to before contacting the corporate office. The manuals are used for training new management staff. _____

21. **Marketing** — All staff are fully informed and rehearsed quarterly on their role in marketing the project. Monthly training in all staff meetings emphasizes this critical issue. _____

22. **Employee opinion survey** — A high level of employee participation is achieved. Survey results are communicated to all employees. Improvement plans are developed and implemented. _____

23. **Performance appraisal process** — All employees understand the appraisal process and receive an annual appraisal before receiving any merit increase. _____

24. **Merit increase process** — All employees understand the merit increase process. Increases are effectively communicated in a timely manner. _____

Departmental Score _____   **Percent** _____   **Rating** _____

■ HOUSEKEEPING/LAUNDRY

KRA	Standard	Score
1. **Job**	All housekeeping staff have current job descriptions and have been given an employee handbook.	_____
2. **Orientation to department**	All staff have been thoroughly oriented to their job expectations and resident relations. Orientation checklists for each employee are on file.	_____
3. **Ancillary revenue**	Ancillary revenue is at or above budget. All staff are fully aware of what work is included and what may be charged to residents. Every effort is being made to maximize this revenue source.	_____
4. **Tasking plan**	All staff consistently follow task lists for apartment cleaning and can communicate the limitations of their services to the resident, when asked.	_____

5. **Master plan**   A written and current master cleaning plan is consistently followed for the entire property.   _____

6. **Cleaning schedules**   Apartment/common area cleaning schedules by individual employees are maintained and posted.   _____

7. **Work schedules**   The staff work schedule is planned at least one week in advance and is posted. Work schedules are approved by the executive director and strictly comply with the labor budget. All overtime is approved in writing.   _____

8. **Nonresident apartments**   All nonresident apartments, including vacant, guest, and model and marketing units, are scheduled for cleaning and consistently cleaned on a routine basis. A monthly status is submitted to the executive director on all vacant apartments, whether leased or not.   _____

9. **Equipment/manuals**   Operating and service manuals and all warranty information are properly filed and are accessible.   _____

10. **Cleaning log**   All resident chargeable housekeeping services are documented by resident, apartment, date, and time and are current as to the end of each shift.   _____

11. **Service contracts**   Copies of all current service contracts are on file and accessible. All service contracts have at least two competitive bids on file and are reviewed annually.   _____

12. **Vendor accounts**   A current ledger is kept on all vendor accounts, outside contractors, and technicians by service area and contact person.   _____

13. **Safety**   OSHA regulations are on file and posted. There is a record of continuing education on chemical use for each employee.   _____

14. **Staff meetings**   Monthly staff meetings are held to discuss issues pertaining to the department and to solicit input from all members of the department. Daily briefing sessions are held with all staff members before beginning the day's schedule.   _____

15. **Deliveries/inventory**   Written procedures are consistently followed for the check-in and security of all deliveries. All supplies are inventoried quarterly and stored in a secure area.   _____

16. **Uniforms**   All staff wear uniforms that are clean and complete.   _____

17. **Key control**   Keys are checked out to each housekeeper only for the rooms for which they have cleaning responsibility. Master keys do not leave the building. Keys are not duplicated without the approval of the executive director.   _____

18. **Tools/equipment**   All facility tools and moveable equipment are marked with facility identification and inventoried.   _____

19. **Budget**   The department consistently meets budgeting guidelines.   _____

20. **Resident survey**   How well did the housekeeping department score on the resident opinion survey? There is a written plan of correction for fair/poor responses.   _____

21. **Training**   There is a training program in place to provide employees with development and growth within their position.   _____

22. **Hazardous waste**

All staff are fully informed regarding infection control and the disposal of hazardous waste.

_____

23. **Goals/objectives**

Departmental prior-period goals and objectives are fully met.

_____

24. **Furnishings**

Cleaning schedules are maintained for all furnishings, fixtures, and equipment in common areas and back-of-the-house areas.

_____

25. **Chemical storage**

All chemicals are properly inventoried, stored, and labeled. Staff are fully trained in safely refilling self-dispensing chemicals. Inventory of and emergency procedures for each chemical are on file and accessible.

_____

26. **Laundry separation**

Clean and dirty linen areas are clearly separated and maintained at all times to assure adequate supplies of linens that are in good condition.

_____

27. **Laundry training**

Staff are trained in the proper use of all laundry equipment and are thoroughly briefed in the operation of all cycles and all aspects of safety. Training includes the proper amounts of detergents and chemicals to be used and the checking of water temperature on a daily basis to assure compliance with all regulations.

_____

28. **Laundry inventory**

Par levels are developed and maintained at all times with a written inventory to assure adequate supplies of linens that are in good condition.

_____

29. **Laundry contract**

For all properties that send laundry out for processing, all items are counted before sending them out and counted again upon their return to confirm proper billing and control. In addition, all items are weighed if weight determines how the property is billed for this service.

_____

30. **Laundry identification**

All linens are clearly marked to facilitate identification whether the items are processed internally or externally.

_____

31. **Marketing**

All housekeeping staff are fully informed and rehearsed in their role in marketing the project.

_____

32. **Resident relations**

All housekeeping staff understand the importance of alerting management to changes in residents' health conditions or any resident dissatisfaction. Housekeepers understand their role in promoting a positive environment within the community and are solution-oriented.

_____

Departmental Score _____ **Percent** _____ **Rating** _____

HUMAN RESOURCES

KRA	Standard	Score
1. **Handbook**	Each employee file contains the handbook's last page signed by the employee and confirming the receipt of a handbook.	_____
2. **Dispute resolution policy**	All employees and management understand the dispute resolution policy.	_____

3. **Discipline policy**

Disciplinary procedures are practiced fairly and consistently. All managers, supervisors, and department heads are constructive when taking disciplinary action. Plans of correction are used to improve performance. All disciplinary decisions are properly documented. There is a proper follow-up to disciplinary discussions. _____

4. **Benefit enrollment**

Benefits are clearly explained to all eligible employees. Employees are enrolled in a timely manner. The benefit plan is perceived as an added value and part of their total compensation. _____

5. **Employee files**

An internal file audit is completed annually. All files have a completed and signed application. All personnel and payroll information is current and kept in a secure area. A separate file is maintained for employee benefits and other miscellaneous information that is inappropriate for an employee personnel file. _____

6. **Interview process**

All applicants are provided an equal opportunity. All new employees have been thoroughly interviewed and have documented reference checks on file. _____

7. **Hiring procedures**

Before being hired, final candidates always receive an executive director interview and authorization. _____

8. **I-9 verification**

No employee works more than three days without presenting proper I-9 identification. Expiration dates on documents are properly tracked. I-9 information is complete, current in compliance with federal law, and filed separately from the personnel file. _____

9. **Orientation**

No employee works more than seven says without receiving a proper orientation. Orientation checklists are complete and on file for all employees. _____

10. **Status change W-4**

All employees on payroll have a completed and authorized status change and W-4 forms. _____

11. **Company property**

Uniforms, keys, tools, manuals, etc. are all distributed with a property receipt form in the personnel file. Company property is returned on separation of employment. _____

12. **Organizational chart**

The facility and corporate organizational chart is explained to new staff in orientation. Direct line and dotted line responsibility is communicated to pertinent staff. _____

13. **Labor notices**

All federal, state, and local labor notices are posted and updated when necessary. _____

14. **Overtime**

All employees understand the overtime policy. All overtime is approved in advance by the employee's supervisor in writing. _____

15. **Time clock**

All employees understand the time clock procedures. Disciplinary action is taken with employees who consistently punch in too early or punch out too late without authorization. _____

16. **Payroll**

All payroll printouts are reviewed and initialed by the executive director before they are submitted to ADP. _____

17. **Risk management**   Risk-management procedures are fully understood and followed. The liability-insurance carrier is known and reporting procedures are followed.   _____

18. **Unemployment compensation**   All terminations, whether voluntary or involuntary, are reported to the corporate office. Reports are reviewed for accuracy and appropriately filed.   _____

19. **Incident reports response**   All employees are aware that injuries/incidents are to be reported to their supervisor immediately. An in-house accident report, state report, and OSHA log are completed.   _____

20. **Workers' compensation**   All employees are aware of the rights of the injured under the Worker's Compensation Act. All supervisory staff are familiar with worker's compensation procedures and reporting.   _____

21. **H.R. reports**   Human resource monthly summary reports are completed and submitted to management each month.   _____

22. **Employee opinion survey**   A high level of participation is achieved. Survey results are communicated to all employees. Improvement plans are developed and implemented.   _____

23. **Performance appraisal**   All employees understand the appraisal process and receive an annual appraisal before receipt of their merit increases.   _____

24. **Merit increase process**   All employees understand the merit increase process. Increases are effectively communicated in a timely manner.   _____

25. **Hourly wage plans**   The wage plan process is updated at least annually and completed for all hourly positions in a timely manner.   _____

Departmental Score _____   **Percent** _____   **Rating** _____

RESIDENT RELATIONS

KRA	Standard	Score
1. **Volunteers**	Volunteers for the building are solicited. There is an annual social event to recognize volunteers. Gifts are given at this event. Residents are encouraged and educated about outside community volunteer opportunities.	_____
2. **Programming manual**	The programming manual is current and is used as a reference and training tool.	_____
3. **Newcomers orientation**	There is a formal orientation of newcomers and a support group to address move-in concerns and relocation trauma. Resident-relations staff make sure that each resident receives a copy of the resident handbook and reviews its contents; meet with each resident and family on the day of move-in to greet and assist where needed; within 24 hours of move-in, review with resident the functions of apartment equipment; provide a tour of the building; and continue to monitor adjustment to living at the community and provide assistance as needed.	_____
4. **Job description**	All staff members have a copy of their job description and an employee handbook. They are oriented and evaluated with their appropriate technical skills supplement.	_____

5. **Budget**	The department consistently meets its budgetary guidelines.	_____
6. **Resident survey**	How well did the resident relations department score on the resident opinion survey? There is a written plan of correction for fair/poor responses.	_____
7. **Training**	Staff members are cross-trained within the resident relations department.	_____
8. **Handling concerns**	All resident concerns are handled in an efficient and timely manner. Concerns are communicated to other cabinet members in writing.	_____
9. **Events**	Resident relations works closely with the marketing Department on marketing events/functions to best promote the community.	_____
10. **Resident communications**	The facility has an organized and consistent way of communicating with residents. Resident meetings are held monthly. Minutes of council meetings and of all resident meetings are on file and current.	_____
11. **Goals**	All department goals and objectives are fully met.	_____
12. **Marketing**	All resident relations staff are fully informed and rehearsed on their role in marketing the project.	_____
13. **Emergency call system**	The emergency call system is checked quarterly, calls are answered promptly, and all activations of the call system are properly documented in the log book.	_____
14. **Library**	The library and all reading areas have a current and accurate inventory of books. Only hardcover books are on display in public areas. All magazines and newspaper subscriptions are kept current, organized, and orderly.	_____
15. **Counseling move outs**	Staff work with families to handle residents who have special needs and problems and begin to recommend a move to greater levels of care when applicable. Staff provide move-out assistance to families, and make sure families receive a move-out package.	_____

Departmental Score _____   **Percent** _____   **Rating** _____

■■■■■ ENGINEERING/MAINTENANCE

KRA	Standard	Score
1. **Job description**	All maintenance staff have current job descriptions and an employee handbook. All current staff and new hires have passed the maintenance skills test.	_____
2. **Orientation to department**	All staff have been thoroughly oriented to their job expectations and resident-relation issues. Orientation checklists for each employee are on file.	_____
3. **Ancillary charges**	Ancillary revenue is at or above budget. All work orders are coded as included or billback. All billbacks are confirmed with the resident before work is performed. Every effort is being made to maximize this revenue source.	_____

4. **Work orders**
Proper work-order procedures are being followed and confirmation of receipt and timing is made to each resident within 24 hours of the order. _____

5. **Preventive maintenance**
A preventive maintenance system is in place, is current, and is in written form, according to company policy and manufacturer instructions. _____

6. **Equipment manuals**
Operating and service manuals are filed and accessible for all major and minor equipment. All warranty information is properly filed and accessible. _____

7. **Service log**
Service logs are kept for all maintenance work by location, date, time, and apartment/service area. Service logs are current as of the end of each shift. _____

8. **Service contracts**
Copies of all current service contracts are on file and accessible. All service contracts have at least two competitive bids on file and are reviewed annually. Certificates of insurance are updated as they expire. _____

9. **Vendor contracts**
A current ledger is kept on all vendor accounts, outside contractors, and technicians by service area and contact person. _____

10. **Emergency/disaster procedures**
A current emergency disaster plan is on file. All department heads are fully aware of their roles in the event of an emergency. The emergency generator is tested monthly. A fire incident log is maintained and periodic fire drills are held. _____

11. **Safety**
OSHA regulations are filed or posted. There is a record of drills and safety training for all employees. _____

12. **Deliveries/inventories**
Written procedures are consistently followed for the check-in and security of all deliveries. All supplies are inventoried quarterly and stored in a secure area. _____

13. **Uniforms**
All staff wear uniforms that are clean and complete. _____

14. **Key control**
A written key-control policy is in place and followed. Master keys do not leave the building. Duplicate keys are not held by residents' families. _____

15. **Tools/equipment**
All facility tools and moveable equipment are marked with facility identification and inventoried. _____

16. **Budget**
The department consistently meets budgetary guidelines. _____

17. **Resident survey**
How well did the maintenance department score on the resident opinion survey? There is a written plan of correction for fair/poor responses. _____

18. **Risk management**
Life safety, fire marshall, and health department surveys are in full compliance or a plan of corrective action exists. Safety/liability consultant reports are in full compliance, or a plan of corrective action exists. _____

19. **Organization**
Engineering files and blueprints/drawings are properly maintained. _____

20. **Conservation**
There is an energy management/conservation plan in use for facility mechanical operations. _____

21. **Training**	There is a training program in place to provide career development for employees.	_____
22. **Goals**	Departmental prior period goals and objectives are fully met.	_____
23. **Marketing**	All maintenance staff are fully informed and rehearsed in their role in marketing the project.	_____

Departmental Score _____   **Percent** _____   **Rating** _____

▄▄▄▄ FOOD AND BEVERAGE

KRA	Standard	Score
1. **Food and beverage manual**	There is a copy of the food and beverage manual in the chef's office. All managers must have working knowledge of all concepts, procedures, and directives.	_____
2. **Health department**	Health department inspections are on file in the chef's office. Department scores must be consistently above 90 percent on all inspections as a minimum standard within the company guidelines. All kitchen staff have current food-handler permits.	_____
3. **Job descriptions**	All food and beverage employees have current job descriptions that outline all aspects of their daily job responsibilities as the accepted standard of performance.	_____
4. **Handbook**	A copy of the handbook is available for review in the chef's office.	_____
5. **Schedules**	All staff work schedules are prepared and calculated in FTE at least one week in advance and posted. Schedules are approved by the executive director and strictly comply with labor budget. All overtime is approved in writing by the executive director.	_____
6. **Food inventory**	Physical inventory of the storeroom and freezer is taken on the last day of the month (or the next working day where applicable) by the chef and the property accountant. Perpetual inventory from the daily food-cost report (book value) and physical count match within 5 percent of each other.	_____
7. **Equipment maintenance**	All kitchen equipment is well maintained and in working order. Work-order procedure is to be followed for any equipment in need of maintenance.	_____
8. **Budget**	The department consistently meets budget guidelines each month.	_____
9. **Uniforms**	Cooks and utility workers are in clean and complete uniforms.	_____
10. **Sanitation**	All cooks, prep persons, and utility workers are completely trained using the company sanitation program and video. Employees are reviewed, tested, and monitored on a quarterly basis as directed by the corporate office.	_____
	All cooks, prep persons, and utility workers have daily sanitation sidework task sheets to assist in maintaining the	

health and sanitation of food products and the kitchen environment. Sidework sheets are distributed by the manager and retained in a file in the food service office. _____

All equipment, such as walk-in/reach-in coolers/freezers, cooking equipment, floors, and food-processing equipment (mixers, slicers, etc.), has regular planned daily/weekly sanitation plans that include how and where food is to be stored, cooked, and held. All of these procedures are identified in task sheets. _____

All cooks, prep persons, and utility workers are trained by managers in the correct health and sanitation maintenance of any and all equipment and procedures prior to the distribution of any tasking sheets. _____

11. **Ware washing**

The dishwasher is cleaned regularly and kept in working order. All cookware is cleaned thoroughly and not allowed to soak overnight. All china and glassware is checked for chips and cracks and taken out of service as needed. Chemical levels and water temperature are to be checked at frequent intervals during the day. The dish machine is drained and cleaned after each meal period. _____

12. **Resident food and beverage satisfaction**

How well did the kitchen score on the resident opinion survey? There is a written plan of correction for the areas where responses were in the fair/poor category. _____

13. **Menu planning**

All menus are planned 30 days in advance and sent to the corporate office for review. Menus include one health smart entree and dessert on each day's plan. _____

Residents with special diet needs are reasonably accommodated by the chef. _____

The menu will include one food and beverage event designed by the food service per month and a minimum of two theme meals per month. _____

14. **Purchasing plan**

Weekly purchasing plans precede all actual orders. All high-cost items such as fish and meat are bid out and ordered at the most competitive price. A purchasing plan is visible in the food service office with all pertinent information available to be used when receiving products. _____

15. **Production plan**

Production plans are done to coordinate with the purchasing plan and menu, giving explicit instructions to all food-service employees involved with the day-to-day production in the kitchen. Production plans are done for the menu on a weekly basis so that staff have the advantage of working on production several days in advance of need. All production and purchasing plans are kept on file. Clear, simple, standard recipes will accompany the production plan where applicable. _____

16. **Reports**

Receiving, payroll, food cost analysis, requisitions, etc. are completed on a daily basis. _____

17. **Implementation: Food temperature**

All food is served at the correct temperature—hot food is on hot plates covered with plate covers, and cold food is on cold plates. _____

Plate presentation	Plates are designed to have color, texture, and variety. All plates are garnished.	_____
Room tray	Room service is always timely and appetizing. All trays, dishes, and glassware are retrieved at the end of each shift.	_____
18. **Banquets**	All banquets are costed out in advance of commitment to ensure that the profit margin is met.	_____
19. **Storage**	All food storage, both dry and refrigerated, is organized to ensure that like items are stored together; cross contamination does not occur; products are appropriately covered, rotated, dated, and priced; and no food product is ever stored on the floor.	_____
20. **Goals**	All departmental prior-period goals and objectives are met.	_____
21. **Resident relations**	Staff routinely visit and maintain liaison with the residents in the dining room, solicit input from residents, and make every effort to implement suggestions within current budgetary limitations.	_____
22. **Marketing**	All kitchen staff are fully informed and rehearsed on their role in marketing the project.	

Departmental Score _____   Percent _____   Rating _____

■■■ DINING ROOM

KRA	Standard	Score
1. **Food and beverage manual**	There is a copy of the food and beverage manual in the chef's office. All managers must have working knowledge of all concepts, procedures, and directives.	_____
2. **Orientation**	All dining room staff are fully oriented to the expectations of their position. The corporate orientation checklist is on file. All employees are trained to understand the specifics of these jobs.	_____
3. **Sanitation**	All dining room staff are completely trained in proper sanitation practices Employees are reviewed, tested, and monitored on a quarterly basis.	_____
4. **Uniforms**	All servers on the floor area are always in complete, clean uniforms. Grooming standards are strictly enforced as part of the uniform. Name tags are always worn.	_____
5. **Work schedules**	All staff work schedules are prepared at least one week in advance and are posted. Schedules are approved by the executive director; they must comply with the labor budget. All overtime is first approved by the department head in writing.	_____
6. **Function sheets**	Function sheets are reviewed daily by the chef and the dining room manager for that day and the following day. Equipment lists and special sidework assignments accompany the function sheets.	_____
7. **Sidework/dining room maintenance**	Individual task sheets are distributed to each person during her scheduled shift. Tasks are identified with predetermined completion times. All employees are checked out by their managers or shift supervisors before the end of their shift.	

The manager and the employee sign off for the work completed each day. Sidework includes vacuuming, wiping down and sanitizing furniture, cleaning side stands, counters and cabinets, removing any and all dishes and serving equipment to the utility area, resetting all tables, restocking all tabletop equipment, and restocking any side stations with nonperishable food or equipment necessary to operate the food service at the next shift. _____

8. **Linen control**

All linen is counted and sorted nightly. If linen is sent to an outside laundry service it is inventoried before it is sent out. All deliveries are counted to verify the delivery receipt. _____

9. **Breakage control**

All broken or chipped items are accounted for daily. All chipped china is retained for reimbursement from the china company. _____

10. **Inventory**

Quarterly inventories of china, glass, silverware, and linen are sent to the corporate office. Operational losses do not exceed 25 percent annually. _____

11. **Walk-through**

The manager walks through the dining room before opening and after closing each meal period to correct any deficiencies. _____

12. **Premeal meetings**

Meetings are held daily to discuss the menu with the manager, chef, and servers. Servers are aware of menu choices and specials. _____

13. **Reservations**

Dinner reservations for guests are reconfirmed with all residents by a return phone call from the shift supervisor. The reservation policy is strictly enforced to ensure that service standards are consistently met. _____

14. **Theme/event meals**

Food service provides a minimum of two theme meals and one food and beverage event per month. The dining room manager and staff work closely with the chef in providing a complementary style of service geared to the theme or event, in addition to any decorations, displays, costumes, or music. _____

15. **Continental**

This breakfast is always appealing, abundant, fresh, and neat and tidy. Second cups of coffee are always poured. Tables are turned immediately and trays of dirty dishes are removed quickly to the kitchen. _____

16. **Resident food and beverage satisfaction**

Surveys are done to find out how well the dining room staff satisfies the residents. There is a written plan of correction for the areas where responses were in the fair/poor categories. _____

17. **Food and beverage meetings**

The executive director, chef, and dining room manager meet weekly. Notes of these meetings are kept on file. _____

18. **Budget**

All supervisors must completely understand how to use the budget in hiring/staffing and purchasing operating supplies and revenue. Monthly labor costs are consistently in line with the budget. _____

19. **Reports**

These reports are completed daily: food checks and check-control sheets, meal count summary, payroll summary, banquet and any other function billings, food and equipment pars and requisitions. _____

20. **Motivation**	Supervisor motivates staff through incentives to achieve better service, less absenteeism, and lower breakage/loss rate of equipment.	_____
21. **Marketing**	All dining room staff are fully informed and rehearsed in their roles to market the project.	_____
22. **Goals**	All departments should strive to meet the goals and objectives of earlier periods.	_____

Departmental Score _____   **Percent** _____   **Rating** _____

■■■■■ TRANSPORTATION

KRA	Standard	Score
1. **Maintenance**	Vehicles are in safe working order. They are regularly maintained, cleaned, and waxed. A daily checklist is used to document deficiencies.	_____
2. **Transportation**	All driving request forms are completed correctly. The resident is notified personally on the day the request is made, and it is strictly followed.	_____
3. **Service**	The driver regularly maintains a punctual record, and nonscheduled drop-offs and pick-ups are strictly prohibited.	_____
4. **Schedule**	The monthly transportation schedule is issued to the residents and is strictly followed.	_____
5. **Records**	Transportation employees' driving records are verified in written form with the state, in accordance with OSHA rules. The drivers are considered safe drivers by the residents.	_____
6. **Assistance**	Residents are always assisted in getting in and out of all vehicles, and are given assistance with their parcels where required.	_____
7. **Deliveries**	Resident-requested deliveries to their room are all labeled and arranged for delivery at convenient times that do not conflict with the driving schedules.	_____
8. **Accidents**	The driver knows how to handle an accident or emergency situation. Proper reporting procedures are kept with the vehicle at all times.	_____
9. **Budget**	The department consistently meets its budgetary guidelines.	_____
10. **Safety**	The driver makes sure that residents use seatbelts in all vehicles at all times and is aware of individual resident needs such as assistance in walking. The driver reports noticeable changes in functioning to the director of resident relations.	_____

Departmental Score _____   **Percent** _____   **Rating** _____

◼◼◼ ACTIVITIES/ENRICHMENT

KRA	Standard	Score
1. **Resident survey**	How well did the activity department score on the resident opinion survey? There is a written plan of correction for all fair/poor responses.	_____
2. **Files**	An activities resource file is maintained and updated.	_____
3. **Participation**	Programs are developed that maximize resident participation. Residents are motivated and encouraged to attend events and programs whenever possible.	_____
4. **Newsletters**	The property publishes a newsletter and calendar of events each month. It is of a quality nature. It is legible for older adults and is used as a marketing tool.	_____
5. **Bulletin boards**	The property is decorated for special events and holidays. Bulletin boards are changed monthly, reflect a theme, and are attractive and current.	_____
6. **Supplies**	The department has all equipment and supplies. Equipment is properly maintained, stored, and inventoried.	_____
7. **Set-up**	There is a variety of common space for the scope of activities such as a card room, exercise room, bar/lounge, and library that are properly set up with assistance from housekeeping and food and beverage at least 30 minutes before an event.	_____
8. **Leisure interests**	All of the residents have had leisure interest interviews. The interview information is being used fully to program activities. There is routine follow-through to invite specific residents to activities in which they have shown interest.	_____
9. **Planning**	All major activities/events are planned at least 60 days in advance and are fully itemized and costed out on a function sheet and distributed to the cabinet.	_____
10. **Continuing education**	Programming for continuing education of the residents is implemented and functioning effectively. It is well received, and marketing prospects are involved in the program.	_____
11. **Transportation**	All resident functions and transportation needs are arranged in advance and appropriately billed to resident accounts where possible.	_____
12. **Budget**	The department consistently meets its budgetary guidelines.	_____
13. **Measurement**	Surveys are given to residents regularly for input and opinions on programs and classes. Resident involvement is encouraged. Participant level in all functions is measured, statistics are kept, and plans are designed to encourage optimal involvement.	_____
14. **Marketing**	All activity staff are fully informed and rehearsed on their role in marketing the project. They work closely with the marketing department on marketing events/functions to promote the community. They are aware of newsmaker and publicity possibilities.	_____

Departmental Score _____   **Percent** _____   **Rating** _____

▨ CONCIERGE

KRA	Standard	Score
1. **Incident reports**	Incident reports are maintained and copies distributed to appropriate cabinet members. A log book is maintained in a complete, professional, and informative manner.	_____
2. **Reception**	The concierge gives a warm, friendly, professional greeting to all who enter the community. The concierge staff have been trained on and are routinely following procedures outlined in the concierge manual.	_____
3. **Guests' rooms**	All guest room check-ins/check-outs are handled properly. Proper procedures are followed, and communication is maintained with the cabinet.	_____
4. **Security**	All concierge staff are informed/trained to handle emergency response. All are knowledgeable in the use of security systems. Keys to property are kept in a locked box and all incoming/outgoing persons are recorded.	_____
5. **Work orders**	Work orders and transportation requests are complete and properly distributed to the appropriate department head. No promises are made that cannot be kept.	_____
6. **Night staff**	Night concierge staff are fully and efficiently used to their maximum potential. Projects are scheduled and completed to ensure maximum productivity on this shift.	_____
7. **Emergency contacts**	Maintains a list of all cabinet staff with emergency phone numbers and a current list of vendors to call in case of an emergency.	_____
8. **"I'm OK"**	The resident "I'm OK" list is carefully completed every day and calls are made and followed up in a timely manner.	_____
9. **Notification**	A log is kept of all packages delivered to the front desk, and residents are notified of their arrival.	_____
10. **Marketing**	All concierge staff are fully informed and rehearsed on their role in marketing the project.	_____
11. **Resources**	The concierge maintains a directory of local area resources including transportation, emergency services, entertainment, hotels and restaurants, and recreational and exercise facilities to serve the needs of residents and their guests off-site.	_____

Departmental Score _____   **Percent** _____   **Rating** _____

▨ SALES/MARKETING

KRA	Standard	Score
1. **Marketing plan**	The department has a current sales/marketing plan in effect that is updated on an ongoing basis.	_____
2. **Job descriptions**	All marketing staff members have current technical-skill descriptions and an employee handbook.	_____

3. **Training** The sales/marketing director has conducted a training needs assessment with the input from the sales staff. A training plan has been developed to address the initial and continuous training needs of the department and carried out in an organized manner at least monthly. _____

4. **Follow-up** The lead-tickler system is used to schedule lead follow-up. All "active" leads are contacted at least monthly. _____

5. **Census** Occupancy and move-in projections are being met. _____

6. **Competition** The department has a current (six months or less) comparative market analysis of the competition. The competition has been mystery shopped within the last six months. _____

7. **Reports** All sales/marketing reports are timely, accurate, and complete. _____

8. **Collateral** The department has a sufficient inventory of all collateral material and supplies. _____

9. **Budget** The department sufficiently meets budgetary guidelines in terms of expenses and rental allowances (if any). _____

10. **Revenue** Monthly fee increases on turnover units are managed to maximize revenue. _____

11. **Communication** Weekly hot lead meetings are conducted that include the executive director. Individual sales representative hot lead meetings occur weekly. _____

12. **Sales** Each sales representative is shadowed monthly by the sales director to determine if relationship selling techniques are used to progress effectively in upgrading leads. _____

13. **Advertising** A competitor ad clipping file is current. The ad-tracking system is current and complete. There is a specific response category assigned to each lead. _____

14. **Referrals** The sales staff works with current residents for referrals. _____

15. **Outreach** There is a community outreach plan in place implemented by all members of the marketing department. _____

16. **Publicity** Publicity opportunities are proactively identified and pursued. _____

17. **Wait list** Wait-list deposit goals are constantly met. _____

18. **Event leads** Event leads are being appropriately followed up during and after all events. _____

19. **Phone-outs** Phone-out goals are consistently being met. This includes phone out-to-appointment conversion ratios as well as phone-out targets by lead classification. _____

20. **Appointments** Appointment goals are consistently being met. This includes appointment-to-sale conversion as well as appointments-kept goals. _____

21. **Operations** Operations staff are fully informed about the role they play in marketing. Operations staff are incorporated into the tour process. _____

22. **Move-ins**   New leases are properly passed on to the move-in coordinator to minimize cancellations. All leases/sales are adequately sold to minimize "not ready yet" cancellations. Average move-ins occur within 60 days.   _____

23. **Resident survey**   How well did the marketing staff score on the resident opinion survey? There is a written plan of correction for fair/poor responses.   _____

Departmental Score _____   Percent _____   Rating _____

■ MOVE-IN COORDINATOR

KRA	Standard	Score
1. **Initial contact**	The move-in coordinator works closely with the marketing department to develop relationships with prospects. Initial contact with a prospect is made within one week of signing the residency agreement.	_____
2. **Ongoing contact**	Consistent (weekly) contact is maintained with future residents. Effective communication exists with approval of family/friends.	_____
3. **Accelerating move-in**	The move-in coordinator is successful at maneuvering residents to move into the community sooner than anticipated (within 60 days).	_____
4. **Transition**	The move-in coordinator provides support to new residents through a formal orientation program.	_____
5. **Communication**	The move-in coordinator communicates the special needs and concerns of future residents with department heads well in advance of move-in dates.	_____
6. **Welcome package**	Correspondence (welcome kit, etc.) is distributed before move-in. Information is current and accurate. The move-in checklist is complete and on file for each new resident before move-in.	_____
7. **Resources**	A resource file is maintained on moving companies, house-sale services, realtors, antique appraiser, decorating services, etc.	_____
8. **Move-in manual**	The move-in manual is followed routinely. The move-in coordinator networks with other move-in coordinators within the company.	_____

Departmental Score _____   Percent _____   Rating _____

■ PERSONAL CARE

KRA	Standard	Score
1. **Regulations**	State regulations are on file. All staff understands their role and follows these regulations.	_____
2. **License**	The facility license is posted and current. All staff are properly licensed and have a copy in their personnel files.	_____

3. **Surveys** Copies of state licensure inspections are on file and posted where required. _____

4. **Resident survey** How well did the assisted-living department score on the resident opinion survey? There is a plan of correction for all fair/poor responses. _____

5. **Job description** All staff members have a current job description and employee handbook. All staff have been fully oriented to management expectations. _____

6. **Work schedules** Staff work schedules are planned in advance and posted. Work schedules are approved by the executive director and strictly comply with the labor budget. _____

7. **Files** All resident files are organized, confidential, and up to date. _____

8. **Records** Records and logs are kept for events and incidents that can be passed on from shift to shift and are current and complete. Any incidents of a serious nature are reported to the insurance carrier. _____

9. **Uniforms** All uniforms are clean and complete. _____

10. **Utilization review** Staff meets to discuss needs and problems of each resident. These needs are properly documented and discussed where appropriate with the resident's family. _____

11. **Family conferences** Staff members hold quarterly conferences with family members to update them on the residents' conditions as they may change. _____

12. **Training/education** All staff members are appropriately trained for their jobs using a training plan that has been developed by the personal care director. The training plan has been created based on the results of a needs assessment. _____

13. **Equipment/supplies** The department has all necessary equipment and supplies. They are properly marked with the community identification and inventoried. _____

14. **Budget** The department consistently meets its budgetary guidelines. _____

15. **Reception** All visitors and guests in the assisted-living unit are greeted immediately and welcomed. A log of all traffic in and out of the unit is kept. _____

16. **Cleanliness** The assisted-living common areas and apartments are clean and odor free. _____

17. **Meals** All meals are served promptly and the dining area is kept immaculate. _____

18. **Special diets** Special diet orders are accommodated and are appropriate for the resident's needs. _____

19. **Medications** All medications taken by residents are documented in the resident's file according to physician, medication, dosage, and expiration date (where appropriate). Prescription medications and treatments are strictly administered according to physician's orders. _____

20. **Testing**

All personal care unit staff have a current T.B. test on file. They have also been provided the option of a hepatitis B series. _____

21. **Wellness program**

Staff members provide ongoing wellness programs and health checks to assisted living and independent apartment residents. _____

22. **Activities**

Social and recreational activities are planned that are appropriate for assisted-living residents. An initial assessment has been completed and is on file for each resident. _____

23. **Policy**

The department has a current policy and procedures manual on hand. If any state regulations apply to the delivery of care in the unit, they are also readily available and routinely followed. _____

24. **Marketing**

All PCU staff are fully informed and rehearsed on their role in marketing the project. _____

25. **CPR**

All staff have current and valid CPR certification and understand the company's resuscitation policy and emergency procedures. A current copy of each certification is on file. _____

26. **Incident reports**

All incident reports are thoroughly investigated, and any suspected client neglect or abuse is reported to the executive director. _____

27. **Quality assurance**

All residents are routinely visited by management to ensure that the personal care plan is consistently implemented as designated. Nurse management visits at-risk residents on a daily basis, and follows up on any need to reassess resident service plans. _____

Departmental Score _____   Percent _____   Rating _____

■ PROPERTY ACCOUNTING

KRA	Standard	Score
1. **Rents**	All rents are proper and agree with the lease.	_____
2. **Billing**	Monthly billings are properly prepared and released prior to the 26th of the month.	_____
3. **Deposits**	Cash collected is properly recorded.	_____
4. **Collections**	After rent due date per the lease, all uncollected balances are resolved and late charges are billed.	_____
5. **Billing**	Copies of monthly billing and supporting documentation are properly filed.	_____
6. **Invoice approval**	All invoices are properly approved.	_____
7. **Payments**	All invoices are paid on a timely basis.	_____
8. **Invoice filing**	Copies of checks and canceled invoices are filed properly and on a timely basis.	_____
9. **Payroll recap**	A monthly recap of payroll by position is prepared and forwarded to corporate on a timely basis.	_____

10. **Food cost** — The food cost report is completed accurately and submitted on a timely basis. _____

11. **Regulations** — All changes in local, state, and federal laws are understood as they relate to payroll issues. _____

12. **Benefits** — Monthly employee contributions are calculated and are accurately withdrawn from paychecks. _____

13. **Reconciliation** — All bank accounts are reconciled on a timely basis. _____

14. **Transactions** — All transactions are properly documented, posted, and filed. _____

15. **Prepaid/accrual** — All prepaid and accruals are calculated, supported, and posted. _____

16. **Month-end schedules** — All supporting month-end schedules are prepared/updated by the 10th of the month. _____

17. **Profit/loss statements** — Profit and loss statements are finalized by the 10th of the month. _____

18. **Cash projections** — By the 9th of the month, a cash projection for the remainder of the month is calculated and a check is cut for the excess or a cash call from ownership is requested. _____

19. **Capital expenditures** — All capital expenditures are processed each month according to the capital expenditure procedure for the site. _____

Departmental Score _____ **Percent** _____ **Rating** _____

Key Result Area
Departmental Operations Audit

▬ TOTAL PROPERTY

Department	Score	Percent	Rating	POC
1. Executive Director	____/240	____	____	____
2. Housekeeping/Laundry	____/320	____	____	____
3. Administration/Human Resources	____/250	____	____	____
4. Resident Relations	____/150	____	____	____
5. Engineering/Maintenance	____/230	____	____	____
6. Food and Beverage	____/220	____	____	____
7. Dining Room	____/220	____	____	____
8. Transportation	____/100	____	____	____
9. Activities/Enrichment	____/140	____	____	____
10. Concierge	____/110	____	____	____
11. Sales/Marketing	____/230	____	____	____
12. Move-In Coordinator	____/80	____	____	____
13. Personal Care	____/270	____	____	____
14. Property Accountant	____/190	____	____	____
Total Property	____/2,750	____	____	____

Financing Alternatives for Assisted Living Communities

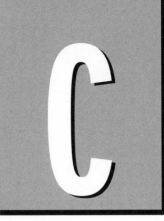

	Commercial banks	Savings and loans	Securities (tax-exempt bonds)	Insurance companies	Credit companies	Real estate investment trusts (REITs)	Fannie Mae/ DUS	Fannie Mae/ PAL	Freddie Mac Conventional Cash Program	HUD 223 (f)	HUD 221 (d) (4)	HUD 232
Description	Construction and mid-term loans: 5–10 years with 20–25 year amortization. Funding is not necessarily senior-oriented.		"Conduit financing" where public agency acts as issuer of tax-exempt bonds if certain eligibility requirements are met. 1. Nonprofit 501(c)(3) bonds. 2. For-profit residential bonds. Can be used for construction and permanent financing.	Specific senior long-term, take-out financing. Usually, but not always, for existing developments with operating history.	Mainly construction financing dealing specifically with tax credit projects.	Construction and acquisition with mortgage loan or sale/lease-back option.	Under DUS, Fannie Mae purchases multifamily mortgages from specially designated lender. These DUS lenders have been delegated responsibility for originating, underwriting, closing, and servicing multifamily mortgages on shared-risk basis.	Individual transactions are submitted by approved Prior Approval Lenders to Fannie Mae regional offices, where they receive full review prior to commitment. Underwriting standards are the same as DUS. Current priority is given to special affordable housing transactions.	This program is a relaunch of a cash program previously offered by Freddie Mac for the finance, acquisition, or moderate rehabilitation loans that demonstrate high investment quality.	This program is for the refinance, acquisition, or moderate renovation of existing apartments and housing cooperative or assisted living facilities, board and care homes, and nursing homes.	This program provides financing for new construction or substantial rehab* of rental or cooperative multi-housing.	This program provides financing for new construction or substantial rehab* of assisted living, board and care homes, or nursing homes.
Eligible projects	All projects, with location as possible restriction.	All projects, with location as possible restriction.	All.	Existing only.	Varies.	All projects.	Completed projects.	Wide range, with priority to special affordable housing; completed projects.	5+ units, garden, mid-rise, high-rise, and co-op properties in good condition.	Multifamily units; all units must have kitchens and baths. ALFs must be licensed by state/local government.	Multifamily properties; units must have kitchens and baths and comply with local building codes.	Assisted living facilities with up to 2 BR units. Kitchens are not required.
Term(s)/ amortization	5–10 / 20–25	5–10 / 20–25	5–10 / 30	10–20 / 20–25	15–25 / 25–30	10–15 / 25–30	25 years, or others by request; 25- or 30-year amortization.	25 years, or others by request.	25 years standard term.	Up to 35 years.	Up to 40 years/ construction period plus up to 40 years.	Up to 40 years/ construction period up to 40 years.
RATES **Construction**	Prime + 1%	Prime + 1%	Same as permanent.		Prime + 1%	Prime + 3%–4%	Priced daily; best prices to most conservative transactions.	Priced daily; special pricing available for special affordable housing transactions.	Fixed for term of loan; competitive rates, based on risk-based pricing.	Based on market conditions. 30-year Treasuries plus 125–150 basis points.	Based on current market conditions. 30-year Treasuries plus 150–200 basis points.	Based on current market conditions. 30-year Treasuries plus 150–200 basis points.
Permanent fixed	150–300 basis points over comparable-term Treasury.	150–300 basis points over comparable-term Treasury.	6.5%–8.5% including enhancements.	150–250 basis points over comparable-term Treasury.	150–250 basis points over comparable-term Treasury.	300–375 basis points over comparable-term Treasury.						
Variable	150–300 basis points over LIBOR.	150–250 basis points over LIBOR.	4.5%–5.5% including enhancements.	100–250 basis points over LIBOR.	100–200 basis points over LIBOR.	Prime + 3%–4%						
Loan-to-value (LTV) / debt service coverage (DSC)	70–80% LTV 1.20–1.30 DSC	70–80% LTV 1.20–1.30 DSC	90–100% LTV fixed 75–90% LTV variable 1.20+ DSC	75% LTV 1.30–1.40 DSC	80–90% LTV 1.10–1.20 DSC	90–100% LTV 1.20–1.30 DSC	80% LTV 1.15 DSC	80%; special pricing available for special affordable housing transactions.	75% based on Freddie Mac value.	85% LTV 1.15 DSC	80–90% LTV 1.10–1.20 DSC	Up to 90% of eligible replacement costs. No BSPRA, but builder's profit can be used.

*Substantial rehab when costs exceed $6,500 per unit adjusted by area high-cost percentage, or when more than one major building component must be replaced.

	Commercial banks	Savings and loans	Securities (tax-exempt bonds)	Insurance companies	Credit companies	Real estate investment trusts (REITs)	Fannie Mae/ DUS	Fannie Mae/ PAL	Freddie Mac Conventional Cash Program	HUD 223 (f)	HUD 221 (d) (4)	HUD 232
Total fees/costs	1%–2%	1%–2%	4%–5%	1%–3%	1%–2%	1%–2%	Vary with DUS lender; 2% Fannie Mae fee refunded at closing (except $10,000, refunded when legally required).	1%–2%; vary with transaction size.	10% application fee.	Application financing and placement, HUD inspection and annual mortgage insurance premium.	Application financing and placement, annual mortgage insurance premium, and inspection fees.	All financeable.
Restrictions	No prepayment; recourse.	Recourse.	Needs issuing agency, bond underwriters.	Nonrecourse.	No prepayment; tax credit only.	No prepayment allowed without yield maintenance.	Yield maintenance.	Yield maintenance.	N/A	Property must be minimum three years old; lease terms must be at least one month; no transient services on the property.	Minimum 30-day leases; no transient services, single asset entity borrower. No congregate housing.	No deposit in excess of one month's rent.
Advantages	Typically local; lower transaction costs; shorter time frame.	Typically local; lower transaction costs; shorter time frame.	Lowest rates available. Variable option is extremely attractive.	Longer terms; may be nonrecourse; pricing is typically better.	Unregulated source; thus flexibility.	High LTVs available, off-balance sheet available through lease structure.	80% LTV, 30-year amortization; Fannie Mae usually in the market with a good price.	Because of direct review by Fannie Mae's Prior Approval, can handle greater complexities than other product lines.	Competitive terms, conditions, process, and rates.	Long-term, fixed-rate, full amortization, nonrecourse, competitive interest rates.	Long-term, fixed-rate, full amortization, nonrecourse, competitive interest rates.	Long-term, fixed-rate, full amortization, nonrecourse, competitive interest rates. Less experience required of management companies.
Disadvantages	Shorter terms; recourse; pricing may be higher.	Shorter terms; recourse; pricing may be higher.	Rental restrictions; high transaction costs; need public issuer; state cap (for profit); set aside requirement 20% @ 50% CMI, 40% @ 60% CMI.	Higher debt service coverage; typically existing properties with good operating history; minimum loan size is $3 million plus.	Typically for tax credit projects only; high LTVs based on restricted value. Thus loan amounts are typically lower.	High financing rates; title or no prepayment flexibility.	Currently unable to lock rate spread until processing is complete.	N/A	DSC is high compared with other conduit programs; small loans have 25% recourse.	Processing time, three-year-old property requirements.	Processing time; prevailing wage rates. Congregate housing is not eligible.	Processing time; prevailing wage rates.

Preopening Critical Path

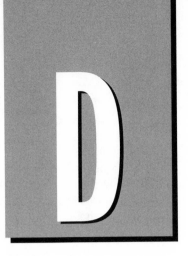

Task no.	Weeks before opening	Area	Task
1	48	Development	Review market feasibility and penetration
2	48	Development	Conduct competitive market analysis
3	48	Development	Develop product pricing and market positioning
4	48	Development	Review plans and evaluate operational efficiency
5	48	Development	Specify phone and emergency call system and number, types, and locations of phones
6	48	Development	Review interior design plan and make recommendations
7	48	Development	Review unit mix and floor plans
8	48	Development	Review and evaluate administrative office plan
9	48	Development	Design and specify central kitchen equipment and layout
10	48	Development	Participate in design development
11	48	Development	Review construction drawings with architect
12	48	Development	Set up preopening accounting procedures
13	48	Development	Create financial projections: pro forma, development budget, 10-year projections, investment returns
14	48	Marketing	Write marketing plan
15	48	Marketing	Develop preopening marketing budget
16	48	Marketing	Hold concept meetings for logo, business papers, brochure
17	36	Development	Create resident lease agreement, application, and financial, medical, and other documents
18	36	Development	Develop preopening budget
19	36	Marketing	Gather media information for market area
20	36	Marketing	Purchase business papers and #10 brochure
21	36	Marketing	Order and install computerized lead management system
22	24	Administration	Set up medical insurance carriers; collect information on each provider for distribution to employees
23	24	Administration	Set up personnel files, to include application, job description, references, copies of licenses, orientation, I9 form
24	24	Marketing	Order display boards for marketing office (floor plans and unit designs)
25	24	Marketing	Create direct mail campaign
26	24	Marketing	Recruit marketing director
27	24	Operations	Recruit executive director
28	24	Operations	Develop resident handbook
29	24	Operations	Set up employee benefit plans
30	24	Operations	Develop employee manual

(continued)

Task no.	Weeks before opening	Area	Task
31	18	Administration	Develop hiring packages and benefits brochure
32	18	Administration	Set up payroll
33	18	Designer	Specify, receive, and set up model furniture
34	18	Development	Evaluate signage needs
35	18	Marketing	Prepare second direct mail campaign
36	18	Marketing	Create advertising concepts
37	18	Marketing	Finalize media schedule
38	18	Marketing	Develop and implement community outreach plan
39	18	Marketing	Begin advertising
40	18	Marketing	Develop move-in coordination manual
41	18	Marketing	Set up temporary sales office
42	18	Marketing	Drop first direct mail pieces
43	18	Operations	Obtain bids for vehicle leasing or purchase
44	16	Operations/marketing	Set up marketing reporting system
45	14	Marketing	Prepare press kit for information center opening
46	14	Operations/marketing	Review start-up budget and progress to date; evaluate and prioritize further needs
47	12	Food and beverage	Acquire permits and licenses
48	12	Marketing	Hold information center opening event
49	12	Operations	Review certificate of occupancy requirements
50	12	Operations	Set up operating accounting procedures; forward copies of management agreements to accounting offices
51	10	Marketing	Set up information session at an appropriate nearby location
52	10	Marketing	Recruit marketing representative
53	8	Accounting	Establish purchase order system
54	8	Accounting	Set up labor reports
55	8	Administration	Set up housekeeping and laundry operations
56	8	Administration	Recruit bookkeeper
57	8	Administration	Establish all service contracts; send notices to all providers, collect certificates of insurance
58	8	Administration	Recruit director of maintenance
59	8	Administration	Recruit director of activities
60	8	Administration	Recruit business office manager
61	8	Administration	Train all managers on interviewing and hiring practices; conduct training and develop manual
62	8	Administration	Hold department head meetings to discuss communications procedures
63	8	Administration	Orient maintenance director on all building systems; obtain all manuals and manufacturer recommendations
64	8	Administration	Develop job descriptions for all positions (may need to customize to suit)
65	8	Administration	Recruit supervisor of assisted living
66	8	Administration	Review health codes
67	8	Food and beverage	Order linen, china, silver, and glassware
68	8	Food and beverage	Establish purchasing practices; set up vendors and pricing; negotiate group discounts
69	8	Food and beverage	Order menu board (framed and glass covered, writable) with easel
70	8	Food and beverage	Develop dining room controls, meal accounting, sanitation procedures, and sidework sheets
71	8	Food and beverage	Order smallware package; arrange delivery date after burnoff of kitchen
72	8	Food and beverage	Review wine and beer licensing (if needed)
73	8	Food and beverage	Create staffing schedules
74	8	Food and beverage	Select uniforms for kitchen and housekeeping staff
75	8	Food and beverage	Establish all work schedules for dining room and kitchen; evaluate job descriptions; review ratios
76	8	Food and beverage	Recruit director of food service
77	8	Food and beverage	Create menus (menus, cycles, and presentations must correspond to budgeted amounts)
78	8	Housekeeping	Establish cleaning schedules and master housekeeping plan
79	8	Maintenance	Develop contact list for local contractors
80	8	Maintenance	Establish key control procedures; distribute policy and review with department heads
81	8	Maintenance	Draw up construction punch list for apartments and common areas; review with architect
82	8	Maintenance	Collect all vendor information and set up accounts

Task no.	Weeks before opening	Area	Task
83	8	Maintenance	Set up maintenance office; order tools and supplies; inventory and mark all equipment
84	8	Maintenance	Arrange utility contracts; investigate deposit requirements
85	8	Maintenance	Recruit housekeeper to clean models; maintenance director to supervise housekeeping
86	8	Marketing	Begin resident assessments, sign leases, collect deposits
87	8	Marketing	Prepare move-in packet
88	8	Operations	Establish EEOC procedures
89	8	Operations	Order property, liability, and general insurance
90	7	Administration	Lease beepers
91	6	Accounting	Set up budget and declining-balance ledgers for each department head (budget should reflect count of actual residents with signed leases)
92	6	Accounting	Set up accounting, ordering, receiving, inventory, production, and reporting systems
93	6	Administration	Create delivery, inventory, and security systems for supplies; inspect supply storage areas and review procedures
94	6	Food and beverage	Recruit kitchen personnel
95	6	Food and beverage	Research local purveyors
96	6	Food and beverage	Assemble training material and food and beverage manual
97	6	Food and beverage	Set up employee lounge
98	6	Maintenance	Arrange for manufacturer training on equipment; record training on video
99	6	Maintenance	Purchase preopening maintenance and housekeeping equipment
100	6	Maintenance	Receive as-built and manuals from architect
101	6	Maintenance	Review maintenance work order procedures; review maintenance log and procedures
102	6	Maintenance	Arrange preopening security if needed
103	6	Maintenance	Accept attic stock of excess materials from general contractor
104	6	Maintenance	Establish preventive maintenance schedules according to manufacturer recommendations
105	5	Accounting	Confirm local tax laws
106	5	Accounting	Set up resident ancillary billing system
107	5	Activities	Confirm vehicle licensing
108	5	Activities	Set up transportation procedures and log
109	5	Administration	Contract with local beautician; obtain beauty shop permit
110	5	Administration	Create emergency plan from master
111	5	Administration	Allocate community storage areas; price resident storage if appropriate
112	5	Food and beverage	Organize storerooms
113	5	Food and beverage	Confirm receivable and storage plans
114	5	Food and beverage	Set up sanitation program; assign responsibility for same
115	4	Accounting	Develop monthly reports and variance summaries; train ED on format and function
116	4	Accounting	Acquire accounting forms from regional accounting office
117	4	Accounting	Set up computer system
118	4	Accounting	Set up accounts payable
119	4	Accounting	Set up file system for contracts
120	4	Accounting	Set up local bank account
121	4	Accounting	Set up petty cash account
122	4	Accounting	Acquire tax identification number
123	4	Accounting	Set up time clock
124	4	Accounting	Create credit information sheet
125	4	Activities	Develop activity calendar of events
126	4	Activities	Order, set up, check out, and inventory activities and craft supplies
127	4	Activities	Develop transportation plan, schedule, and staffing
128	4	Activities	Review activity and recreation manual
129	4	Activities	Develop leisure interest surveys
130	4	Administration	Perform operations audit (see Appendix B); meet with department heads to discuss purpose and implementation
131	4	Administration	Recruit personal care aides (consider a job fair for rapid recruitment)
132	4	Administration	Orient all employees (six-hour orientation and video training)

(continued)

Task no.	Weeks before opening	Area	Task
133	4	Administration	Recruit receptionist (orient to marketing materials and procedures)
134	4	Assisted living	Acquire assisted living manual
135	4	Assisted living	Set up quality assurance program; create quality assurance and safety committee
136	4	Assisted living	Hold training program for CNAs; formal training for aides
137	4	Food and beverage	Acquire food service manual; set up systems and procedures
138	4	Food and beverage	Receive dry and frozen goods
139	4	Food and beverage	Order supplies and paper goods
140	4	Food and beverage	Review order of service; set up sidework sheets for all dining rooms and assign ongoing responsibility for them
141	4	Food and beverage	Recruit dining room staff (consider a job fair for rapid recruitment)
142	4	Food and beverage	Set up sanitation control
143	4	Food and beverage	Place initial dry goods order
144	4	Food and beverage	Recruit and train lead server
145	4	Human resources	Train local human resources person on employee orientation
146	4	Human resources	Train concierge and implement lobby control procedures; set up training for all shifts and part-timers
147	4	Human resources	Review OSHA requirements with regional human resources office
148	4	Human resources	Acquire risk management manual and train staff
149	4	Maintenance	Develop log system for work orders
150	4	Maintenance	Test emergency call system
151	4	Maintenance	Test sprinkler and fire alarm systems; establish monitoring or testing contracts if appropriate
152	4	Maintenance	Confirm chemical set-up and training; post Material Safety Data Sheets; install eyewash stations
153	4	Maintenance	Stock maintenance supplies; create master inventory for all supplies
154	4	Maintenance	Recruit housekeeping staff
155	4	Marketing	Prepare press kit for grand opening
156	4	Marketing	Send out invitations to preview opening ("sneak peek")
157	3	Food and beverage	Organize all coolers
158	3	Food and beverage	Turn over kitchen equipment
159	3	Food and beverage	Burn off kitchen
160	3	Food and beverage	Set up cooking line
161	3	Food and beverage	Place opening perishable order
162	3	Food and beverage	Train dining room staff with manual, video, and skill practice sessions
163	3	Food and beverage	Start cook and utility training
164	3	Food and beverage	Break out smallwares and utility equipment
165	3	Food and beverage	Receive dining room uniforms; develop cost, inventory, and control systems; install purchasing manual
166	3	Maintenance	Supervise final cleaning
167	3	Maintenance	Review emergency call system condition and installation
168	2	Activities	Develop newsletter
169	2	Administration	Establish resident advisory committee
170	2	Administration	Establish relationship for in-house banking services
171	2	Food and beverage	Deep-clean kitchen
172	2	Human resources	Post required personnel posters
173	2	Human resources	Create all employee rosters and organization charts, including rate of pay, hire date, and date of next review
174	2	Maintenance	Review landscaping issues with builder
175	2	Marketing	Counsel initial move-ins; schedule elevator use
176	1	All	Preview opening event for prospects
177	1	All	Preview event for referral sources
178	1	Marketing	Coordinate grand opening
179	1	Maintenance	Complete punch list with general contractor and architect
180	0	All	Enjoy your success!

Albrecht, K., and R. Zemke. *Service America! Doing Business in the New Economy.* Homewood, Ill.: Dow Jones-Irwin, 1985.

Aronson, M. K. *Understanding Alzheimer's Disease.* New York: Macmillan, 1988.

Bloodborne Compliance Program. Zee Medical Service Co., 747 Church Road, Suite G-7, Elmhurst, Ill. 60126, (708) 832-9850.

Desatnick, R. L. *Managing to Keep the Customer.* San Francisco: Jossey-Bass, 1987.

Dychtwald, K., and J. Flowers. *Age-Wave: The Challenges and Opportunities of an Aging America.* New York: Bantam Books, 1990.

Elliot, W. H., J. L. Beck, and D. S. Schless. *Seniors Housing Finance: Trends and Prospects.* Washington, D.C.: American Seniors Housing Association (ASHA), June 1992.

Hayflick, L. *How and Why We Age.* New York: Ballantine Books, 1994.

Leary, M. G., and B. W. Pearce. "Offensive versus Defensive Marketing." *Retirement Community Business* 3(3) (May 1994): 10.

Mace, N. L., and P. V. Rabins. *The 36-Hour Day: A Family Guide to Caring for Persons with Alzheimer's Disease, Related Dementing Illnesses and Memory Loss in Later Life.* Baltimore: Johns Hopkins University Press, 1991.

Moore, J. "Strategic Industry Focus Needed." *Contemporary Long-Term Care* 16(2) (March 1993): 94.

Pearce, B. W. "How to Slow the Revolving Door." *Contemporary Long Term Care* 15(5) (September 1992): 36.

———. "Resident Turnover." *Retirement Community Business* 1(2) (Summer 1992): 12.

———. "Resident Satisfaction." *Inside Assisted Living* 3(1) (February 1996): 3.

———. "Market Fill-up Rates and Financial Performance." *Inside Assisted Living* 4(1) (February 1997): 3.

Pearce, B. W., and T. Grape. "Checks and Balances." *Assisted Living Today* 4(2) (Winter 1997): 30.

Peters, T. J., and N. Austin. *A Passion for Excellence.* New York: Random House, 1985.

Peters, T. J., and R. H. Waterman, Jr. *In Search of Excellence.* New York: Random House, 1982.

Powell, A. V., and H. E. Winklevoss. *Continuing Care Retirement Communities: An Empirical, Financial, and Legal Analysis.* Homewood, Ill.: Pension Research Council, 1984.

"Residents on the Board." *D&O Forum—FORCE Financial Publication,* Fall 1994, 5.

Resource Directory for Older People. Bethesda, Md.: National Institute on Aging, 1993.

Robinson, A., B. Spencer, and L. White. *Understanding Difficult Behaviors.* Ypsilanti, Mich.: Eastern Michigan University, 1992.

Rogers, W. W. *General Administration in the Nursing Home.* Waco, Tex.: Davis Brothers, 1971.

Schiffman, S. S. "Taste and Smell in Disease." *New England Journal of Medicine* 308 (1983): 1275–79, 1337, 1343.

Schiffman, S. S., and Z. S. Warwick. "Effect of Flavor Enhancement of Foods for the Elderly on Nutritional Status: Food Intake, Biochemical Indices, and Anthropometric Measures." *Physiology and Behavior* 53 (1992): 395–402.

Simonson, W. *Medications and the Elderly: A Guide for Promoting Proper Use.* Rockville, Md.: Aspen Publications, 1984.

Strauss, W., and N. Howe. *Generations.* New York: Morrow, 1990.

Winsor, A. B. *Retirement Communities with the "Catered Lifestyle."* Fort Walton Beach, Fla.: Seacoast Productions, 1983.

Wolfe, D. B. *Serving the Ageless Market.* New York: McGraw-Hill, 1990.

Wolfe, S. M., L. Fugate, E. P. Hulstrand, et al. *Worst Pills, Best Pills.* Washington, D.C.: Public Citizen Health Research Group, 1988.

Zemke, R., and D. Schaaf. *The Service Edge.* New York: New American Library, 1989.

Index

Where an entry refers to a subject discussed on several pages, only the number of the page on which the discussion begins is listed in this index.

ABOUT THE AUTHOR

BENJAMIN W. PEARCE is the president and chief operating officer of Potomac Homes Holding Corporation. Potomac Homes provides management, development, and consulting services to communities that provide assisted living, Alzheimer's disease and related dementia care, and other care services for seniors. Potomac Homes is composed of Potomac Group Home Corporation and Antioch Construction.

Mr. Pearce brings a rich set of skills and accomplishments to the assisted living arena from his extensive experience. Formerly senior vice president of Senior Housing for Genesis Health Ventures, Mr. Pearce was responsible for planning, implementing, and directing all facets of operations and marketing for new and existing projects. He also served as senior vice president of operations for A•D•S Senior Housing, a wholly owned subsidiary of the Multicare Companies, which was acquired by Genesis Health Ventures in October of 1997. Prior to that he was vice president of operations for Classic Residence by Hyatt in Chicago, Illinois; regional director of operations for the Hillhaven Corporation in Tacoma, Washington; director of operations for the Careage Corporation in Bellevue, Washington; and vice president of operations for International Care Centers in Bellevue, Washington.

Retirement communities under Mr. Pearce's management have been awarded the prestigious Contemporary Long Term Care Order of Excellence Award on three separate occasions. Mr. Pearce is a former director of the National Association of Senior Living Industries (NASLI) and Assisted Living Federation of America (ALFA). He teaches graduate level classes on senior housing and is a faculty member of the Real Estate Institute at New York University and the Johns Hopkins University. Mr. Pearce has also published widely and serves on the editorial advisory boards of *Resident Life/Assisted Living Success* magazine, *Briefings on Assisted Living*, and *Assisted Living Executive Report*. Mr. Pearce enjoys sailing and is an accomplished triathlete.

Library of Congress Cataloging-in-Publication Data

Pearce, Benjamin W.
    Senior living communities : operations management and marketing for assisted
living, congregate, and continuing care retirement communities / Benjamin W.
Pearce.
        p.   cm.
    Includes bibliographical references (p.   ) and index.
    ISBN 0-8018-5961-1 (alk. paper)
    1. Congregate housing—United States—Management. 2. Life care
communities—United States—Management. 3. Aged—Care—United States.
    4. Frail elderly—Care—United States. I. Title.
HD7287.92.U54P4   1998
362.1'6'088—dc21

                                         98-8731
                                            CIP